MYOCARDIAL ISCHEMIA
From mechanisms to therapeutic potentials

BASIC SCIENCE FOR THE CARDIOLOGIST

1. B. Swynghedauw (ed.): *Molecular Cardiology for the Cardiologist.* Second Edition. 1998 ISBN 0-7923-8323-0
2. B. Levy, A. Tedgui (eds.): *Biology of the Arterial Wall.* 1999 ISBN 0-7923-8458-X
3. M.R. Sanders, J.B. Kostis (eds.): *Molecular Cardiology in Clinical Practice.* 1999 ISBN 0-7923-8602-7
4. B.Ostadal, F. Kolar (eds.): *Cardiac Ischemia: From Injury to Protection.* 1999 ISBN 0-7923-8642-6
5. H. Schunkert, G.A.J. Riegger (eds.): *Apoptosis in Cardiac Biology.* 1999 ISBN 0-7923-8648-5
6. A. Malliani, (ed.): *Principles of Cardiovascular Neural Regulation in Health and Disease.* 2000 ISBN 0-7923-7775-3
7. P. Benlian: *Genetics of Dyslipidemia.* 2001 ISBN 0-7923-7362-6
8. D. Young: *Role of Potassium in Preventive Cardiovascular Medicine.* 2001 ISBN 0-7923-7376-6
9. E. Carmeliet, J. Vereecke: *Cardiac Cellular Electrophysiology.* 2001 ISBN 0-7923-7544-0
10. C. Holubarsch: *Mechanics and Energetics of the Myocardium.* 2002 ISBN 0-7923-7570-X
11. J.S. Ingwall: *ATP and the Heart.* 2002 ISBN 1-4020-7093-4
12. W.C. De Mello, M.J. Janse: *Heart Cell Coupling and Impuse Propagation in Health and Disease.* 2002 ISBN 1-4020-7182-5
13. P.P.-Dimitrow: *Coronary Flow Reserve – Measurement and Application: Focus on transthoracic Doppler echocardiography.* 2002 ISBN 1-4020-7213-9
14. G.A. Danieli: *Genetics and Genomics for the Cardiologist.* 2002 ISBN 1-4020-7309-7
15. F.A. Schneider, I.R. Siska, J.A. Avram: *Clinical Physiology of the Venous System.* 2003. ISBN 1-4020-7411-5
16. Can Ince: *Physiological Genomics of the Critically Ill Mouse.* 2004 ISBN 1-4020-7641-X
17. Wolfgang Schaper, Jutta Schaper: *Arteriogenesis.* 2004 ISBN 1-4020-8125-1 eISBN 1-4020-8126-X
18. Nico Westerhof, Nikos Stergiopulos, Mark I.M. Noble: *Snapshots of Hemodynamics: An aid for clinical research and graduate education.* 2005 ISBN 0-387-23345-8 eISBN 0-387-23346-6
19. Toshio Nishikimi: *Adrenomedullin in Cardiovascular Disease.* 2005 ISBN 0-387-25404-8 eISBN 0-387-25405-6
20. Edward D. Frohlich, Richard N. Re: *The Local Cardiac Renin Angiotensin-Aldosterone System. 2005* ISBN 0-387-27825-7 eISBN 0-387-27826-5
21. D.V. Cokkinos, C. Pantos, G. Heusch, H. Taegtmeyer: *Myocardial Ischemia: From mechanisms to therapeutic potentials.* 2005 ISBN 0-387-28657-8 eISBN 0-387-28658-6

MYOCARDIAL ISCHEMIA
From mechanisms to therapeutic potentials

Edited by

Dennis V. Cokkinos, MD, PhD
University of Athens
Athens, Greece

Constantinos Pantos, MD, PhD
University of Athens
Athens, Greece

Gerd Heusch, MD, PhD
University of Essen
Essen, Germany

Heinrich Taegtmeyer, MD, DPhil
The University of Texas Medical School
Houston, Texas, USA

Springer

Dennis V. Cokkinos
Prof. of Cardiology
University of Athens
Chairman Cardiology Dept.
Onassis Cardiac Surgery Center
Athens, Greece

Constantinos Pantos
Assistant Professor of Pharmadcology
Depart. Of Pharmacology, Medical School
University of Athens
Athens, Greece

Gerd Heusch
Professor of Medicine
Director, Institute of Pathophysiology
Department of Internal Medicine
University of Essen
Essen, Germany

Heinrich Taegtmeyer
Professor of Medicine
Co-Director, Division of Cardiology
The University of Texas
Houston Medical School
Houston, Texas
USA

Library of Congress Cataloging-in-Publication Data

Myocardial ischemia: from mechanisms to therapeutic potentials / edited by D.V. Cokkinos, C. Pantos, G. Heusch and H. Taegtmeyer
p. ; cm. – (Basic science for the cardiologist ; 21)
Includes bibliographical references and index.
ISBN-13: 978-0-387-28657-0 (alk. paper)
ISBN-10: 0-387-28657-8 (alk. paper)
1. Coronary heart disease—Pathophysiology. 2. Coronary heart disease—Treatment. I. Cokkinos, Dennis V. II. Series
[DNLM: 1. Myocardial Ischemia—physiopathology. 2. Myocardial Ischemia—therapy. WG 300 M99764 2005]
RC685.C6M9585 2005
616.1'23—dc22

2005051640

ISBN -10 1-4899-7358-3　　ISBN 0-387-28658-6 (eBook)
ISBN -13 978-1-4899-7358-0　　ISBN 978-0-387-28658-7 (eBook)

Printed on acid-free paper.

9 8 7 6 5 4 3 2 1　　SPIN 11316282

springeronline.com

CONTENTS

PREFACE

Effective new treatments of heart disease are based on a refined understanding of cellular function and the heart's response to environmental stresses. Not surprisingly therefore, the field of experimental cardiology has experienced a phase of rapid exponential growth during the last decade. The acquisition of new knowledge has been so fast that textbooks of cardiology or textbooks of cardiovascular physiology are often hard-pressed to keep up with the most important conceptual advances. Witness the explosive increase in knowledge about signaling pathways of cardiac growth, transcriptional regulation of cardiac metabolism, hormonal signaling, and the complex responses of the heart to ischemia, reperfusion, or ischemic preconditioning. This book is meant to bridge the gap between original literature and textbook reviews. It brings together investigators of various backgrounds who share their expertise in the biology of myocardial ischemia. Each chapter is a self-contained mini-review, but it will soon become apparent to the reader that there is also a common thread: Molecular and cellular cardiology has never been more exciting than now, but ever more exciting times are yet to come.

The Editors

ACKNOWLEDGEMENTS

– Publication of this book was generously supported by Sanofi-Aventis Hellas.

– Eikon creative team provided the technical assistance in preparing the manuscripts.

– We thank Dr. Bernard Swynghedauw for all his scientific support.

INTRODUCTION

FROM FETAL TO FATAL

Metabolic adaptation of the heart to environmental stress

Heinrich Taegtmeyer MD, DPhil*

The year 2004 marked the centenary of two important discoveries in the field of metabolism: The discovery of beta-oxidation of fatty acids by Franz Knoop (1904),[1] and the discovery of the oxygen dependence for normal pump function of the heart by Hans Winterstein (1904).[2] The year 2004 also marked the 50th anniversary of the discovery, by Richard Bing and his colleagues, that the human heart prefers fatty acids for respiration.[3]

These early studies support the concept that the heart is well designed, both anatomically and biochemically, for uninterrupted, rhythmic aerobic work. Although heart muscle has certain distinctive biochemical characteristics, many of the basic biochemical reaction patterns are similar to those of other tissues. In short, metabolism and function of the heart are inextricably linked (Fig. 1).

In spite of, or perhaps because of the intricate network of metabolic pathways, heart muscle is an efficient converter of energy. The enzymatic catabolism of substrates results in the production of free energy, which is then used for cell work and for various biosynthetic activities including the synthesis of glycogen, triglycerides, proteins, membranes, and enzymes. Here I highlight the many actions of cardiac metabolism in energy transfer, cardiac growth, gene expression, and viability.

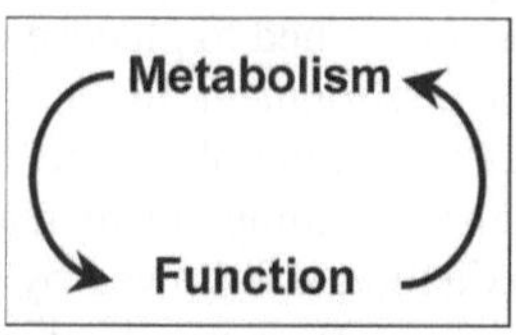

Figure 1. The coupling of metabolism and function. H. Taegtmeyer, *Circulation* **110**, 895 (2004).

* University of Texas Houston Medical School, Department of Medicine, Division of Cardiology, 6431 Fannin Street, MSB 1.246, Houston, Texas 77030, e-mail: heinrich.taegtmeyer@uth.tmc.edu

1. THE LOGIC OF METABOLISM

The heart makes a living by liberating energy from different oxidizable substrates. The logic of metabolism is grounded in the first law of thermodynamics, which states that energy can neither be created nor destroyed (the law of the conservation of energy). In his early experiments on the chemistry of muscle contraction, Helmholtz observed that "during the action of muscles, a chemical transformation of the compounds contained in them takes place".[4] The work culuminated in the famous treatise "On the Conservation of Force." The first law of thermodynamics forms the basis for the stoichiometry of metabolism and the calculation of the efficiency of cardiac performance.[4]

2. SUBSTRATE SWITCHING AND METABOLIC FLEXIBILITY

Heart muscle is a metabolic omnivore with the capacity to oxidize fatty acids, carbohydrates and also (in certain circumstances) amino acids either simultaneously or vicariously. Much work has been done in the isolated perfused rat heart to elucidate the mechanisms by which substrates compete for the fuel of respiration. In their celebrated studies in the 1960s, Philip Randle and his group established that, when present in sufficiently high concentrations, fatty acids suppress glucose oxidation to a greater extent than glycolysis, and glycolysis to a greater extent than glucose uptake; these observations gave rise to the concept of a "glucose-fatty acid-cycle".[5] The concept was later modified with the discovery of the suppression of fatty acid oxidation by glucose[6] through inhibition of the enzyme carnitine-palmitoyl transferase I (CPTI).[7] CPTI is, in turn, regulated by its rate of synthesis (by acetyl-CoA carboxylase, ACC) and its rate of degradation (by malonyl-CoA decarboxylase, MCD). Of the two enzymes, MCD is transcriptionally regulated by the nuclear receptor peroxisome proliferator activated receptor α (PPARα),[8] while ACCβ, the isoform that predominates in cardiac and skeletal muscle, is regulated both allosterically and covalently.[9, 10] High-fat feeding, fasting, and diabetes all increase MCD mRNA and activity in heart muscle. Conversely, cardiac hypertrophy, which is associated with decreased PPARα expression[11] and a switch from fatty acid to glucose oxidation[12, 13] results in decreased MCD expression and activity, an effect that is independent of fatty acids. Thus, MCD is regulated both transcriptionally and post-transcriptionally, and, in a feedforward mechanism, fatty acids induce MCD gene expression. The same principle applies to the regulation of other enzymes governing fatty acid metabolism in the heart, including the expression of uncoupling protein 3 (UCP3).[14] Here, fatty acids upregulate UCP3 expression, while UCP3 is downregulated in the hypertrophied heart that has switched to glucose for its main fuel of respiration.

For a given physiologic environment, the heart selects the most efficient substrate for energy production. A fitting example is the switch from fatty acid to carbohydrate oxidation with an acute "work jump" or increase in workload.[15] The transient increase in rates of glycogen oxidation is followed by a sustained increase in rates of glucose and lactate oxidation (Fig. 2). Because oleate oxidation remains unaffected by the work jump, the increase in O_2 consumption and cardiac work are entirely accounted for by the increase in carbohydrate oxidation.

The enzymes of glucose and glycogen metabolism are highly regulated by either allosteric activation or covalent modification. The regulation of glycogen phosphorylase by the metabolic signals AMP and glucose is a case in point (Fig. 3). The acute increase

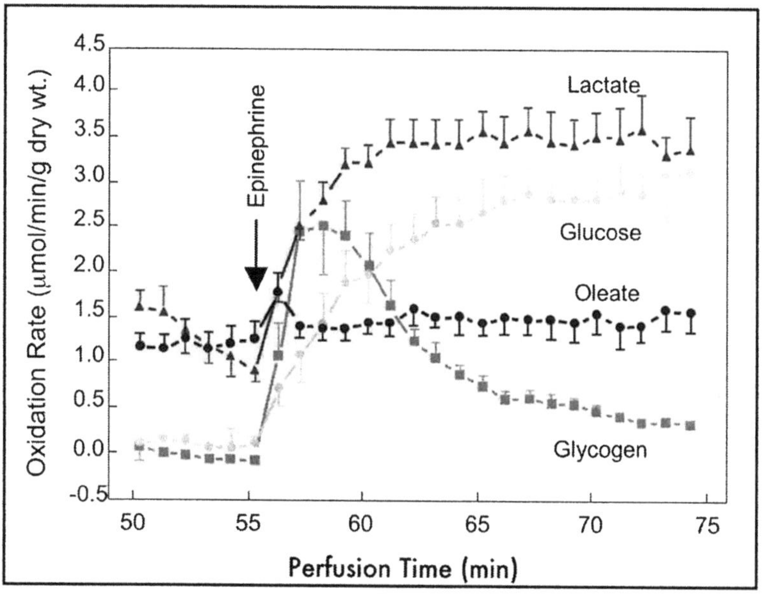

Figure 2. Substrate oxidation rates before and after contractile stimulation. G. W. Goodwin et al. *J Biol Chem* **273**, 29530-9 (1998).

in workload of the heart is accompanied by increases in [AMP] and intracellular free [glucose]. While AMP activates phosphorylase and promotes glycogen breakdown, free glucose inhibits phosphorylase and promotes glycogen synthesis (via an increase in glucose 6-phosphate and inhibition of glycogen synthase kinase). Thus, the metabolite measurements depicted in Figure 3 serve as illustrations for metabolic signals regulating fluxes through metabolic pathways and, hence, determining metabolic flexibility.

However, adaptations to sustained or chronic changes in the environment induce changes of the metabolic machinery at a transcriptional and/or translational level of the enzymes of metabolic pathways. We proposed earlier that metabolic remodeling precedes, triggers, and maintains structural and functional remodeling of the heart.[16] Here the nuclear receptor PPARα and its coactivator PGC-1 need to be mentioned again, because they have been identified as master-switches for the metabolic remodeling of the heart.[16-18] For example, pressure overload[19] and unloading of the heart,[20] hypoxia,[21] and, unexpectedly, also insulin-deficient diabetes[22] all result in the downregulation of genes controlling fatty acid oxidation and in reactivation of the fetal gene program (Fig. 4). These recent observations are in line with earlier work showing increased glucose metabolic activity in the pressure overloaded heart,[23] even before the onset of hypertrophy.[24] They are also in line with work showing impaired fatty acid oxidation by failing heart muscle in vitro,[25] and in vivo.[26, 27] We have proposed that metabolic flexibility is lost in diseased heart.[28] Richard Shannon's group has recently presented evidence for the development of myocardial insulin resistance in conscious dogs with advanced dilated cardiomyopathy induced by rapid ventricular pacing.[29]

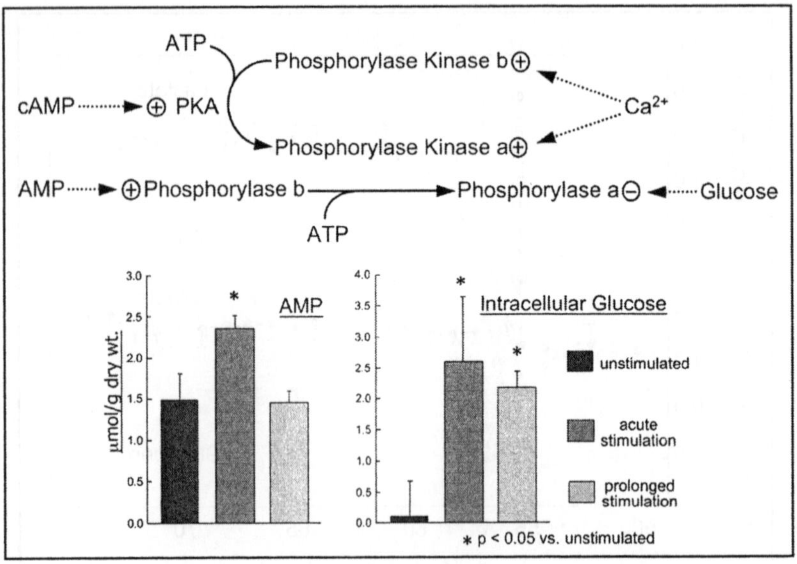

Figure 3. Metabolic regulating phosphorylase activity.

	Hypertrophy	Atrophy	Diabetes
Contractile proteins			
α-MHC	↓	↓	↓
β-MHC	↑	↑	↑
Cardiac α-actin	↓	↓	↓
Skeletal α-actin	↑	↑	↑
Ion pumps			
α_2 Na/K-ATPase	↓	↓	↓
SERCA 2a	↓	↓	↓
Metabolic proteins			
GLUT4	↓	↓	↓
GLUT1	=	=	↓
Muscle CPT-1	↓	↓	=
Liver CPT-1	=	=	=
mCK	↓	↓	↓
PPARα	↓	↓	↓
PDK4	↓	↓	↑
MCD	↓	↓	↑
UCP2	↓	↓	=
UCP3	↓	↓	↓
Protooncogenes			
c-fos	↑	↑	↓

Figure 4. Coordinated transcriptional responses of the heart in hypertrophy, atrophy, and diabetes.

3. PLEIOTROPIC ACTIONS OF METABOLISM

From the above discussion it becomes apparent that the actions of metabolism are more diverse than those found in the network of energy transfer and function of the heart. In addition to function, metabolism provides signals for growth, gene expression, and viability.

Metabolic Signals for Cardiac Growth. A case in point is the mammalian target of rapamycin (mTOR), an evolutionary conserved kinase and regulator of cell growth that serves as a point of convergence for nutrient sensing and growth factor signaling. In preliminary studies with the isolated working rat heart, we found that both glucose and amino acids are required for the activation of mTOR by insulin (Sharma et al., unpublished observations). In the same model we observed an unexpected dissociation between insulin stimulated Akt and mTOR activity, suggesting that Akt is not an upstream regulator of mTOR. We found that, irrespective of the stimulus, nutrients are critical for the activation of mTOR in the heart (Sharma et al., unpublished observations). The studies are ongoing.

Metabolic Signals of Cardiac Gene Expression. A single factor linking myosin heavy chain (MHC) isoform expression in the fetal, hypertrophied, and diabetic heart is intracellular free glucose. Compared to fatty acids, relatively little is known about the effects of glucose metabolism on cardiac gene expression.[30] The mechanisms by which glucose availability affects the DNA binding of transcription factors are not known precisely, although glucose availability and/or insulin affect the expression of specific genes in the liver.[31] A number of candidate transcription factors have been identified that are believed to be involved in glucose-mediated gene expression, mainly through investigations on the glucose/carbohydrate responsive elements. Carbohydrate responsive element-binding protein (ChREBP),[32] sterol regulatory element binding proteins (SREBPs), stimulatory protein 1 (Sp1), and upstream stimulatory factor 1 (USF1)[33] have all been implicated in glucose sensing by non-muscle tissues.[30] We have begun to investigate whether glucose-sensing mechanisms exist in heart muscle.

In preliminary experiments, we observed that altered glucose homeostasis through feeding of an isocaloric low carbohydrate, high fat diet completely abolishes MHC isoform switching in the hypertrophied heart (Young et al., unpublished observations). One mechanism by which glucose affects gene expression is through O-linked glycosylation of transcription factors. Glutamine: fructose-6-phosphate amidotransferase (gfat) catalyzes the flux-generating step in UDP-N-acetylglucosamine biosynthesis, the rate determining metabolite in protein glycosylation (Fig. 5). In preliminary studies we observed that overload increases the intracellular levels of UDP-N-acetylglucosamine and the expression of gfat2, but not gfat1, in the heart (McClain et al., unpublished work). Thus, there is early evidence for glucose-regulated gene expression in the heart and, more specifically, for the involvement of glucose metabolites in isoform switching of sarcomeric proteins. This work is ongoing.

Viability and Programmed Cell Survival. Perhaps the most dramatic example of chronic metabolic adaptation is the hibernating myocardium. Hibernating myocardium represents a chronically dysfunctional myocardium most likely the result of extensive

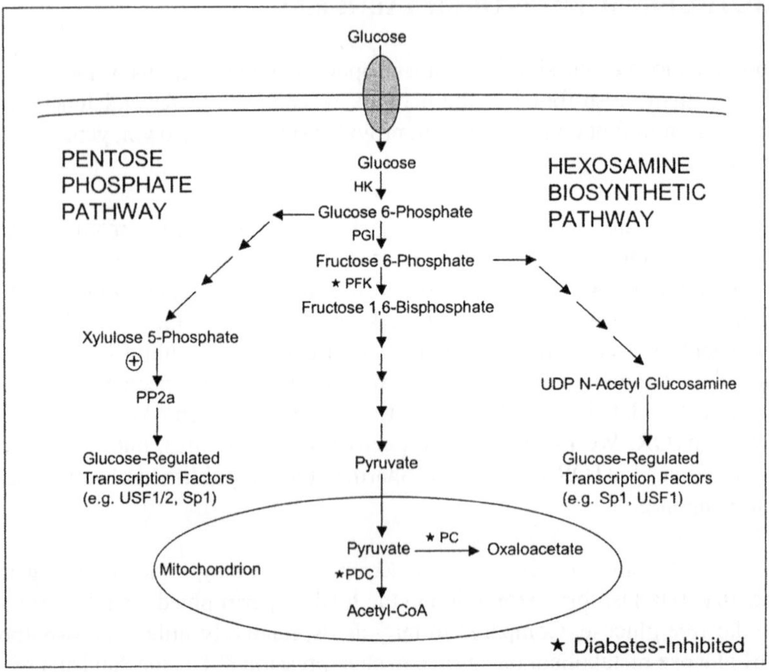

Figure 5. Mechanisms for glucose sensing in heart. Young et al., *Circulation* **105**, 1861-70 (2002).

cellular reprogramming due to repetitive episodes of ischemia. The adaptation to reduced oxygen delivery results in the prevention of irreversible tissue damage. A functional characteristic of hibernating myocardium is improved contractile function with inotropic stimulation or reperfusion. A metabolic characteristic of hibernating myocardium is the switch from fat to glucose metabolism, accompanied by reactivation of the fetal gene program. Because glucose transport and phosphorylation is readily traced by the uptake and retention of [18F] 2-deoxy, 2-fluoroglucose (FDG), hibernating myocardium is readily detected by enhanced glucose uptake and glycogen accumulation in the same regions.[34, 35] Like in fetal heart, the glycogen content of hibernating myocardium is dramatically increased. There is a direct correlation between glycogen content and myocardial levels of ATP,[36] and one is tempted to speculate that improved "energetics" may be the result of improved glycogen metabolism in hibernating myocardium. The true mechanism for "viability remodeling" of ischemic myocardium is likely to be much more complex.

The vast literature on programmed cell death, or apoptosis,[37, 38] and our own observations on programmed cell survival[36] support the idea of a direct link between metabolic pathways and the pathways of cell survival and destruction. Striking evidence for a link between cell survival and metabolism is found in cancer cells. Cancer cells not only possess an increased rate of glucose metabolism,[39] they are also less likely to "commit suicide" when stressed.[40] The same general principle appears to apply to the hibernating myocardium, where the downregulation of function and oxygen consumption is viewed as an adaptive response when coronary flow is impaired.[41] In other words, metabolic reprogramming initiates and sustains the functional and structural feature of hibernating myocardium.

Recently, the hypothesis has been advanced that insulin promotes tolerance against ischemic cell death via the activation of innate cell-survival pathways in the heart.[42] Specifically, activation of PI3 kinase, a downstream target of the insulin receptor substrate (IRS), and activation of protein kinase B/Akt, are mediators of antiapoptotic, cardioprotective signaling through activation of p70s6 kinase and inactivation of proapoptotic peptides. The major actor is Akt (pun not intended). Akt is located at the center of insulin and insulin-like growth factor 1 (IGF1) signaling. As the downstream serine-threonine kinase effector of PI3 kinase, Akt plays a key role in regulating cardiomyocyte growth and survival.[43] Overexpression of constitutively active Akt raises myocardial glycogen levels and protects against ischemic damage in vivo and in vitro.[44] Akt is also a modulator of metabolic substrate utilization.[45] Phosphorylation of GLUT4 by Akt promotes its translocation and increases glucose uptake. Although the "insulin hypothesis" is attractive, there is good evidence showing that the signaling cascade is dependent on the first committed step of glycolysis and translocation of hexokinase to the outer mitochondrial membrane.[46, 47] These few examples illustrate the fact that signals detected by metabolic imaging of stressed or failing heart are the product of complex cellular reactions – truly only the tip of an iceberg.

Concluding remarks

Energy substrate metabolism and function of the heart are inextricably linked. For a given change in its environment the heart oxidizes the most efficient fuel. Substrate switching and metabolic flexibility are therefore features of normal cardiac function. Loss of metabolic flexibility and metabolic remodeling precede, trigger, and sustain functional and structural remodeling of the stressed heart. Here I highlight the pleiotropic actions of metabolism in energy transfer, cardiac growth, gene expression, and viability. Examples are presented to illustrate that signals of stressed and failing heart are the product of complex cellular processes.

ACKNOWLEDGEMENTS

I thank past and present members of my laboratory for their many contributions to the ideas discussed in this review. Work in my laboratory is supported by grants from the National Institutes of Health of the U. S. Public Health Service.

REFERENCES

1. F. Knoop, Der Abbau aromatischer Fettsaeuren im Tierkoerper, *Beitr chem Physiol Pathol* **6**,150–162 (1904).
2. H. Winterstein, Ueber die Sauerstoffatmung des isolierten Saeugetierherzens, *Z Allg Physiol* **4**, 339–359 (1904).
3. R. J. Bing, A. Siegel, I. Ungar, and M. Gilbert, Metabolism of the human heart. II. Studies on fat, ketone and amino acid metabolism, *Am J Med* **16**, 504–15 (1954).

4. F. L. Holmes, Between Biology and Medicine: The Formation of Intermediary Metabolism. Berkeley, CA: University of California at Berkeley; p. 114 (1992).
5. P. J. Randle, P. B. Garland, C. N. Hales, and E. A. Newsholme, The glucose fatty-acid cycle. Its role in insulin sensitivity and the metabolic disturbances of diabetes mellitus, *Lancet* **1**, 785–789 (1963).
6. H. Taegtmeyer, R. Hems, and H. A. Krebs, Utilization of energy providing substrates in the isolated working rat heart, *Biochem J* **186**, 701–711 (1980).
7. J. D. McGarry, S. E. Mills, C. S. Long, and D.W. Foster, Observations on the affinity for carnitine and malonyl-CoA sensitivity of carnitine palmitoyl transferase I in animal and human tissues. Demonstration of the presence of malonyl-CoA in non-hepatic tissues of the rat, *Biochem J* **214**, 21–28 (1983).
8. M. E. Young, G. W. Goodwin, J. Ying, P. Guthrie, C. R. Wilson, F. A. Laws, and H. Taegtmeyer, Regulation of cardiac and skeletal muscle malonyl-CoA decarboxylase by fatty acids, *Am J Physiol Endocrinol Metab* **280**, E471–E479 (2001).
9. D. G. Hardie, and D. Carling, The AMP-activated protein kinase--fuel gauge of the mammalian cell? *Eur J Biochem* **246**, 259–273 (1997).
10. N. B. Ruderman, A. K. Saha, D. Vavvas, and L. A. Witters, Malonyl-CoA, fuel sensing, and insulin resistance, *Am J Physiol* **276**, E1–E18 (1999).
11. P. M. Barger, J. M. Brandt, T. C. Leone, C. J. Weinheimer, and D. P. Kelly, Deactivation of peroxisome proliferator-activated receptor-alpha during cardiac hypertrophic growth, *J Clin Invest* **105**, 1723–1730 (2000).
12. M. F. Allard, B. O. Schonekess, S. L. Henning, D. R. English, and G. D. Lopaschuk, Contribution of oxidative metabolism and glycolysis to ATP production in hypertrophied hearts, *Am J Physiol* **267**, H742–H750 (1994).
13. T. Doenst, G. W. Goodwin, A. M. Cedars, M. Wang, S. Stepkowski, and H. Taegtmeyer, Load-induced changes in vivo alter substrate fluxes and insulin responsiveness of rat heart in vitro, *Metabolism* **50**, 1083–1090 (2001).
14. M. E. Young, S. Patil, J. Ying, C. Depre, H. S. Ahuja, G. L. Shipley, S. M. Stepkowski, P. J. Davies and H. Taegtmeyer, Uncoupling protein 3 transcription is regulated by peroxisome proliferator-activated receptor (alpha) in the adult rodent heart, *FASEB J* **15**, 833–845 (2001).
15. G. W. Goodwin, C. S. Taylor, and H. Taegtmeyer, Regulation of energy metabolism of the heart during acute increase in heart work, *J Biol Chem* **273**, 29530–29539 (1998).
16. H. Taegtmeyer, Genetics of energetics: transcriptional responses in cardiac metabolism, *Ann Biomed Eng* **28**, 871–876 (2000).
17. P. M. Barger, and D. P. Kelly, PPAR signaling in the control of cardiac energy metabolism, *Trends Cardiovasc Med* **10**, 238–45 (2000).
18. D. P. Kelly, PPARs of the heart: three is a crowd, *Circ Res* **92**, 482–4 (2003).
19. J. J. Lehman, and D. P. Kelly, Gene regulatory mechanisms governing energy metabolism during cardiac hypertrophic growth, *Heart Fail Rev* **7**, 175–85 (2002).
20. C. Depre, G. L. Shipley, W. Chen, Q. Han, T. Doenst, M. L. Moore, S. Stepkowski, P. J. Davies and H. Taegtmeyer, Unloaded heart in vivo replicates fetal gene expression of cardiac hypertrophy, *Nature Medicine* **4**, 1269–1275 (1998).
21. P. Razeghi, M. E. Young, S. Abbasi, and H. Taegtmeyer, Hypoxia in vivo decreases peroxisome proliferator-activated receptor alpha-regulated gene expression in rat heart, *Biochem Biophys Res Commun* **287**, 5–10 (2001).
22. M. E. Young, P. Guthrie, S. Stepkowski, and H. Taegtmeyer, Glucose regulation of sarcomeric protein gene expression in the rat heart, *J Mol Cell Cardiol* **33**, A181 (abstract) (2001).
23 S. Bishop, and R. Altschuld, Increased glycolytic metabolism in cardiac hypertrophy and congestive heart failure, *Am J Physiol* **218**, 153–159 (1970).
24. H. Taegtmeyer, and M. L. Overturf, Effects of moderate hypertension on cardiac function and metabolism in the rabbit, *Hypertension* **11**, 416–426 (1988).
25. B. Wittels, and J. F. Spann, Defective lipid metabolism in the failing heart, *J Clin Invest* **47**, 1787–1794 (1968).
26. M. N. Sack, T. A. Rader, S. Park, J. Bastin, S. A. McCune, and D. P. Kelly, Fatty acid oxidation enzyme gene expression is downregulated in the failing heart, *Circulation* **94**, 2837–2842 (1996).

27. V. G. Davila-Roman, G. Vedala, P. Herrero, L. de las Fuentes, J. G. Rogers, D. P. Kelly and R. J. Gropler, Altered myocardial fatty acid and glucose metabolism in idiopathic dilated cardiomyopathy, *J Am Coll Cardiol* **40**, 271–7 (2002).
28. H. Taegtmeyer, S. Sharma, L. Golfman, M. Van Arsdall, and P. Razeghi, Linking gene expression to function: metabolic flexibility in normal and diseased heart, *Ann N Y Acad Sci* **1015**, 1–12 (2004).
29. L. A. Nikolaidis, A. Sturzu, C. Stolarski, D. Elahi, Y. T. Shen, and R. P. Shannon, The development of myocardial insulin resistance in conscious dogs with advanced dilated cardiomyopathy, *Cardiovasc Res* **61**, 297–306 (2004) .
30. M. E.Young, P. McNulty, and H. Taegtmeyer, Adaptation and maladaptation of the heart in diabetes: Part II: potential mechanisms, *Circulation* **105**, 1861–1870 (2002).
31. P. Ferre, Regulation of gene expression by glucose, *Proc Nutr Soc* **58**, 621–3 (1999).
32. K. Uyeda, H. Yamashita, and T. Kawaguchi, Carbohydrate responsive element-binding protein (ChREBP): a key regulator of glucose metabolism and fat storage, *Biochem Pharmacol* **63**, 2075–80 (2002).
33. J. Girard, P. Ferre, and F. Foufelle, Mechanisms by which carbohydrates regulate expression of genes for glycolytic and lipogenic enzymes, *Annu Rev Nutr* **17**, 325–352 (1997).
34. M. Maki, M. Luotolahti, P. Nuutila, H. Iida, L. Voipio-Pulkki, U Ruotsalainen, M. Haaparanta, O. Solin, J. Hartiala, R. Harkonen and J. Knuuti, Glucose uptake in the chronically dysfunctional but viable myocardium, *Circulation* **93**, 1658–66 (1996).
35. C. Depre, J. L. Vanoverschelde, B. Gerber, M. Borgers, J. A. Melin, and R. Dion, Correlation of functional recovery with myocardial blood flow, glucose uptake, and morphologic features in patients with chronic left ventricular ischemic dysfunction undergoing coronary artery bypass grafting, *J Thorac Cardiovasc Surg* **113**, 82–87 (1997).
36. C. Depre, and H. Taegtmeyer, Metabolic aspects of programmed cell survival and cell death in the heart, *Cardiovasc Res* **45**, 538–548 (2000).
37. R. A. Gottlieb, Mitochondria: ignition chamber for apoptosis, *Mol Genet Metab* **68**, 227–231 (1999).
38. J. Downward, Metabolism meets death, *Nature* **424**, 896–7 (2003).
39. O. Warburg, On the origin of cancer cells, *Science* **123**, 309–314 (1956).
40. D. Hanahan, and R. A. Weinberg, The Hallmarks of cancer, *Cell* **100**, 57–70 (2000).
41. J. A. Fallavollita, B. J. Malm, and J. M. J. Canty, Hibernating myocardiam retains metabolic and contractile reserve despite regional reductions in flow, function, and oxygen consumption at rest, *Circ Res* **92**, 48–55 (2003).
42. M. N. Sack, and D. M. Yellon, Insulin Therapy as an Adjunct to Reperfusion After Acute Coronary Ischemia, A Proposed Direct Myocardial Cell Survival Effect Independent of Metabolic Modulation, *J Am Coll Cardiol* **41**,1404–07 (2003).
43. T. Matsui, T. Nagoshi, and A. Rosenzweig, Akt and PI 3-kinase signaling in cardiomyocyte hypertrophy and survival, *Cell Cycle* **2**, 220–3 (2003).
44. T. Matsui, L. Li, J. Wu, S. Cook, T. Nagoshi, M. Picard, R. Liao and A. Rosenzweig, Phenotypic spectrum caused by transgenic overexpression of activated Akt in the heart, *J Biol Chem* **277**, 22896–901 (2002).
45. E. Whiteman, H. Cho, and M. Birnbaum, Role of Akt/protein kinase B in metabolism, *Trends Endocrinol Metab* **13**, 444–51 (2002).
46. K. Gottlob, N. Majewski, S. Kennedy, E. Kandel, R. B. Robey, and N. Hay, Inhibition of early apoptotic events by Akt/PKB is dependent on the first committed step of glycolysis and mitochondrial hexokinase, *Genes Dev* **15**, 1406–1418 (2001).
47. N. Majewski, V. Nogueira, R. B. Robey, and N. Hay, Akt inhibits apoptosis downstream of BID cleavage via a glucose-dependent mechanism involving mitochondrial hexokinases, *Mol Cell Biol* **24**, 730–40 (2004).

CHAPTER 1

MYOCARDIAL ISCHEMIA

Basic Concepts

Constantinos Pantos*, Iordanis Mourouzis*, Dennis V. Cokkinos**

1. THE PATHOPHYSIOLOGY OF ISCHEMIA AND REPERFUSION INJURY

1.1. Cellular injury

An imbalance between oxygen supply and demand due to compromised coronary flow results in myocardial ischemia. In theory, the process is very simple; lack of adequate oxygen and metabolic substrates rapidly decreases the energy available to the cell and leads to cell injury that is of reversible or irreversible nature. In practice, the process is very complex. The extent of injury is determined by various factors; the severity of ischemia (low-flow vs zero–flow ischemia), the duration of ischemia, the temporal sequence of ischemia (short ischemia followed by long ischemia), changes in metabolic and physical environment (hypothermia vs normothermia, preischemic myocardial glycogen content, perfusate composition) as well as the inflammatory response. Reperfusion generally pre-requisite for tissue survival may also increase injury over and above that sustained during ischemia. This phenomenon named reperfusion injury leads in turn to myocardial cell death.

Two major forms of cell death are recognized in the pathology of myocardial injury; the necrotic cell death and the apoptotic cell death. The exact contributions of the necrotic and apoptotic cell death in myocardial cell injury is unclear. Both forms of cell death occur in experimental settings of ischemia and reperfusion. Necrotic cell death was shown to peak after 24h of reperfusion and apoptotic cell death was increased up to 72 h of reperfusion, in a canine model of ischemia and reperfusion.[1] Furthermore, apoptotic cell death can evolve into necrotic cell death and pharmacological inhibition of the apoptotic signaling cascade during the reperfusion phase is able to attenuate both the apoptotic and necrotic components of cell death.[2, 3] Apoptosis and necrosis seem to share common

*Department of Pharmacology, University of Athens, 75 Mikras Asias Ave. 11527 Goudi, Athens, Greece
**Professor of Cardiology, Medical School, University of Athens Greece and Chairman, department of cardiology, Onassis Cardiac Surgery Center
Correspondence: Ass. Professor Constantinos Pantos, Department of Pharmacology, University of Athens, 75 Mikras Asias Ave. 11527 Goudi, Athens, Greece, Tel: (+30210) 7462560, Fax: (+30210) 7705185, Email: cpantos@cc.uoa.gr

mechanisms in the early stages of cell death. The intensity of the stimulus is likely to determine the apoptosis or necrosis.

Necrosis is characterized by membrane disruption, massive cell swelling, cell lysis and fragmentation, and triggers the inflammatory response. The primary site of irreversible injury has been a subject of intense investigation and several hypotheses are postulated. These include the lysosomal, the mitochondrial, the metabolic end-product, calcium overload, the phospholipase, the lipid peroxidation and the cytoskeleton hypotheses, reviewed by Ganote.[4]

Apoptosis is a programmed, energy dependent process that results in chromatin condensation, DNA fragmentation and apoptotic body formation, preserved cell membrane integrity and does not involve the inflammatory response. Apoptosis occurs during the ischemic phase and can be accelerated during reperfusion[5] or can be triggered at reperfusion.[6] Apoptosis can progress to necrosis by the loss of ATP in severely ischemic tissue. The cellular processes by which the apoptotic signal is transduced are divided into two basic pathways; the extrinsic and the intrinsic pathway. Figure 1. Both pathways are executed by proteases known as caspases. The extrinsic pathway is a receptor–mediated system activated by tumor necrosis factor–α (TNF-α) and Fas receptors and executed through the activation of caspase–8 and caspase-3.[7] Figure 1. Cardiomyocytes have Fas and TNF-α receptors, and cardiac cells produce Fas ligand and TNF-α, which can activate the death receptor mediated pathway.[8] Fas ligand and TNF-α are involved in late apoptosis after reperfusion. In hearts from mice lacking functional Fas, apoptosis was reduced 24h later following 30 min of ischemia.[9] Fas ligand and TNF-α have not been implicated in apoptosis induced by hypoxia alone. The intrinsic pathway of apoptosis signaling is mediated through the mitochondria and is activated by stimuli such as hypoxia, ischemia and reperfusion and oxidative stress.[10] Figure 1. These pro-apoptotic signals induce mitochondrial permeability transition, which is characterized by increased permeability of the outer and inner mitochondrial membranes. The mitochondrial permeability transition pore (MPTP) is a protein complex that spans both membranes and consists of the voltage anion channel (VDAC) in the outer membrane, the adenine nucleotide translocase (ANT) in the inner membrane and cyclophilin–D in the matrix.[11] MPTP opening occurs by mitochondrial calcium overload particularly in the presence of oxidative stress, depletion of adenine nucleotides, increase in phosphate levels and mitochondrial depolarization while low pH is a restraining factor for MPTP opening. In fact, with correction of acidosis at reperfusion this restrain is removed and MPTP opens. MPTP opening occurs mainly at reperfusion but there is an increasing evidence that can also occur during ischemia.[12] Opening of the MPTP leads to the release of cytochrome c, Smac/DIABLO, endonuclease G (EndoG) and apoptosis–inducing factor (AIF) all of which facilitate the apoptosis signaling.[13, 14] Figure 1. Cytochrome c is a catalytic scavenger for the mitochondrial superoxide and loss of cytochrome c results in inactivation of mitochondrial respiratory chain, reactive oxygen species (ROS) production and initiation of apoptosis. Cytochrome c binds to the cytosolic protein Apaf-1 and results in caspase-9 and caspase-3 activation.[15] Figure 1. This process can only be executed when sufficient ATP is available. Therefore, cytochrome c release may have little or no consequences on apoptosis with severe ischemia as ATP depletion will limit caspase activation and cause necrosis. Smac/DIABLO indirectly activates caspases by sequestering caspase–inhibitory proteins while EndoG and AIF translocate to nucleus where they facilitate DNA fragmentation. Figure 1. It appears that MPTP converts the mitochondrion from an organelle that provides ATP to sustain cell life to an instrument of programmed cell death if the insult is mild and necrosis if the insult is severe. Interventions which inhibit MPTP opening and enhance pore closure, either directly in the form of cyclosporin A or sanglifehrin A, or indirectly, in the form of propofol, pyruvate, or ischemic preconditioning are shown to provide protection against ischemia and reperfusion injury.[12]

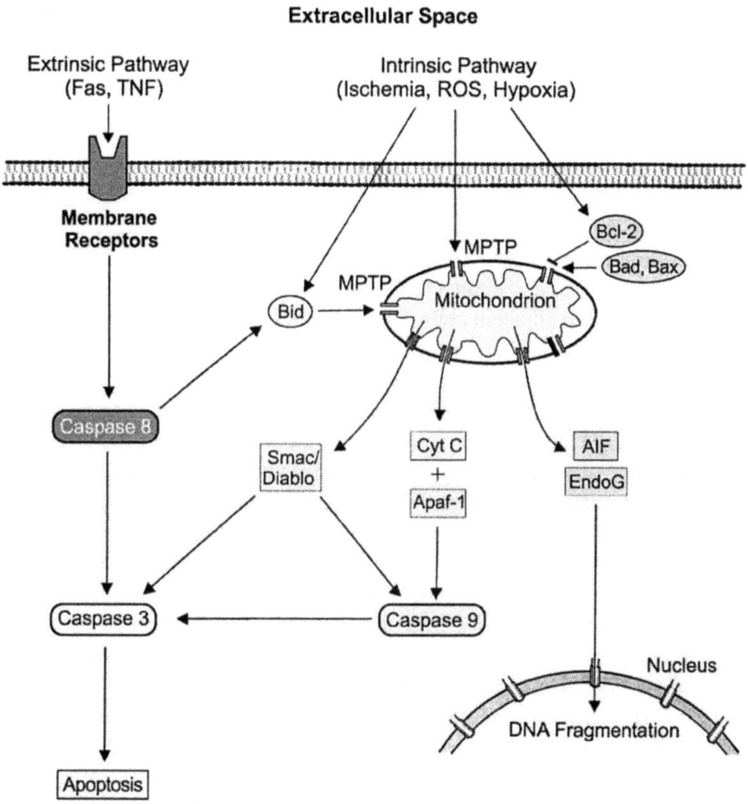

Figure 1. Schematic of the apoptotic signaling pathways. The intrinsic apoptotic pathway consists of the mitochondrial pathway. The extrinsic pathway mediates apoptosis through activation of the death receptors, TNF-α/Fas receptors. Apoptosis is executed by activation of proteases, known as caspases. ATP is essential for apoptosis. Bcl-2 family proteins are apoptosis regulating proteins; Bcl-2 inhibits while Bid, Bax, Bad facilitate apoptosis. An interaction between these two apoptotic pathways exists. See text for a more detailed explanation.

The Bcl-2 family of proteins are considered as apoptosis regulating proteins. Members of this family are the Bcl-2 and Bcl-xL which are anti-apoptotic while Bax, Bad, Bid, Bim are pro-apoptotic. Pro-apoptotic and anti-apoptotic Bcl-2 proteins can bind directly to the components of mitochondrial pore, leading to either its opening or closure respectively.[16] Figure 1. Alternatively, pro-apoptotic members, such as Bak or Bax, insert into the outer mitochondrial membrane where they oligomerize to form a permeable pore.[17] Furthermore, an interaction between the intrinsic and the extrinsic pathway can occur through Bcl-2 proteins. Bid is cleaved by caspase–8 and translocates to the mitochondria and induces permeability pore transition.[18] Figure 1. Bcl-2 proteins are regulated through various processes. For instance, phosphorylation of Bad by kinases results to its inactivation while phosphorylaton of Bim leads to its proteosomal degradation.[19,20]

1.2. Spread of cell injury

1.2.1 Gap junctions; cell to cell communication

While much has been learned about mechanisms of cell death in cultured cardiomyocytes, heart muscle cells in vivo form a functional syncytium and do not exist in isolation. The communication between cells occurs through Gap junctions (GJ). Gap junctions are specialized membrane areas containing a tightly packed array of channels. Each channel is formed by the two end to end connected hemichannels (also known as connexons) contributed by each of the two adjacent cells. Hemichannels are formed by six connexins. Gap junctions are not connected to other cytoskeletal filaments and are not considered part of the cytoskeletal system.[21] GJ are now recognized to play an important role in progression and spread of cell injury and death during myocardial ischemia and reperfusion.[22] Closure of gap junctions during ischemia was initially thought to occur as a protective mechanism preventing spreading of injury across the cardiomyocytes. However, it is now realized that persistent cell to cell communication can exist during ischemia and reperfusion. In fact, gap junction communication allows cell to cell propagation of rigor contracture and equalization of calcium overload in ischemic myocardium. Although the mechanism of propagation of ischemic contracture is not clear, it can be speculated that cells developing rigor contracture and consuming ATP in an accelerated way may steal gap junction permeable ATP from adjacent cells, decreasing their ATP levels to the critical values at which rigor contracture develops, reviewed by Garcia-Dorado.[22]

The role of GJ in ischemia and reperfusion injury has been shown in studies using GJ blockers; reduction of necrosis after ischemia and reperfusion was observed in in situ rabbit hearts and in isolated rat hearts with administration of halothane (presumed to be a GJ uncoupling agent).[23,24] Furthermore, regulation of the phosphorylation of connexin 43 (non phosphorylated Cx43 increases the opening of GJ) resulted in modification of ischemic injury. In fact, ischemic preconditioning (brief episodes of ischemia and reperfusion) induced cardioprotection was associated with preservation of connexin 43 phosphorylation.[25]

GJ opening may also contribute to cardioprotection. Survival signals can be transferred from one cell to another. In fact, cell to cell interaction through GJ has been described to prevent apoptosis in neonatal rat ventricular myocytes.[26] The intensity of the stimulus is likely to determine the beneficial or detrimental role of GJ communication. See also chapter 4.

1.2.2 The inflammatory response

Myocardial ischemia is associated with an inflammatory response that further contributes to myocardial injury and ultimately leads to myocardial healing and scar formation. Myocardial necrosis has been associated with complement activation and free radical generation that trigger cytokine cascades and upregulate chemokines expression. Mononuclear cell chemoattractants, such as the CC chemokines CCL2/Monocyte

Chemoattractant Protein (MCP)-1, CCL3/Macrophage Inflammatory Protein (MIP)-1 alpha, and CCL4/MIP-1 beta are expressed in the ischemic area, and regulate monocyte and lymphocyte recruitment. Chemokines have also additional effects on healing infarcts beyond their leukotactic properties. The CXC chemokine CXCL 10/Interferon–y inducible Protein (IP)-10, a potent angiostatic factor with antifibrotic properties, is induced in the infarct and may prevent premature angiogenesis and fibrous tissue deposition. Chemokine induction in the infarct is transient, suggesting that inhibitory mediators, such as transforming growth factor (TGF)-beta may be activated suppressing chemokine synthesis and leading to resolution of inflammation and fibrosis, reviewed by Frangogiannis.[27] Daily repetitive episodes of brief ischemia and reperfusion in mice resulted in chemokine upregulation followed by suppression of chemokine synthesis and interstitial fibrosis, in the absence of myocardial infarction.[28]

Interleukin–8 and C5a are released in the ischemic myocardium and may have a crucial role in neutrophil recruitment.[29] Neutrophils are cells rich in oxidant species and proteolytic enzymes and can cause cell injury. In fact, annexin 1, a potent inhibitor of neutrophil extravasation in vivo was shown to protect the heart against ischemia and reperfusion injury.[30] However, the importance of neutrophil in causing myocardial damage in the context of ischemia and reperfusion is now questioned. Experimental evidence shows that the time course of neutrophil accumulation in postischemic myocardium seems to be different from the time course of injury, myocardial injury is observed in neutrophil free conditions and anti-inflammatory interventions do not consistently limit infarct size, reviewed by Baxter.[31]

Cytokines also exert direct negative inotropic effects via paracrine and autocrine modulation. This negative inotropic effect appears early (2-5min) and at later stages.[32] Tumor necrosis factor (TNF-α), interleukin (IL-6) and (IL-1) are all shown to reduce myocardial contractility acting in synergistic and cascade–like reactions.

The heart is a tumor necrosis factor-α producing organ (TNF-α). TNF-α is produced in response to stress. Macrophages and cardiac myocytes themselves synthesize TNF-α and TNF-α is also released by mast cells. TNF-α is an autocrine contributor to myocardial dysfunction and cardiomyocyte death in ischemia and reperfusion injury. Ischemia-reperfusion induced activation of p38 MAPK results in activation of the nuclear factor kappa B (NFkB) and leads to TNF-α production. During reperfusion, TNF-α release occurs early (from mast cell activation) as well as at a later phase as a result of de novo synthesis possibly induced by TNF-α itself and /or intracellular oxidative stress. Antioxidant treatment and mast cell stabilizers have been shown to prevent TNF-α release.[33] TNF-α depresses myocardial function by nitric oxide independent (sphingosine dependent) (early effect) and nitric oxide dependent (later effect) mechanisms. Sphingosine is produced by the sphingomyelin pathway which inhibits calcium release from sarcoplasmic reticulum (SR) by blocking the ryanodine receptor. Activation of TNF-α receptor or Fas also induces apoptosis. However, TNF-α at low doses before ischemia and reperfusion is shown to be cardioprotective through a reactive oxygen species dependent signaling pathway.[34]

IL-1 increases nitric oxide (NO) production by upregulating the synthesis of iNOS.[35] This cytokine acts also via an NO-independent mechanism and causes downregulation of calcium regulating genes with subsequent depressed myocardial contractility.[36]

IL-6 levels are elevated in patients with acute myocardial infarction. IL-6 is secreted by mononuclear cells in the ischemic area and is also produced by cardiac myocytes. IL-6 apart from its inflammatory effect regulates contractile function by its acute effect on calcium transients.[37]

Complement activation also contributes to ischemic injury. Current evidence indicates that ischemia leads to the expression of neoantigen or ischemia antigen on cellular surfaces, and this induces binding of circulating IgM natural antibody. This immune complex causes C1 binding, complement activation and the formation of C3a and C3b. C3b activates the remainder of the complement cascade leading to the formation of the membrane attack complex, which is the principal mediator of injury. Complement inhibition results in less myocardial ischemia and reperfusion injury, reviewed by Chan.[38]

Platelet-activating factor (PAF) is released during ischemia and reperfusion injury from non cardiac cells and cardiomyocytes. PAF is rapidly synthesized during ischemia and reperfusion from membrane phospholipids after sequential activation of phospholipase A2 and acetyl-transferase. The effect of PAF is mediated through specific PAF cell surface receptors that belong to G protein–coupled receptors. It depresses cardiac contractility by negatively regulating calcium handling. Furthermore, PAF stimulates the release of other biologically active mediators such as eicosanoids, superoxide anions and TNF-α that can further enhance myocardial injury. An adverse effect of PAF is also mediated by the induction of vascular constriction and capillary plugging.[39]

Despite the potential injurious effect, the reperfusion inflammatory response also triggers the healing process. Accumulation of monocyte derived macrophages and mast cells increase expression of growth factors inducing angiogenesis and fibroblast accumulation. Inflammatory mediators may induce recruitment of blood derived primitive stem cells in the healing infarct which may differentiate into endothelial cells and even lead to myocardial regeneration.[40]

Matrix metalloproteinases (MMPs) and their inhibitors regulate extracellular matrix deposition and play an important role in ventricular remodeling. Three MMPs (MMP-1, MMP-2, and MMP-9) appear to be of importance, with each enzyme being generated from different sources and most likely responsible for different aspects of the pathological process of tissue necrosis and healing. MMP-1, which is activated through a p38 MAPK dependent pathway (either directly or indirectly), can induce cardiomyocyte death that might contribute to the immediate lethal injury observed within the first few minutes of reperfusion. MMP-2, which could be present intracellularly or possibly released from platelets activated by ischemia, appears to play a very early role following myocardial reperfusion, where, it is involved in the breakdown of the contractile apparatus, resulting in cellular injury and in the functional consequence of impaired myocardial contractility. MMP-9 is most closely associated with neutrophils, which are known to infiltrate injured tissue later at reperfusion, where, it is likely to contribute to the extension of cellular death, reviewed by Wainwright.[41] MMP effects can be modulated by the tissue inhibitors of MMP, the TIMPs and the extent of injury seems to be determined by TIMP/MMP balance during ischemia and reperfusion. In fact, angiotensin II is shown to modulate this balance and in an in vivo dog model of regional ischemia and reperfusion, inhibition of angiotensin II type 1 receptor by valsartan resulted in protection by increasing TIMP-3 expression and improving the balance of TIMP-3 /MMP-9.[42]

1.3. Microvascular injury

Endothelial dysfunction and microvascular injury start at the interphase of the endothelium with the bloodstream. Reperfusion of ischemic vasculature results in production of excessive quantities of vasoconstrictors, oxygen–free radical formation and neutrophil activation and accumulation. Neutrophils and macrophages further increase the formation of reactive oxygen species and act as an amplifier of the ischemic injury. Severe microvascular dysfunction can arrest the microcirculation, a phenomenon known as the "no reflow phenomenon". Capillaries may be occluded by extravascular compression, endothelial swelling or intravascular plugs, such as platelet aggregates and thrombi. In experimental models of temporary coronary artery occlusion, tissue perfusion at the microvascular level remains incomplete even after the patency of the infarct related epicardial coronary artery is established, and distinct perfusion defects develop within the risk zone. A major determinant of the extent of no reflow seems to be the infarct size itself. Reperfusion related expansion of no reflow zones occurs within the first hours following reopening of the coronary artery with a parallel reduction of regional myocardial flow. On a long–term basis, tissue perfusion after ischemia and reperfusion remains markedly compromised for at least 4 weeks, reviewed by Reffemann.[43]

1.4. Biochemical aspects of ischemia-reperfusion

The heart is a metabolic omnivore that is able to use a variety of substrates to generate energy, including exogenous glucose, fatty acids, lactate, amino acids and ketone bodies as well as endogenous glycogen and triglycerides. Glucose taken up by the myocardium is rapidly phosphorylated and either is catabolized or incorporated into glycogen. Myocardial glucose uptake is facilitated by transport via the glucose transporters GLUT1 (basal glucose uptake) and GLUT4 (insulin or stress mediated glucose uptake). Glucose is converted to pyruvate by sequential series of reactions, termed the glycolytic pathway. Figure 2. The enzymes hexokinase and 6-phospho-fructo-kinase-1 are among the major sites regulating flux through this pathway. Pyruvate which may also be derived from glycogen or lactate is converted to acetyl-CoA in the mitochondria, and pyruvate dehydrogenase determines the extent of this reaction. Figure 2. Acetyl-CoA enters the tricarboxylic acid cycle (TCA) for oxidation (i.e. generation of H^+) and combustion (i.e. generation of CO_2). Long chain fatty acids uptake is facilitated by membrane–bound and cytosolic fatty acid–binding proteins. They are esterified with coenzyme-A prior to incorporation into triacylglycerols or transport to mitochondrial matrix (regulated by carnitine palmitoyltransferase-1, CPT-1). Figure 2. In the mitochondria, fatty acid oxidation occurs by means of the β-oxidation spiral (FAO) and tricarboxylic acid cycle (TCA). Figure 2. The $NADH_2$ and $FADH_2$ formed from glycolytic pathway, TCA cycle and fatty acid oxidation are oxidized in the respiratory chain and the energy generated from the transport of electrons to oxygen is the driving force for ATP production. Figure 2. This process is known as oxidative phosphorylation.

In response to ischemic stress, several changes in the metabolic pathways and energy production are observed in cytosol and mitochondria followed by changes in membrane ion homeostasis and morphological alterations in subcellular organelles (See chapter 1). These changes might contribute to cell survival under anaerobic conditions. Glucose uptake is increased either by the translocation of glucose transporters to the membrane or by the orientation of the transporters within the sarcolemma. Glycogen breakdown is enhanced. The glycolytic rate increases (the key enzyme 6-phospho-fructokinase-1 is activated). However, pyruvate cannot entry the TCA cycle because pyruvate dyhydrogenase (PDH) is inhibited. Instead, it is converted to lactate and alanine. Figure 2. Accumulation of $NADH_2$ in cytosol is increased due to its reduced removal by mitochondria (inhibition of the malate–aspartate cycle) and is counterbalanced by $NADH_2$ conversion to NAD through the formation of lactate from the pyruvate. Figure 2. Mild acidosis develops from

ATP hydrolysis and this could be seen as beneficial; competes with calcium and decreases contractility, inhibits nucleotidases and prevents further breakdown of AMP. AMP activates AMP kinase with subsequent increase in the rate of glycolysis and fatty acid oxidation. Figure 2. AMPK is responsible for the activation of glucose uptake and glycolysis during low-flow ischemia and seems to play an important protective role in limiting damage and apoptotic activity associated with ischemia and reperfusion in the heart.[44]

Glucose derived ATP preserves sarcolemmal pump function and membrane integrity while glycogen breakdown derived ATP (present at myofibrils and possibly at the sarcoplasmic reticulum) supports cell contractile function. Under normoxia these functions are supported by oxidative phosphorylation derived ATP. With more severe ischemia, the progressive accumulation of the end-products of anaerobic metabolism inhibits glucose uptake and glycolysis. Thus, severe ATP depletion and acidosis occur. Fatty acyl-CoA derivatives accumulate resulting in cell damage of irreversible nature, reviewed by Opie.[45]

Loss of the activity of the respiratory complexes occurs during ischemia. Progression of the ischemic damage is shown to progressively inhibit the respiratory chain with complex I activity to be lower in less severe ischemia and complex IV activity to be reduced in severe ischemia.[46] Mitochondrial changes during ischemia and reperfusion result in increased production and accumulation of reactive oxygen species. The energy transport from mitochondria to cytosol is also impaired. Adenine nucleotide translocase and mitochondrial creatine kinase activity (enzymes that are required for transportation of ATP from the mitochondria to the cytosol) is reduced with subsequent impaired ATP transportation into the sites of utilization. ATP in the mitochondrial matrix is hydrolyzed by the reversal of the ATP synthase, reviewed by Opie.[45]

Selective inhibition of TCA cycle enzymes aconitase and α-ketoglutarate dehydrogenase, both known to be sensitive to in vitro oxidative modification occurs at reperfusion. TCA enzymes activation does not decline with ischemia. As a consequence the production of $NADH_2$ and a rise in reactive oxygen production occurs.[47,48] Glucose metabolism is limited to the cytosolic pathway (increased glycolysis and glycogen synthesis) while fatty acids are oxidized at high rates. Malonyl-coenzyme (CoA) production is decreased and facilitates fatty acid transport to mitochondria. Increased fatty acid metabolism by β-oxidation represses glucose metabolism due to its inhibitory effect on the pyruvate dehydrogenase activation. The imbalance between glucose and fatty acid oxidation leads to the decrease in cardiac efficiency, reviewed by Lopaschuk.[49]

Energy depletion and acidosis result in several changes in ion homeostasis with important physiological consequences. Sodium enters the cell due to the inhibition of the sodium pump (Na^+/K^+-ATPase) and enhanced activation of the sodium–proton exchanger (NHE). NHE is important for correcting cell acidosis. NHE activity is regulated by a variety of G-protein coupled receptor systems. An increase in NHE activity occurs in response to the activation of the α_1-adrenergic, angiotensin (AT_1), endothelin and thrombin receptors. β_1-adrenergic stimulation inhibits NHE activity while stimulation of adenosine A_1 and angiotensin (AT_2) receptors have a modulatory effect and attenuates NHE activation induced by other ligands, reviewed by Avkiran.[50] In the setting of ischemia and reperfusion most of these stimulatory and inhibitory systems are operated and ultimately modulate NHE activity with detrimental or protective effects. NHE1 mRNA is increased after global ischemia (30 min) and apoptosis is induced in a mitochondrial calcium-dependent manner.[51, 52] However, the expression of NHE1 is found to be decreased in the non infarcted myocardium in a rat model of acute myocardial infarction.[53] Furthermore, mice with a null mutation in the NHE1 exchanger are resistant to ischemia and reperfusion injury.[54]

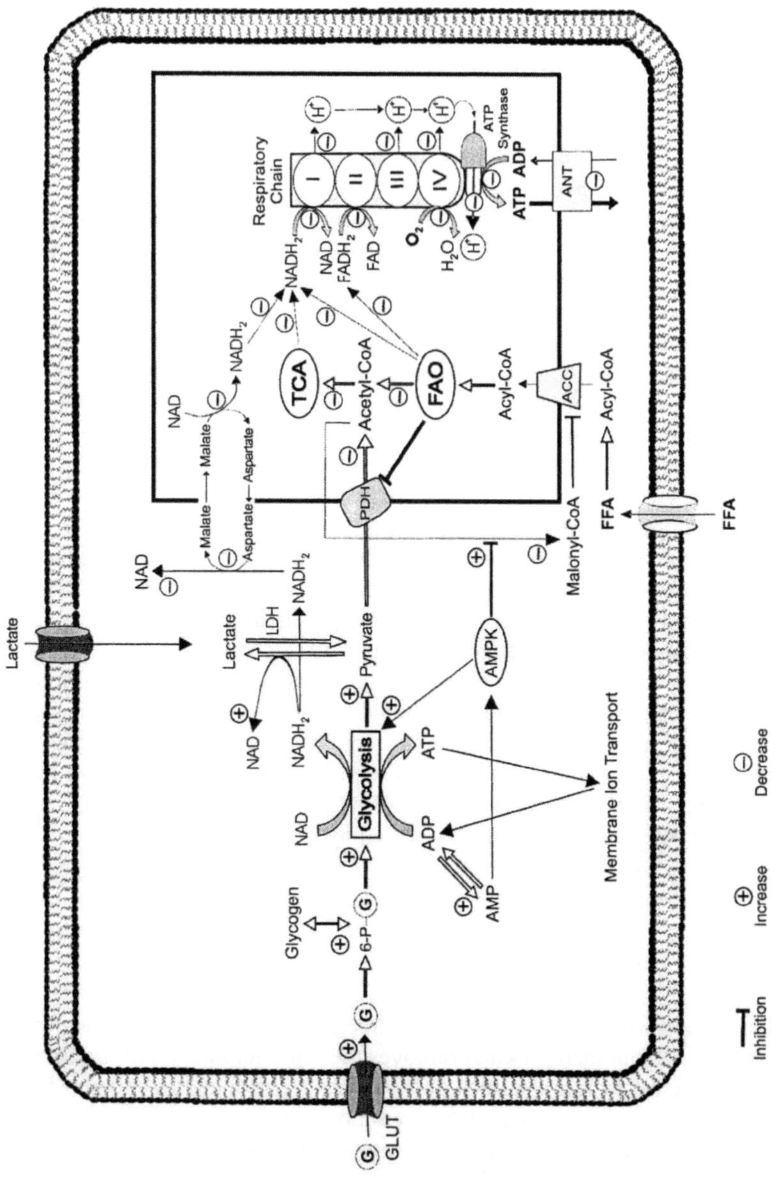

Figure 2. Schematic of metabolic changes in myocardial ischemia. Lack of oxygen slows mitochondrial activity (-). Consequently, slowing and then cessation of both TCA and FAO cycles occurs (-). Cytosolic glucose metabolism is enhanced (+). Glucose increases due to the enhanced glucose uptake and glycogen breakdown (+). The regulatory enzyme PDH is inhibited (-) so that less pyruvate enters the TCA cycle. Enhanced glycolysis provides the ATP required for maintaining cell membrane integrity. Intermediates of fatty acid metabolism accumulate and damage heart cell membranes. Breakdown of ATP to AMP results in AMPK activation. AMPK stimulates glycolysis while inhibits the malonyl-CoA synthesis and removes its negative regulatory effect on FFAs transport to mitochondria. FFAs use the residual oxygen instead of the energy friendly glucose substrate. See text for a more detailed explanation.

"G"=Glucose

Intracellular sodium excess results in enhanced osmotic pressure and swelling as well as in calcium overload. In fact, sodium leaves the cell in exchange with calcium due to the activated sodium-calcium exchanger (in the reverse direction). Figure 3. Calcium reuptake by the sarcoplasmic reticulum is reduced (due to energy depletion) and further contributes to calcium overload. Figure 3. Calcium overload leads to cell damage by activating membrane phospholipases, depresing mitochondrial respiration and increasing mitochondrial permeability, reviewed by Carmeliet.[55]

Loss of intracellular potassium occurs early during ischemia. Depletion of the cytosolic ATP and ADP and adenosine, breakdown products of ATP, leads to opening of the membrane potassium channel with subsequent potassium loss. Figure 3. These channels serve as metabolic sensors and respond to the decreased sub-sarcolemmal ATP. Furthermore, potassium moves out the cell together with negatively charged lactate and phosphate ions while inhibition of the Na^+/K^+-ATPase also contributes to potassium leakage. Potassium loss causes membrane action potential shortening and may prevent excessive calcium entry into the cell, reviewed by Carmeliet.[55] Cytosolic potassium also decreases due to the opening of mitochondrial ATP depended potasium channels (K_{ATP}). Mitochondrial K_{ATP} channels are activated during ischemia and may serve an important role in the adaptive response of the cell to ischemic stress. [56]

Magnesium increases in cytosol due to the hydrolysis of ATP to which magnesium is bound and from inadequate removal of magnesium via the magnesium-ATPase and sodium–magnesium exchanger. Magnesium exerts stabilizing effects but can also cause (via effects on phosphorylation) changes in sodium and calcium channels (blocking the pores) and inward rectification in the case of potassium channels, reviewed by Carmeliet.[55]

Several changes in ion membrane homeostasis also occur from fatty acid and long chain acylcarnitines (LCAC) accumulation or from the formation of lysophosphadylcholine (LPC) and arachidonic acid (AA) due to phospholipid breakdown by lipases. In fact, fatty acids and AA favor activation of K^+ outward current while LCAC and LPC favor inward over outward current, reviewed by Carmeliet.[55]

1.5. Contractile dysfunction

1.5.1 Ischemic contracture

Under normoxic conditions, the interaction between actin–myosin starts when intracellular calcium increases and removes the inhibitory action of troponin I. Myosin heads are attached to actin and flex at the expense of the energy produced by ATP hydrolysis. This results in myocardial contraction. ATP then binds to myosin heads and detaches them from actin filaments resulting in myocardial relaxation.[57] Figure 4. During severe and prolonged ischemia, the strong interaction between the myosin heads and actin is maintained due to ATP depletion and ischemic contracture develops. Increased ADP levels seem to be the early trigger of rigor contracture development. Interestingly, ADP further increases myosin ATPase activity leading to ATP depletion.[58] Rigor bridges exert a cooperative effect on the thin filament and calcium sensitivity is increased. However, calcium sensitivity can be reduced when hydrogen ions and phosphate are accumulated. Ischemic contracture is moderate in its extent and does not actually cause major structural damage but it leads to cytoskeletal defects and cardiomyocytes become more fragile and susceptible to mechanical damage. In perfused heart models, the development of contracture has been correlated to pre-ischemic myocardial glycogen content

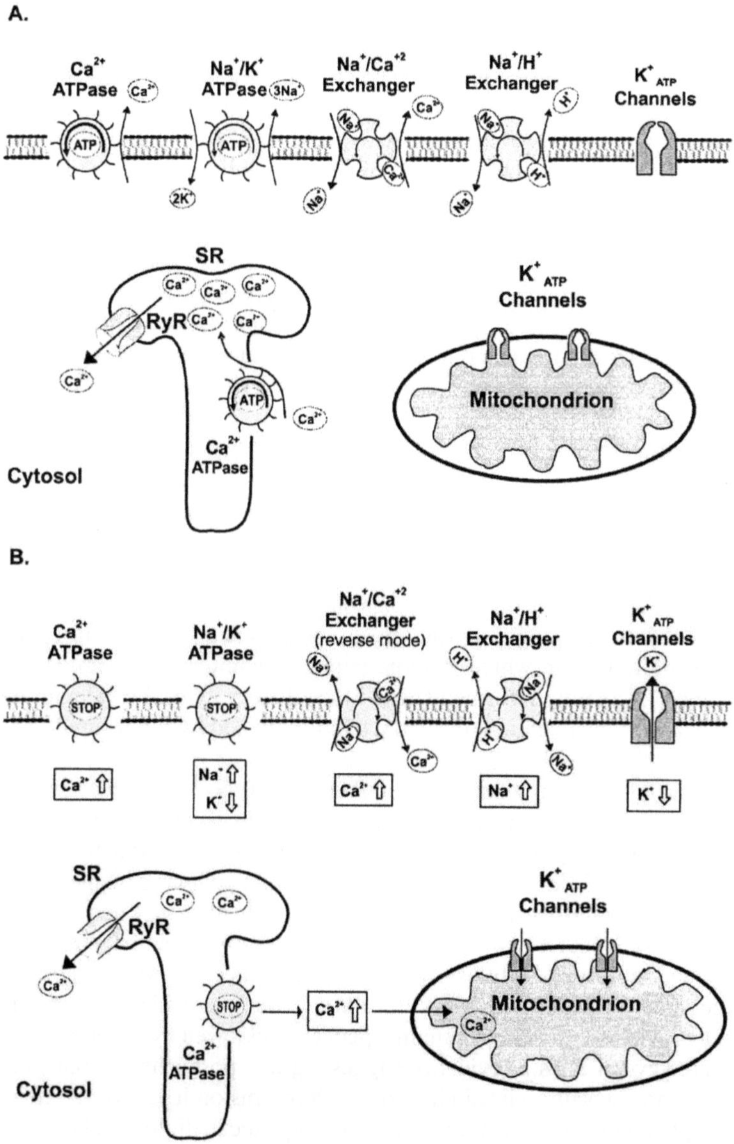

Figure 3. Ion homeostasis under normoxia (A) and hypoxia or ischemia (B). Ion gradients for Na^+ and K^+ are maintained by the operation of Na^+/K^+-ATPase. The increased intracellular Ca^{2+} following triggered Ca^{2+} release from the sarcoplasmic reticulum (SR) is reduced from Ca^{2+} reuptake by the SR, and outward Ca^{2+} transport by the Na^+/Ca^{2+} exchanger and Ca^{2+} pump. (B). In hypoxia or ischemia, Na^+/K^+-ATPase activity declines and intracellular sodium increases whereas potassium decreases. A further increase in sodium occurs due to the operation of Na^+/H^+ exchanger aiming to correct acidosis. Sodium is removed in exchange to Ca^{2+} by the operation of Na^+/Ca^{2+} exchanger in reverse mode. Ca^{2+} reuptake by SR and outward Ca^{2+} transport by Ca^{2+} pump is inhibited and intracellular calcium increases. Sodium and calcium overload induces cell damage. Opening of the sarcolemmal and mitochontrial ATP dependent potassium channels occurs and potassium leakage is increased.

"RyR"=Ryanodine receptor, ⬆= Increase, ⬇= Decrease

particularly in the setting of zero-flow global ischemia. The time of the development of contracture seems to coincide with the decrease in ATP availability and corresponds to fully depleted glycogen. Glycogen–derived ATP is present mainly at the myofibrils, and possibly at the sarcoplasmic reticulum (SR), thereby influencing ischemic contracture. Furthermore, glycogen and glycogen–metabolizing enzymes appear to co-locate with the sarcoplasmic reticulum, the main site of Ca^{2+} regulating proteins.[59] Ischemic contracture occurs earlier in glycogen depleted hearts such as the hyperthyroid or ischemic preconditioned hearts and is delayed in hearts in which myocardial glycogen content is increased.[60, 61] The profile of ischemic contracture is not necessarily related to the postischemic recovery of function. A dissociation between ischemic contracture and cardioprotection has been observed. Interventions such as ischemic preconditioning or chronic thyroid hormone treatment although reduce preischemic glycogen content and exacerbate contracture, increase postischemic recovery of function. [60, 61] Figure 25.

1.5.2 Hypercontracture

Hypercontracture develops immediately upon reperfusion. Figure 5. Reperfusion-induced hypercontracture might either originate from calcium overload or it is of rigor type. Figure 4. Following the ischemic period, cells are calcium overloaded and this is aggravated upon reperfusion by the persistence of the reverse mode of action of the sodium–calcium exchanger. Furthermore, re-oxygenation causes re-energizing of the sarcoplasmic reticulum which in turn starts to accumulate calcium and once full, releases calcium. Calcium movements lead to oscillatory cytosolic calcium elevations that provoke an uncontrolled myofibrilar activation fuelled by the resupply of ATP, reviewed by Piper.[62] Figure 4.

Reoxygenated cardiomyocytes are in acute jeopardy of the calcium overloaded contracture as long as mitochondrial energy production recovers rapidly upon reperfusion. However, after prolonged ischemia, this mechanism of contracture development is less likely to occur. With the progression of ischemic cellular damage, the ability of the mitochondria to rapidly restore a normal cellular state of energy upon reoxygenation is reduced. Cardiomyocytes, during the early phase of reoxygenation, may contain very low ATP concentrations that provoke rigor contracture. In cases where rigor contracture prevails, therapeutic actions aiming at cytosolic calcium overload are not effective since rigor contracture is essentially calcium independent, reviewed by Piper.[62]

There are several lines of evidence suggesting that postischemic necrosis and hypercontracture are causally related phenomena. Reperfusion injury of the myocardium is a complex phenomenon consisting of several independent etiologies. During the earliest phase of reperfusion (minutes), the development of cardiomyocyte hypercontracture seems to be the primary cause of cardiomyocyte necrosis. Thereafter, lasting for hours, various additional causes can lead to cell death by necrosis or apoptosis. Furthermore, vascular failure may aggravate cardiomyocyte injury. In cardiac surgery, when hearts are reperfused after prolonged ischemia or unsatisfactory intra-operative cardioplegia, reperfusion provokes the "stone heart" phenomenon i.e. a stiff and pale heart resulting from massive muscle contracture. Histologically, stone hearts present hypercontracted myofibrils and ruptured cellular membranes. A similar pattern of contracture and necrotic cell injury, termed 'contraction band necrosis" is also observed after regional ischemia and reperfusion.[4] In the heart in situ, exposed to transient coronary occlusion, the area of necrosis is shown to be composed almost exclusively of contraction band necrosis.[63, 64]

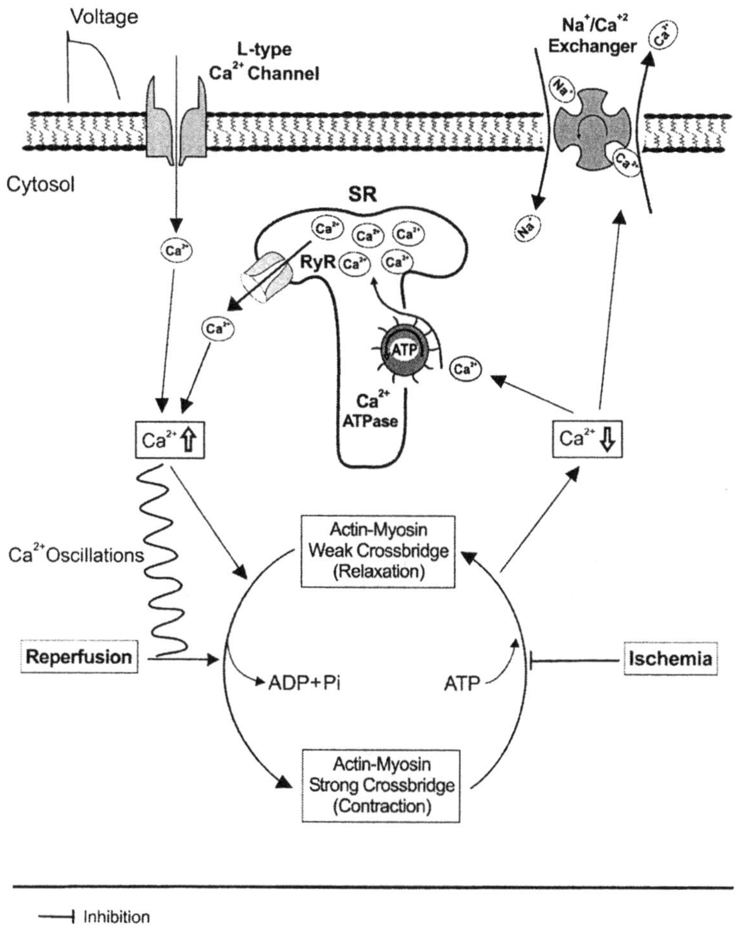

Figure 4. Contraction results when the heads of the thick myosin filaments interact with the thin actin filaments (strong cross-bridge). This process is initiated by triggered release of calcium from SR at the expense of ATP. Reduced calcium and ATP resupply result in myosin–actin detachement (weak cross-bridge) and relaxation. Upon ischemia, the strong cross-bridge state is maintained due to the low levels of ATP and ischemic contracture of rigor type develops. At the time of reperfusion, despite ATP resupply, a state of a strong cross-bridge between actin and myosin can occur due to calcium oscillations (calcium overload hypercontracture). Hypercontracture of a rigor type can develop at reperfusion following prolonged ischemia where severe ATP depletion occurs.

"RyR"=Ryanodine receptor, ⬆= Increase, ⬇= Decrease "SR"= Sarcoplasmic Reticulum

The extent of contraction band necrosis is shown to correlate well with the magnitude of macroscopic myocardial shrinkage during the first minutes of reperfusion, and with the magnitude of the enzyme release occurring during the initial minutes of reflow.[65]

1.5.3 Myocardial Stunning

Myocardial stunning is defined as transient contractile dysfunction that appears after reperfusion despite the absence of irreversible damage and restoration of normal or near normal coronary flow.[66] In rat models, stunning has been induced by global ischemia in isolated heart preparations. In rabbit models, multiple, completely reversible episodes of regional ischemia result in stunning. In large animals, a single or multiple, completely reversible episode(s) of regional ischemia or prolonged coronary stenosis (without necrosis) were shown to induce myocardial stunning, reviewed by Kim.[67] Although the pathogenesis of myocardial stunning has not been definitively established, the two major hypotheses are that it is caused by the generation of oxygen derived free radicals and by calcium overload during reperfusion. These two hypotheses are not mutually exclusive and are likely to represent different facets of the same pathophysiological cascade.[68]

The first hypothesis was primarily tested in large animals and has been proved by experimental evidence such as the increase in reactive oxygen species (ROS) production in stunned myocardium,[69] the protection against stunning by antioxidants[70] and the contractile dysfunction induced by direct exposure to ROS.[71] Calcium overload is thought to be the possible mechanism through which ROS can induce stunning.[72] The calcium hypothesis postulates that stunning is due to calcium overload that occurs during the early phase of reperfusion secondary to intracellular sodium overload following metabolic inhibition of the sodium–potassium ATPase. In fact, NMR measurements show an increase in intracellular sodium during ischemia and reperfusion[73] and reperfusion with perfusates containing low calcium concentration resulted in attenuation of stunning.[74] Another possible mechanism through which calcium can be implicated in stunning is the activation of calcium dependent proteases. These proteins, known as calpains are enzymes that cleave other proteins when calcium is elevated. This might lead to proteolysis of the troponin I (TnI) that together with the damage to other contractile proteins (a-actinin, myosin light chain–1) result in decrease in calcium responsiveness.[75] Direct exposure of cardiac myofilaments to activated calpain I is shown to reproduce the phenotype of stunned myocardium with blunted sensitivity and depressed maximal force. Furthermore, these effects were prevented by coincubation with excess calpastatin, the natural inhibitor of calpain.[76] A phenotype of stunning, characterized by reduced myofilament calcium sensitivity has been also produced in transgenic mice expressing the major degradation product of TnI induced by calpain.[77] However, in vivo studies in large animals do not confirm the presence of TnI degradation, indicating that this is not a universal feature of myocardial stunning.[78] It is likely that the proteolysis of TnI observed in the isolated rat heart preparations might be the effect of the increased diastolic pressure and not that of the calcium mediated proteolysis.

The absence of irreversible cellular damage in stunned myocardium may correspond to an increased resistance of the heart to ischemia. Myocardial stunning may trigger the expression of different sets of genes acting to protect the myocardium against irreversible injury. In fact, it has been recently shown that in a swine model of regional reversible ischemia, stunned and normal areas within the same heart corresponded to different gene expression. Interestingly, more than 30% of the genes which were upregulated in the stunned myocardium are known to be involved in different mechanisms of cell survival including resistance to apoptosis, cytoprotection and cell growth. It seems that gene response matches the flow reduction.[79]

Stunning resolves spontaneously and it can be viewed as a protective mechanism which should be given sufficient time to recover. However, in clinical settings where stunning impairs myocardial function to the extent that compromises other organ perfusion it requires treatment.

1.5.4 Myocardial Hibernation

Myocardial hibernation is an adaptation caused by chronic or intermittent reduction in coronary flow characterized as reduced regional contractile function that recovers after removal of the artery stenosis. A "subacute downregulation" of contractile function in response to reduced regional myocardial blood flow can occur, which normalizes regional energy and substrate metabolism but does not persist more than 12-24 h. Chronic hibernation develops in response to episodes of myocardial ischemia and reperfusion, progressing from repetitive stunning with normal blood flow to hibernation with reduced blood flow, reviewed by Heusch.[80]

Salient features of the hibernating myocardium are the increase in glucose uptake out of proportion to coronary flow (metabolism/perfusion mismatch)[81] and the increase in myocardial glycogen content with ultrastructural characteristics resembling those of the fetal heart.[82]

Morphological changes are observed in long-term hibernation. The morphology of hibernating myocardium is characterized by both adaptive and degenerative features. The number of myofibrils is reduced while the number of mitochondria and glycogen deposits are increased after 24 h and these changes are reversed in a week following the release of the coronary stenosis. Other morphological changes include a variable degree of fibrosis and expansion of the interstitium by increased infiltration of macrophages and fibroblasts together with collagen deposition. Extracellular matrix proteins (such as desmin, tubulin and vinculin) are increased, indicating disorganization of the cytoskeleton. Mitochondria are small and doughnut like. Depletion of sarcomeres and sarcoplasmic reticulae is observed and glycogen is seen to fill the place previously occupied by filaments. These changes result in myocytes that appear to be de-differentiated. Apoptosis has also been identified in biopsies taken from hibernating myocardium at the time of surgical revascularization. It is suggested that cellular de–differentiation may lead to apoptosis but this finding has not been documented in humans, reviewed by Heusch.[80]

The pathophysiology of hibernation remains under intense investigation. In short term hibernation, the only possible mechanism that has been identified is reduced calcium responsiveness.[83] In long-term hibernation, changes seem to correspond to a genetic program of cellular survival that is induced probably from repetitive episodes of ischemia and reperfusion. Heat shock protein 70 and hypoxia-inducible factor–1α are upregulated in the hibernating myocardium.[84] Furthermore, iNOS and cyclooxygenase–2 immunoreactivity are increased in hibernating human myocardium resembling the survival gene program of delayed preconditioning.[85] Enhanced expression of chemokines at the level of mRNA accompanied by extensive macrophage infiltration and fibrosis has been observed in a mouse model with repeated brief episodes of ischemia and reperfusion (with absence of infarction and decreased regional contractile function).[28] Similarly, in human hibernating myocardium, tumor necrosis factor–α (TNF-α) and iNOS mRNA were higher than in the remote control myocardium.[86] Interestingly, these features of inflammation are also found with microembolization where a contractile

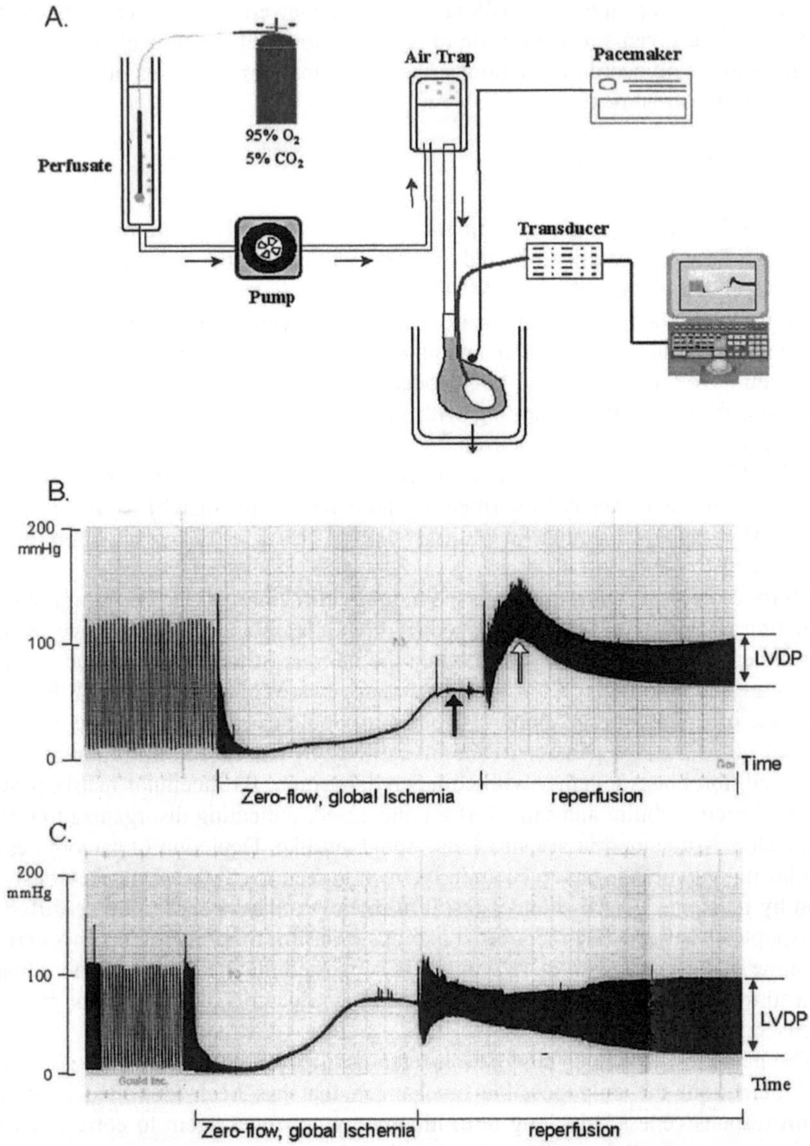

Figure 5. A. Schematic of a Langendorff perfused rat heart model. Retrograde perfusion is established through the aorta. Perfusate oxygenated with 95% O_2 and 5% CO_2 is circulated by a peristaltic pump and the flow can be adjusted. Left ventricular pressure is monitored through a balloon which is inserted into the empty left ventricle. Heart rhythm is controlled by pacing.

B. Recording of left ventricular developed pressure (LVDP is defined as the difference between systolic and diastolic left ventricular pressure) from Langendorff perfused heart after stabilization followed by complete flow cessation (zero-flow global ischemia) and flow re-establishment (reperfusion). Note the development of ischemic contracture (black arrow) and hypercontracture early at the time of reperfusion (white arrow).

C. Left ventricular pressure recording of a perfused rat heart model of zero-flow global ischemia and reperfusion. A progressive increase in LVDP occurs at reperfusion. This corresponds to myocardial stunning (data from our laboratory).

dysfunction is induced through an inflammatory signal cascade.[87] Thus, it is suggested that microembolization (derived from subclinical plaque fissuring and rapture) is likely in hibernation. Alterations in calcium handling and adrenergic control are also seen in hibernation but their causal role remains to be elucidated.[80] See also chapter 6.

Hibernating myocardium is prone to arrhythmias. Scar formation and reduction and inhomogeneity of connexin 43 expression in human myocardium may contribute to alterations in electrical impulse propagation and re-entry. Furthermore, cardiomyocytes from hibernating myocardium in pigs are hypertrophied and have reduced contraction and striking prolongation of the action potential rendering them more prone to after depolirizations.[88, 89]

1.6. Ischemia–reperfusion induced arrhythmias

Under ischemic conditions, increase in extracellular potassium and the existence of inward currents result in increased depolarization of the resting membrane potential while the increased outward currents through potassium and chloride channels result in shortening of the action potential. Figure 6. Potassium currents which are activated under physiological conditions are inhibited under ischemic conditions and several other new channels come to the operation (IK_{ATP}, IK_{Na}, IK_{FFA}). Figure 6. Shortening of the action potential also occurs from injury currents generated from current differences between ischemic and non ischemic areas. This is mainly observed in the border zone of the ischemic area. At reperfusion, shortening of the action potential is mainly due to the excessive stimulation of the sodium pump (Na^+/K^+-ATPase). Under ischemia, membrane action potential is altered due to the accumulation of metabolites, such as fatty acids, free oxygen radical species production, the release of endogenous molecules, such as catecholamines, acetylcholine and adenosine as well as the stretch and the changes in cell volume. Changes in action potential and its conductance constitute the basis of ischemia and reperfusion arrhythmias, reviewed by Carmeliet.[55]

Arrhythmias are observed during the ischemic phase as well as at reperfusion in most of the animal models. In the first 2-10 min of ischemia, a burst of irregular ventricular tachycardia occurs but evolution to ventricular fibrillation is rare. These arrhythmias are mainly of a reentry nature. A second phase of arrhythmias is evident after 20-30 min of ischemia. The percentage of animals that show this delayed phase of arrhythmias is small and the evolution to ventricular fibrillation is more frequent and the animals can die. This phase is associated with a massive release of catecholamines, changes in calcium overload and an increase in extracellular potassium, reviewed by Carmeliet.[55]

Arrhythmias occur within a few seconds after reperfusion, following ischemic periods of 10-30 min long. They start by a spontaneous stimulus in the reperfused zone and change afterward in a re-entry multiple wavelet type of ventricular tachycardia (VT) or ventricular fibrillation (VF). Extremely short action potential, short refractory period and slow conduction are the main contributing factors. Increased hyperpolarization and elevated intracellular calcium that act negatively on gap conductance impair conduction. Unidirectional conduction is favored by the marked heterogeneity in extracellular potassium, action potential and refractory period. The extra stimulus is initiated in the reperfused zone, probably by early (EAD) and late (DAD) afterdepolirizations.

Delayed reperfusion arrhythmias appear as a second phase of irregular rhythm when the occlusion period has been longer than 10-20 min. Extrasystoles and runs of

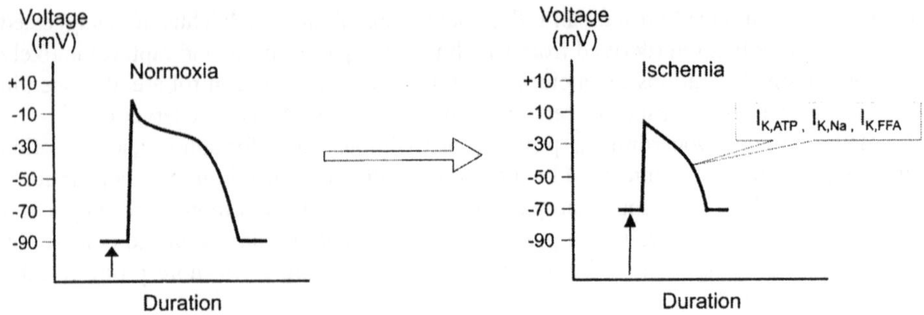

Figure 6. Resting membrane potential under normoxia (left) and ischemia (right). Increased outward potassium current during ischemia causes shortening of the resting membrane potential. Potassium currents activated under physiological conditions are inhibited under ischemia and several other new channels come to the operation (IK_{ATP}, IK_{Na}, IK_{FFA}). Resting membrane potential is less negative due to the increased extracellular potassium and inward currents.

tachycardia probably originate in surviving Purkinje system due to the abnormal automaticity. Oscillatory release of calcium or even stretch depolarizations may also be involved, reviewed by Carmeliet.[55]

Concluding remarks

Lack of oxygen availability and metabolites result in myocardial ischemia and cellular injury of reversible or irreversible nature. Reperfusion, generally pre-requisite for tissue survival may also increase injury over and above that sustained by ischemia, a phenomenon known as reperfusion injury. Necrotic and apoptotic cell death are the two major forms of cell death recognized in the pathology of myocardial injury. Apoptosis is an energy dependent process, executed through the mitochondrial and/or death receptor pathways and does not involve an inflammatory response. Cell to cell communication (Gap junctions) contributes to spread of injury but survival signals can also be transferred depending on the intensity of stimulus. Myocardial ischemia is accompanied by the inflammatory response that further contributes to myocardial injury and ultimately leads to myocardial healing and scar formation. Myocardial necrosis is associated with complement activation and reactive oxygen species triggering cytokine cascades and resulting in chemokine upregulation. Cytokines exert direct negative inotropic effects via paracrine and autocrine modulation and induce apoptosis. Chemokine expression may play a role in the pathogenesis of non-infarctive ischemic cardiomyopathy, where early ischemia-induced chemokine expression may be followed by activation of inhibitory mediators that suppress inflammation, but induce fibrosis. Endothelial dysfunction and microvascular injury start at the interphase of the endothelium with the bloodstream. During reperfusion severe microvascular dysfunction can arrest the microcirculation, a phenomenon known as the no–reflow phenomenon.

Metabolism is altered during myocardial ischemia contributing to cell survival or cell death depending on the severity of the ischemic insult. Mitochondrial activity decreases and slowing and ultimately cessation of TCA and FAO cycles occurs. Glucose increases due to the enhanced glucose uptake and glycogen breakdown. The activity of the regulatory enzyme PDH declines and less pyruvate enters the TCA cycle. Enhanced glycolysis provides the ATP that is required for maintaining cell membrane integrity. Intermediates of fatty acid metabolism accumulate and damage heart cell membranes. AMPK is stimulated due to the breakdown of ATP to AMP. AMPK stimulates glycolysis but also inhibits the malonyl-CoA synthesis, removes the negative regulatory effect of malonyl-CoA on FFAs transport to mitochondria and facilitates FFA metabolism. As a consequence FFAs use residual oxygen, instead of the energy-friendly glucose substrate. Energy depletion and acidosis change ion homeostasis causing potassium leakage and calcium and sodium overload. Calcium and sodium excess results in cell damage.

During prolonged ischemia, ATP levels decline and the strong cross-bridge between myosin heads and actin is maintained resulting in the development of the ischemic contracture. Ischemic contracture has been related to preischemic myocardial glycogen content, at least in the setting of zero-flow global ischeamia and reperfusion. Severity of contracture does not correlate to postichaemic recovery of function. At the time of reperfusion, hypercontracture develops due to calcium oscillations or to severe ATP depletion (rigor type). Hypercontracture can contribute to cell death at early reperfusion.

Myocardial stunning is defined as transient contractile dysfunction that appears after reperfusion despite the absence of irreversible damage and restoration of normal or near normal coronary flow. Although the pathogenesis of stunning has not been definitively established, the two major hypotheses are that it is caused by the generation of oxygen free radicals or by calcium overload. The absence of irreversible cellular damage in stunned myocardium may correspond to an increased resistance of the heart to ischemia. Survival genes are upregulated in stunned myocardium. Stunning may explain much delayed contractile recovery after thrombolytic therapy in acute myocardial infarction.

Myocardial hibernation is an adaptation caused by chronic or intermittent reduction in coronary flow characterized as reduced regional contractile function that recovers after removal of the artery stenosis. Two current hypotheses are perfusion–contraction matching with downgraded myocardial energy requirements and repetitive cumulative stunning. Salient features of the hibernating myocardium are the increase in glucose uptake out of proportion to coronary flow (metabolism/perfusion mismatch) and the increase in myocardial glycogen content with ultrastructural characteristics resembling those of the fetal heart. In long-term hibernation, changes seem to correspond to a genetic program of cellular survival that is induced probably by the repetitive episodes of ischemia and reperfusion. Hibernation is searched for and diagnosed in efforts to improve left ventricular contractile function by revascularization.

Increased outward potassium currents during ischemia cause shortening of membrane potential. Potassium currents activated under physiological conditions are inhibited under ischemia and several other new channels come to the operation (IK_{ATP}, IK_{Na}, IK_{FFA}). Resting membrane potential is less negative due to the increased extracellular potassium and inward currents. Changes in action potential and its conductance constitute the basis of ischemia and reperfusion arrhythmias.

2. STRESS SIGNALING IN MYOCARDIAL ISCHEMIA

Complex cell signaling pathways exist in the cell involved in growth, cell survival or cell death. Intracellular signaling is considered as an important transducer of both adaptive and maladaptive responses of the cell to stress. Signaling pathways are activated by ligand-receptor interaction or receptor independent stimuli such as mechanical stress, osmotic and oxidative stress or haemodynamic loading. Activation of intracellular signaling includes phosphorylations by tyrosine kinases and/or serine/threonine kinases while phosphatases are physiological negative feedback regulators of these pathways. Protein phosphorylations change enzyme activities and protein conformations. The eventual outcome is changes in gene expression and in the function of the responding cells. The intracellular signaling system consists of cell surface signal transduction receptors, intracellular signaling pathways and end-effectors. Signal pathways are not clear cut in their sequences; not all the intermediates are known while unknown feedback loops and signaling cross-talk exist. They can converge or diverge and are more like a web than straight lines.

2.1. Membrane bound receptors

Signal transduction receptors are of different classes:

a) Receptors with intrinsic enzymatic activity. These receptors are capable of autophosphorylation as well as phosphorylation of other substrates. Receptors with intrinsic enzymatic activity include those that are tyrosine kinases (e.g PDGF, insulin, EGF, FGF receptors), tyrosine phosphatases (e.g CD45 protein of T cells and macrophages), guanyl cyclases (e.g natriuretic peptide receptors) and serine/threonine kinases (e.g TGF-β). Receptors with intrinsic enzymatic activity can interact with intracellular proteins; insulin receptor is associated with a protein termed IRS–1 which in turn is associated with the PI3K signaling. This protein acts as a docking or adapter protein. Growth factor receptor binding protein 2 (Grb2) is another common adapter protein through which receptors with intrinsic enzymatic activity can interact with Ras signaling. Figure 7.

b) Receptors lacking intrinsic enzymatic activity. These receptors are coupled to intracellular non receptor tyrosine kinases, such as Src and Lck protein and Janus kinase (JAK). This class of receptors includes all of the cytokine receptors, e.g IL-2 receptor. Figure 8.

c) Receptors (GPCRs) which are coupled, inside the cell, to GTP-binding and hydrolyzing proteins, collectively termed G-proteins. GPCRs modulate adenyl cyclase activity and the production of c-AMP with a negative regulation to occur by binding of the receptor to Gi-protein, e.g β_2-adrenergic receptor, figure 9 and positive regulation by binding to Gi-protein, e.g β_1-adrenergic or β_2-adrenergic receptor. Figure 10. Table 1. c-AMP diffuses to protein kinase A (PKA) which phosphorylates glycogen synthase, phosphorylase and the trancription factor CREB (transcribes genes for gluconeogenesis). ERK or Akt intracellular signaling can be regulated through receptors bound to Gi. Figure 9. GPCRs which are bound to Gq activate phospholipase C (PLC) leading to hydrolysis of polyphosphoinositides (e.g PIP2) generating the second messengers diacylglycerol (DAG) and inositol-triphosphate (IP3). IP3 increases the release of stored calcium. Calcium together with DAG activate PKC dependent signaling. Figure 11. This class of receptors include the angiotensin (AT_1), the α_1-adrenergic and endothelin receptors. Table 1.

d) Receptors which are found intracellularly and upon ligand binding migrate to the nucleus where the ligand–receptor complex directly affects gene transcription. Figure 12.

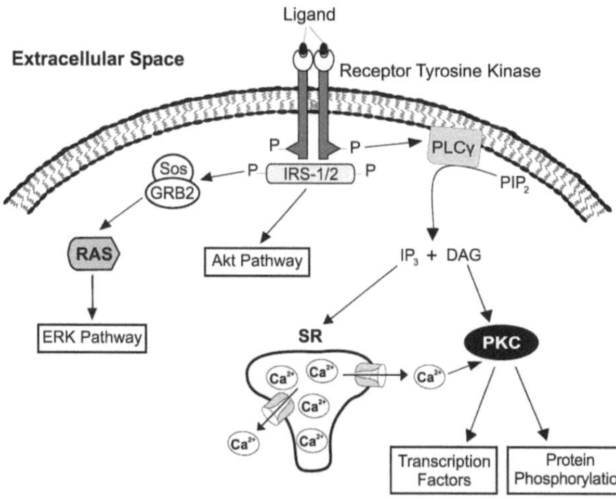

Figure 7. Schematic of a receptor with intrinsic enzymatic activity. Ligand mediated activation results in phosphorylation of phospholipase C (γ isoform) leading to hydrolysis of polyphosphoinositides (PIP2). Diacyl-glycerol (DAG) and inositol-triphosphate (IP3) are formed. IP3 increases the release of stored calcium. Calcium together with DAG can activate PKC signaling pathway. Association of this type of receptor with adapter proteins results in activation of Ras/Raf/ERK signaling or in activation of PI3K/Akt signaling.

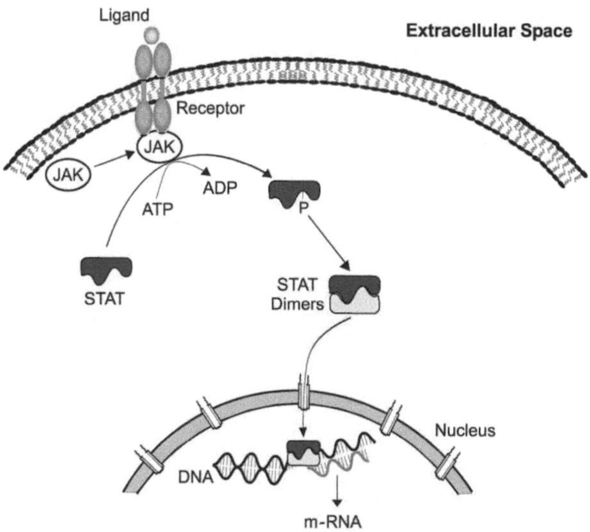

Figure 8. Schematic of membrane receptors lacking intrinsic enzymatic activity. Intracellular signaling is initiated by coupling of the receptor to an intracellular kinase (e.g JAK kinase). These receptors mediate cytokine signaling (prosurvival protective and maladaptive pathways leading to apoptosis). JAK/STAT signaling is involved in the cellular response to ischemia. Activation of STAT3 reduces ischemia induced apoptosis, whereas activation of STAT1 has the opposite effect.

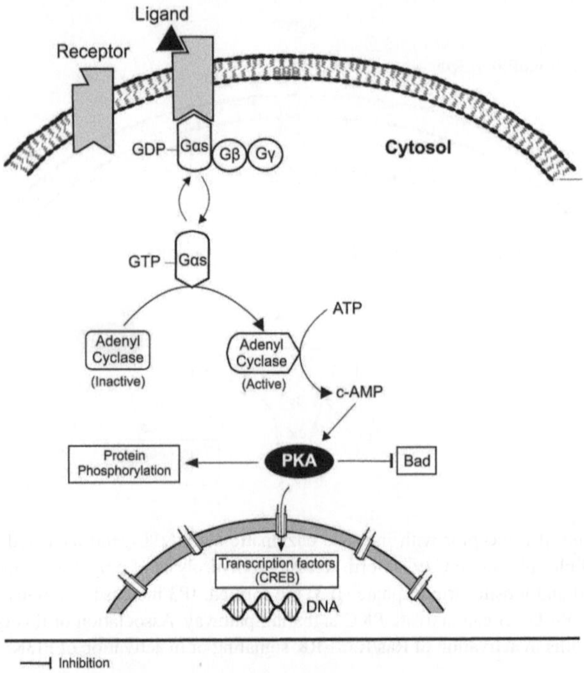

Figure 9. Schematic of Gs-coupled receptors. This type of receptor is coupled to adenyl cyclase (AC) via the activated stimulatory Gs protein and leads to the formation of c-AMP. c-AMP in turn activates protein kinase A (PKA). PKA regulates calcium homeostasis and may induce apoptosis due to the elevation of intracellular calcium levels or prevent apoptosis by inactivating the proapoptotic Bad. β_1 and β_2 adrenergic signaling pathways are mediated through this receptor. For PKA targeted proteins, see figure 17.

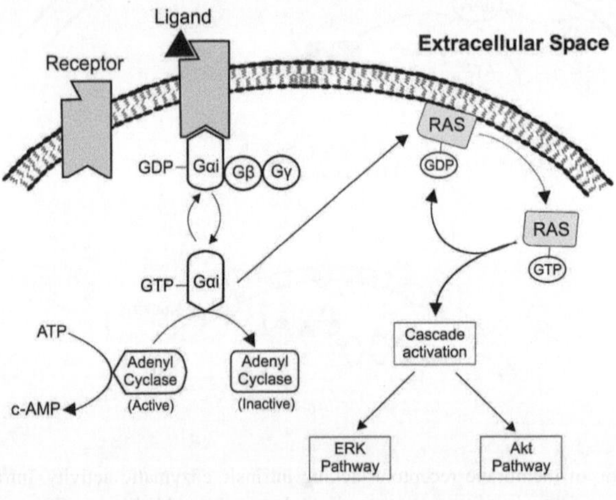

Figure 10. Schematic of Gi-coupled receptors. Adenyl cyclase (AC) activity is inhibited by the Gi protein. Ras signaling is activated by Gi-coupled receptors. Acetylcholine, adenosine, opioid or β_2-adrenergic signaling is mediated through this type of receptor. Gi-coupled receptors are able to trigger the preconditioned state in the heart (see chapter 3). For ERK and Akt signaling pathway, see figure 19.

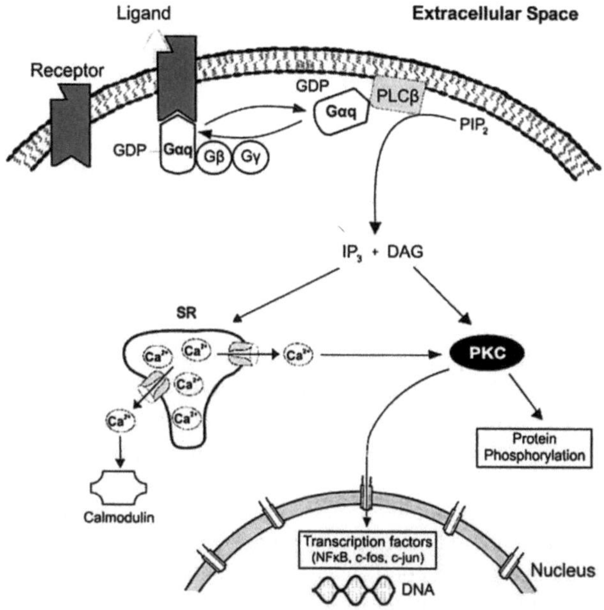

Figure 11. Schematic of Gq-coupled receptors. Activation of phospholipase C (PLC isoform β) results in hydrolysis of polyphosphoinositides (PIP2) generating the diacyl-glycerol (DAG) and inositol-triphosphate (IP3). IP3 increases the release of stored calcium. Calcium together with DAG activate PKC signaling. The angiotensin AT_1 receptor, α_1-adrenergic and endothelin-1 signaling is mediated through this type of receptor. For PKC targeted proteins, see figure 18.

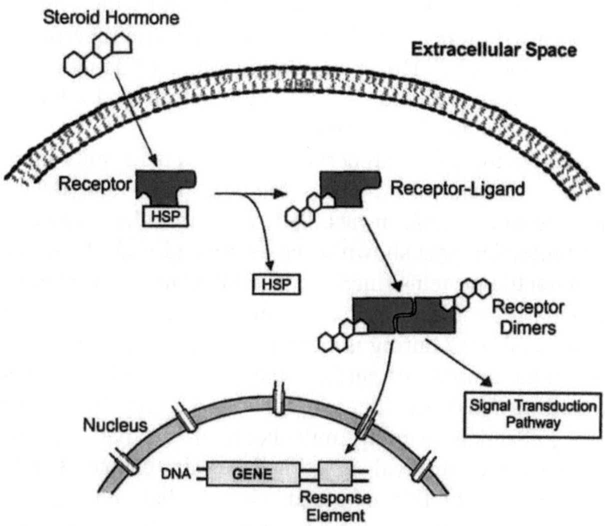

Figure 12. General receptor pattern for steroid hormones action. Ligand binding dissociates receptor from heat shock proteins (e.g Hsp90). Receptor dimers are formed and translocate to nucleus. This results in gene transcription (genomic effects). Activation of intracellular signaling with immediate physiological effects can also occur (non genomic effects).

2.2. Triggers of cell signaling

2.2.1. Receptor dependent endogenous triggers

Several endogenous mediators are released during ischemia and reperfusion that could potentially modulate intracellular signaling by acting on surface membrane receptors or on intracellular components of signaling pathways. See Table 1 and figures 9, 10, 11. Depending on their site of origin the mediators are termed autocrine when they act on the cell that produces them and paracrine when they act on a neighboring cell. The potential cardioprotective role of autocrine and paracrine mediators in the context of ischemia and reperfusion has been intensively investigated.

An increase in presynaptic release of endogenous catecholamines with concomitant regulation of the adrenergic signaling at various levels occurs during ischemia and reperfusion. The density of α and β receptors and the activity of adenyl cyclase are increased early in the course of subacute ischemia. In prolonged ischemia, adenyl cyclase activity gradually declines resulting in reduced responsiveness of the adrenergic system. Furthermore, energy depletion and intracellular acidosis differentially regulate β-adrenergic receptors, adenyl cyclase and protein kinase C; energy depletion induces an increase in β-adrenergic receptors, yet fails to activate adenyl cyclase and protein kinase C. Acidosis leads to the activation of protein kinase C and sensitization of cardiac adenyl cyclase activity without affecting the density of β-adrenergic receptors.[90]

β-adrenergic receptor activation results in stimulation of most plasma membrane currents (inward and outward), gap junction channels, and SR Ca^{2+}-ATPase. β_1 and β_2-receptors exert opposite effects on apoptosis; in adult ventricular myocytes activation of β_2 adrenergic receptor attenuates apoptosis while activation of β_1 adrenergic receptors induces apoptosis.[91] A possible beneficial effect of beta adrenergic signaling has been suggested. Exogenous preischemic activation of β-receptor with isoproterenol increased tolerance of the perfused rat heart subjected to ischemia and reperfusion, an effect that was abolished by β_1 blockade.[92] However, administration of dobutamine at reperfusion, (an agent with dominant β_1 receptor action) had a detrimental effect on postischemic recovery of function in perfused rat hearts.[93]

Preischemic activation of α-adrenergic signaling also results in cardioprotection. Pretreatment with norepinephrine induces bimodal (early and delayed) myocardial functional adaptation to ischemia in rats. PKC appears to be involved in the early response. Delayed protection was shown to be associated with the expression of genes encoding fetal contractile proteins (increase in β-MHC mRNA).[94] However, α-receptor agonists can trigger arrhythmias in the setting of ischemia and reperfusion.[55]

Acetylcholine is released during ischemia. Acetylcholine can induce cardioprotection by its action on the muscarinic surface receptors with subsequent activation of the PI3K signaling pathway and Src–kinases. Table 1. Figures 10, 11. This leads to the mitochondrial K_{ATP} channels opening, mitochondrial reactive oxygen species (ROS) production and induction of survival signaling.[95] See also chapter 3 and figures 3, 4.

Cardiac tissue angiotensin II is increased in myocardial ischemia and seems to serve an important physiological role. Figure 13. Angiotensin II can induce oxidative stress through the activation of NADH/NADPH oxidase system thereby generating reactive oxygen species (ROS) with subsequent induction of cardioprotective genes adapting the heart to the angiotensin detrimental effects.[96] Angiotensin II activates Akt, an effect that is blocked by either wortmannin, a PI3K inhibitor or by the overexpression of catalase.[97] A beneficial role for angiotensin has been identified in the context of ischemia and reperfusion. Exogenous angiotensin II limited infarct size in a concentration–dependent manner in the perfused rat heart without having an effect on contractile stunning.[98]

Bradykinin, endothelin and prostacyclin are released in myocardial ischemia. Bradykinin acts through B_2 and B_1 receptor and is inactivated by ACE and NEP (cell surface zinc metalloprotease). Figure 13. Activation of B_2 receptor can confer protection through activation of the nitric oxide/protein kinase C pathway or through the activation of PI3K/Akt prosurvival pathway (see figures 10,11). Furthermore, activation of B_1 receptor mediates protection to endothelium, limits noradrenaline outflow and reduces the occurrence of arrhythmias induced by ischemia and reperfusion.[99]

Endothelin–1 is a potent vasoconstrictor peptide derived from endothelial cells.[100] Its physiological function is mediated by two receptors the ET-A and ET-B. Table 1. Figure 11. ET-A and ET-B receptors are located in vascular smooth muscle and their activation causes vasoconstriction, whereas ET-B receptor is also located in the endothelium and its activation results in vasodilation by increasing nitric oxide or prostacyclin. Endothelin is released following myocardial ischemia and reperfusion. Endothelin reduces infarct size in a perfused rat heart model of ischemia and reperfusion through activation of protein kinase C and K_{ATP} channel.[101] Furthermore, in neonatal rat ventricular myocytes, endothelin is shown to activate the calcineurin–NFAT (nuclear factor of activated cells) pathways and enhance the expression of Bcl-2.[102] However, endogenous blockade of endothelin at the level of the ET-A receptor reduced infarct size in a pig model of coronary occlusion and reperfusion.[103]

Prostacyclin is increased in response to ischemia and reperfusion through activation of the cyclooxygenase–2 pathway. Inhibition of cyclooxygenase-2 by celecoxib or meloxicam resulted in a concentration dependent exacerbation of the myocardial dysfunction and damage in a perfused rabbit heart model of ischemia and reperfusion, indicating a cardioprotective role for prostacyclin.[104]

Endogenous opioid peptides are increased in myocardial ischemia. Their effect is mediated through presynaptic and postsynaptic mechanisms. Opioids limit the release of stimulating catecholamines by its presynaptic action while opioid receptor agonists act via Gi –linked pathways postsynaptically and alter myocardial channel activity and intracellular activities of protein kinases. Table 1. Figure 10. Blockade of δ and ϰ–opioid receptors reduced the tolerance of the isolated rabbit heart to ischemia and reperfusion.[105] Furthermore, blockade of δ–opioid receptor abrogated the ischemic preconditioning mediated cardioprotective effect while activation of δ–opioid receptor by morphine decreased infarct size and apoptosis in a rabbit model of coronary occlusion and reperfusion.[106]

Adenosine is released during ischemia and can exert several effects on the myocardium.[107] It can interact with three receptors; the A_1 receptor (myocardium, mast cell), the A_2 receptor (vascular) and the A_3 receptor (myocardium). See table 1 and figures 9, 10, 11. Adenosine induces opening of the potassium channel (A_1 receptor) with subsequent bradycardia (sinus node, AV node), induces vasodilation (vascular K_{ATP}, A_2 receptor) and increases calcium channel closing time (negative inotropic effect, A_1 receptor). Its cardioprotective role has been identified in several studies.[108] Adenosine is released during the brief episodes of ischemia and reperfusion of the preconditioning protocol and triggers cardioprotective signaling. This effect is mediated through the A_1 and/or A_3 receptors.[109, 110] See also chapter 3.

Histamine is released in the setting of ischemia and reperfusion. The mast cell degranulates during ischemia and the wash out of mast cells releases histamine dur-

Table 1. List of important G-protein membrane-bound receptors involved in cardiovascular physiology

Membrane receptors coupling to G-proteins	
Receptors	G-proteins
α_1 adrenergic receptor	Gq, Gs
α_2 adrenergic receptor	Gi
β_1 adrenergic receptor	Gs
β_2 adrenergic receptor	Gs, Gi
Dopamine receptor 1	Gs
Dopamine receptor 2	Gi
Adenosine receptor (A_1)	Gi
Adenosine receptor (A_2)	Gs
Adenosine receptor (A_3)	Gi, Gq
Muscarinic receptor (M_1)	Gi, Gq
Muscarinic receptor (M_2)	Gi
Muscarinic receptor (M_3)	Gi, Gq
Angiotensin receptor type 1 (AT_1)	Gq
Angiotensin receptor type 2 (AT_2)	Gi
Endothelin receptor	Gq
Histamine receptor type 2	Gq, Gs
Bradykinin receptors	Gq, Gi
Opioid receptors	Gi
PTH receptor	Gs, Gq

ing reperfusion. Alternatively, it has been suggested that reperfusion induces mast cell degranulation and histamine release during this period. Adenosine can induce mast cell degranulation and histamine release through the adenosine A_1 receptor. Histamine acts on the myocardium via the H_1, H_2 and the presynaptic H_3 receptors. Transgenic mice lacking H_3, display a greater incidence of ischemia induced arrhythmias, indicating a possible cardioprotective role of histamine. This effect has been attributed to the histamine presynaptic inhibitory effect on catecholamine release.[111]

2.2.2. Non receptor triggers; reactive oxygen species and nitric oxide

Reactive oxygen species are generated during ischemia and particularly during reperfusion. They can act as triggers or intermediates of both cell survival or cell death. Reactive oxygen species (ROS) are molecules with one or more misdonated unpaired electrons. Singlet oxygen is an oxygen molecule with an unpaired electron moved to a higher orbital. The unpaired electron alters the chemical reactivity of an atom or mole-

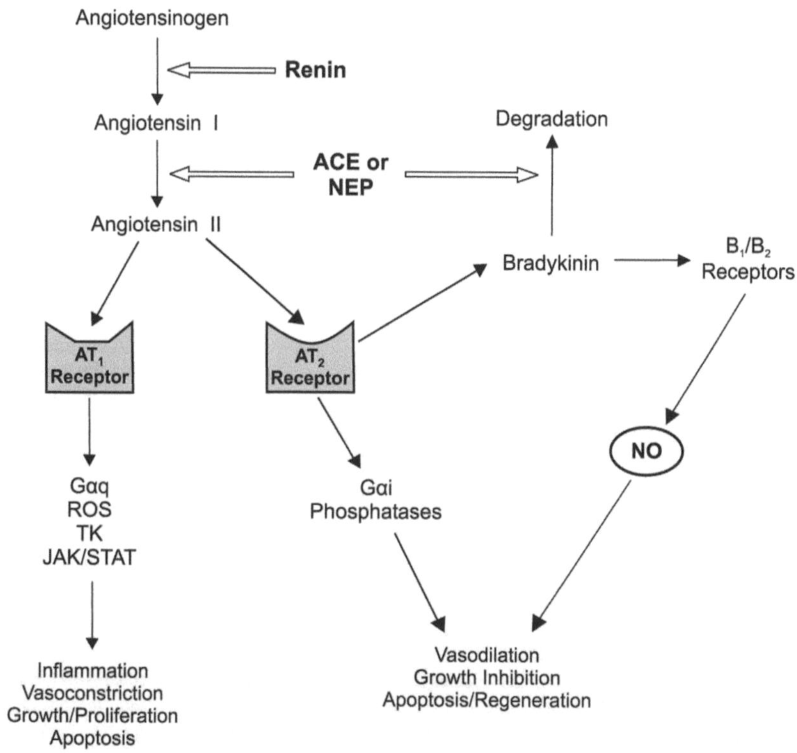

Figure 13. Schematic of angiotensin and bradykinin cellular actions. Note that angiotensin and bradykinin actions can be differentiated at the receptor level; e.g activation of AT_1 causes vasoconstriction, while activation of AT_2 results in vasodilation. Both angiotensin and braykinin have been linked to cardioprotection against ischemia and reperfusion injury. See text for a more detailed explanation.

cule and makes it more reactive. To some extent, reactive oxygen species are normal products of oxidative metabolism of physiological importance. Superoxide, which is converted to hydrogen peroxide (H_2O_2) by superoxide dismutase (SOD), is produced in the respiratory chain or from other sources shown in figure 14. The copper–zinc SOD is located in cytosol while the manganese SOD (MnSOD) is located in mitochondria. Cells have a well adapted mechanism that can control excess of free radical formation by the reduction of H_2O_2 to H_2O via the catalase or the glutathione system. Antioxidants exist as a network to remove oxidant stress; myocardial hydrophilic antioxidants such as ascorbate and glutathione are utilized first, while with more severe stress, lipophilic antioxidants are also involved.[112] In addition, ROS production can be regulated by mitochondrial uncoupling. Figure 14.

Mitochondria are the site of ROS production during ischemia. Arachidonic acid, eNOS, NADPH oxidase and xanthine oxidase are sources of reactive oxygen species at reperfusion. Cytochrome P450 monooxygenases (CYPs) have also been implicated. CYP catalyzes arachidonic acid oxidation to a variety of biologically active eicosanoids and generates reactive oxygen species.[113]

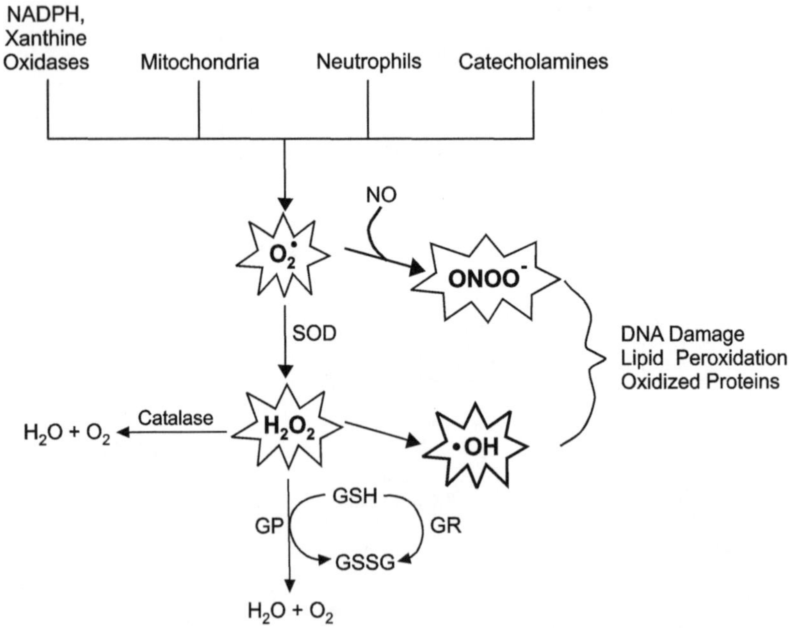

Figure 14. Schematic of reactive oxygen species production and cellular defense mechanisms (antioxidant enzymes; catalase, SOD, GSH). Reactive oxygen species (ROS) production is detrimental for the cell. However, ROS, in small amounts and for short periods, can act as intermediates of cardioprotective signaling.

ROS can cause direct cell membrane damage, lipid peroxidation and damage to proteins and sulfhydryl bonds. The detrimental role of reactive oxygen species in ischemia and reperfusion has been shown by studies using antioxidants or removing endogenous antioxidant defense. Antioxidant administration resulted in reduced infarct size.[114] Furthermore, mice with reduced expression of the mitochondrial SOD had a potent deficit in postischemic myocardial function compared with wild–type or mice with diminished expression of cytosolic SOD.[115] However, no protection is demonstrated with antioxidant administration in rabbit hearts.[116] Patients treated with streptokinase and N–acetylcysteine (NAC), a precursor of GSH synthesis, showed improved functional recovery.[117] Furthermore, inhibition of cytochrome P450 monooxygenases by chloramphenicol reduced infarct size in perfused rat and rabbit heart models of ischemia and reperfusion.[118]

Paradoxically, ROS are not only injurious but may also be protective. ROS are shown to upregulate survival signaling.[119] Furthermore, the cardioprotective abilities of ischemic preconditioning are completely abolished with the administration of N-acetylcysteine indicating that ROS can act as important mediators of the preconditioning response.[120] (See also chapter 3).

Nitric oxide is a molecule with pleiotropic effects on the cardiovascular system. Figure 15. Nitric oxide (NO) is produced when NO synthase (NOS) converts L-arginine to citrulline. The major target of NO in the cardiovascular system is the NO sensitive soluble guanyl cyclase that converts guanosine triphosphate (GTP) to c-GMP.

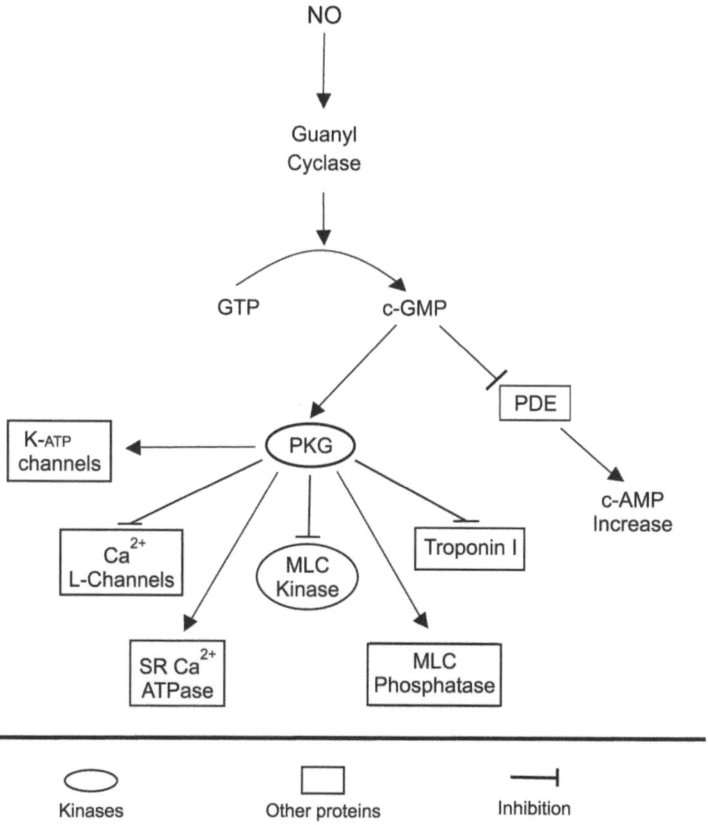

Figure 15. Schematic of nitric oxide mediated signaling. Protein kinase G (PKG) responds to c-GMP, much as PKA responds to c-AMP. An interaction between c-GMP and c-AMP signaling also occurs. See text for a more detailed explanation.

"PDE"= Phosphodiesterase, "MLC"= Myocin light chain

Figure 15. Dose dependently c-GMP inhibits PDE or activates PKG, thereby mediating its effects on the vasculature, platelets and myocytes. The cardiac interstitial NO concentration during early ischemia and early reperfusion is increased. The increase in NO concentration is derived from activated NO synthase (NOS) isoforms (species specific) and from NOS independent pathways. Cardiac c-GMP concentration during ischemia is somewhat increased while upon reperfusion is decreased. NO seems to mediate protective as well as deleterious effects which are critically dependent on the specific experimental conditions. NO at lower concentrations preserves blood flow and attenuates platelet aggregation and neutrophil–endothelium interaction following ischemia and reperfusion. In small amounts might also be beneficial by nitration of the cardioprotective PKCε. Furthermore, NO increases cardiomyocyte function. Figure 16. At higher concentrations, NO depresses cardiomyocyte function, mediates inflammatory processes following ischemia and reperfusion, impairs mitochondrial respiration

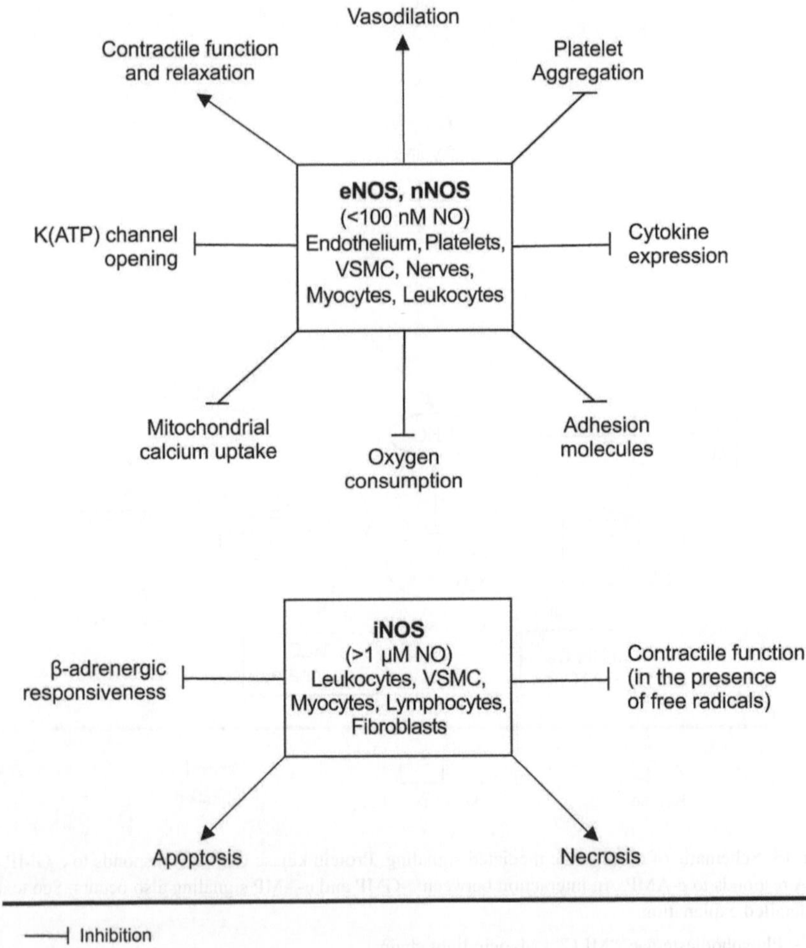

Figure 16. Schematic representation of NO mediated cellular effects. NO mediated beneficial or detrimental effects are dependent on NO concentration (modified by Schulz[121]).

and even induces cardiomyocyte death. Formation of the toxic free radical peroxynitrite contributes to cardiac damage, reviewed by Schulz.[121] Figure 16.

The importance of endogenous NO on the postischemic recovery of function after ischemia and reperfusion appears to be species–specific. In guinea pigs and mice, endogenous NO mediates beneficial effects. Blockade of endogenous NO improves and exogenous NO worsens the postischemic function in rabbits and dogs. In rats, a dose dependent effect of NOS inhibitors is observed with low or high concentrations being ineffective or even aggravating myocardial stunning while intermediate concentration of NOS inhibitors are beneficial.[121]

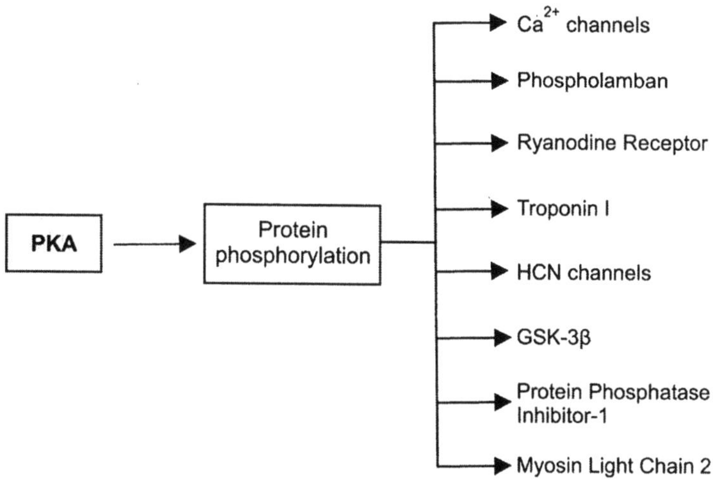

Figure 17. Schematic of protein kinase A targeted proteins. Protein kinase A serves important physiological role in contractile function. The role of PKA in the context of ischemia and reperfusion remains elusive.

2.3. Intracellular Pathways and End-Effectors

2.3.1. Protein kinase A

Protein kinase A (PKA) is regulated by G-protein coupled receptors and plays an important role in growth and cardiac contractility. Figure 9. A pro-apoptotic role of PKA has been demonstrated in in vivo and in vitro studies. PKA activation by isoproterenol or c-AMP analogues induces apoptosis in rat ventricular myocytes.[122] Overexpression of Gs receptor, which would enhance PKA activity, also induces myocyte apoptosis.[123] PKA has a profound effect on calcium homeostasis (Figure 17) and calcium secondarily can affect apoptosis. It is suggested that increased calcium entry through the L-type calcium channel is responsible for β-adrenergic/PKA induced apoptosis.[124] However, PKA is also localized to mitochondria, binding to mitochondrial specific designated kinase A anchoring proteins and can phosphorylate and inactivate the pro-apoptotic Bcl-2 family protein, Bad.[125] Evidence for a potential cardioprotective role of PKA derives from studies in an in vivo dog model of coronary occlusion showing that pharmacological activation of PKA can result in infarct size limitation. Furthermore, ischemic preconditioning effect is abrogated by the inhibition of PKA.[126] However, inhibition of PKA by H-89 (presumed to be a PKA inhibitor) further decreased infarct size beyond preconditioning or forskolin in the perfused rat heart model of global ischemia and reperfusion.[127]

2.3.2. Protein kinase C

Protein kinase C (PKC) is an non receptor serine/threonine kinase which serves important subcellular functions and has an important role in a spectrum of adaptive and maladaptive cardiac responses. PKC is involved in the regulation of cardiac contractility,

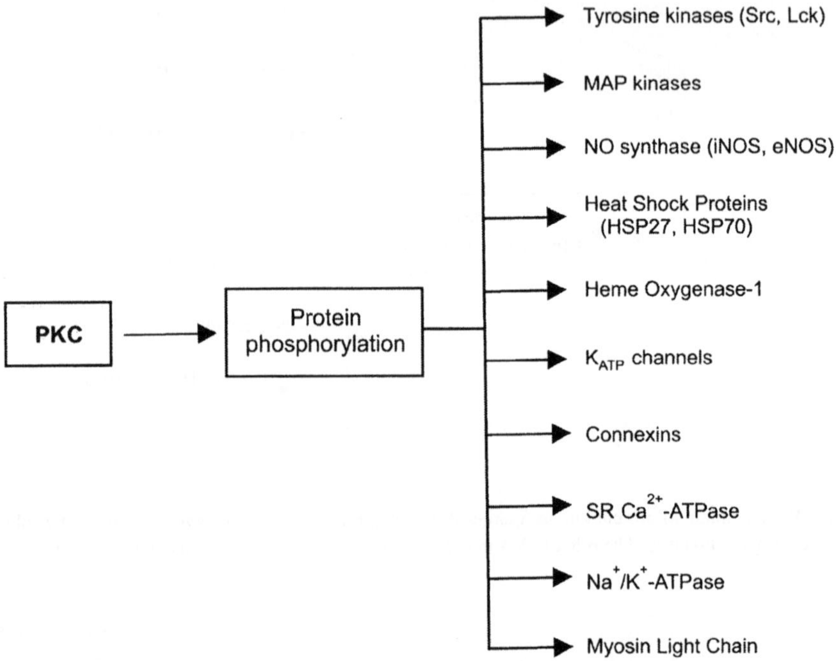

Figure 18. Schematic of protein kinase C targeted proteins. Protein kinase C serves important physiological role in cellular response to stress, growth, inflammatory processes and contractile function.

growth and response to stress as well as in the inflammatory response. Figure 18. Its action is differentiated by various isoforms. Cardiomyocytes co–express the following PKC isoforms; calcium sensitive isoforms (PKCα, PKCβ), novel isoforms (PKCδ, PKCε, PKCη) and atypical isoforms (PKC λ/ι). PKC is normally activated as a result of G receptor–dependent activation of phospholipase C and hydrolysis of membrane phosphoinositides. Figure 11. Nitric oxide or reactive oxygen species can also induce PKC activation in a non receptor manner.

For all PKC isoforms, translocation to membrane structures provides a mechanism to regulate access to substrate and has been taken as the hallmark of activation. Distinct substrate specificity in vivo has been ascribed to isoform–selective interactions with membrane–associated anchoring proteins, known as RACKs.[128] PKCε and PKCδ isoforms have been mostly linked to cardioprotection. PKCε appears to exert an anti-apoptotic effect. ERK1/2 (activation), Akt (activation), Bad and Bax (inactivation), as well as mitochondrial transition pore (closure) are some of the targets of PKCε that have been identified in relation to its anti-apoptotic action.[129] PKCδ has been linked to a pro-death action. Translocation of PKCδ to the mitochondria is essential for apoptosis and is associated with mitochondrial permeability transition and activation of the mitochondrial death pathway. The pro-apoptotic JNK and p38 MAPK pathways can be regulated by PKCδ. Overexpression of active PKCδ results in activation of the JNKs and p38 MAPK.[129]

During ischemia and reperfusion PKC translocation occurs with concomitant increase in its phosphorylation. Translocation of α and ε PKC isoforms from the cytosol to membrane and nuclei and PKCδ from membrane to cytosol has been observed during ischemia in perfused rat heart models.[130] However, with brief episodes of ischemia and reperfusion, PKCδ translocates to the sarcolemma.[131]. The role of the PKCs in lessening ischemia and reperfusion injury has been addressed by several studies. Translocation of PKCε occurs during the ischemic component of the preconditioning cycles[132] and targeted deletion of the protein kinase C epsilon gene abolished the infarct size reduction induced by preconditioning in perfused mouse hearts.[133] Furthermore, hearts from transgenic animals overexpressing PKCε are more tolerant to ischemia.[134]

The role of PKCδ in the context of ischemia and reperfusion is somewhat controversial. Activation of PKCδ by pharmacological agents (opioids, diazoxide) is shown to increase resistance of the heart to ischemic stress.[135, 136] Overexpression of active PKCδ in cells or hearts (e.g pretreated with thyroxine) resulted in protection against ischemic injury through a negative regulation of ischemia induced p38 MAPK activation.[137, 138] Conversely, ischemic preconditioning exaggerated cardiac damage in PKCδ null-mice.[139] Furthermore, pharmacological activation of PKCδ resulted in phosphorylation of HSF1 and overexpression of Hsp72 and induced protection against ischemia and reperfusion injury.[140] However, activation of PKCδ by specific peptide activators increased ischemic damage in perfused rat hearts and cardiomyocytes.[141]

2.3.3. The Rho signaling

Rho signaling is activated by receptors with intrinsic enzymatic activity or GPCR (G-protein coupled receptors), as well as by non receptor stimuli. Activation of small G proteins of the Rho family (Rac and Cdc42) activates MKK4/7 and MKK3/6 followed by sequential activation of JNK1/2 and p38 MAPKα/β respectively. Important end-effectors including transcription factors and proteins are activated through this cascade; c-jun and ATF-2 (by JNK), Elk-1, ATF-2, MEF-2 and CREB (by p38 MAPK), heat shock proteins –Hsp27 (by p38 MAPK), alpha-B crystallin (by p38 MAPK) and several other cellular substrates. Figure 19. This signaling facilitates apoptosis through various targets.[129] p38 MAPK directly phosphorylates Bcl-2 inactivating its anti-apoptotic effects, increases p53 protein levels with subsequent increased expression and mitochondrial translocation of Bax and induces caspase–3 cleavage. However, the antiapoptotic chaperone alpha-B crystallin is also phosphorylated and activated by p38 MAPK.[142]

JNKs induce apoptosis through transcription dependent mechanisms that involve c-jun activation and the induction of pro-apoptotic genes. JNKs phosphorylate Bcl-2 and inactivate it, while activate the pro-apoptotic Bad, Bim and Bmf. JNKs can directly activate Bid independently of the caspase–8. Furthermore, JNKs have a direct action on mitochondria and induce cytochrome c release.[143] Figure 19.

p38 MAPK is activated at the time of ischemia followed by a further activation during reperfusion. JNKs are not activated by ischemia alone but only after ischemia and reperfusion. Activation of these kinases can occur by reactive oxygen or reactive nitrogen species. The role of p38 MAPK and JNKs as pro- vs anti-apoptotic signals in the context of ischemia and reperfusion is a matter of controversy. However, there is some consensus that sustained activation of p38 MAPK or JNKs during prolonged ischemia and reperfusion increases cell death and apoptosis while transient activation seems to be protective. In cell based models of simulated ischemia, activation of p38 MAPK was detrimental while blockade with SB203580 (presumed to be p38 MAPK inhibitor) dur-

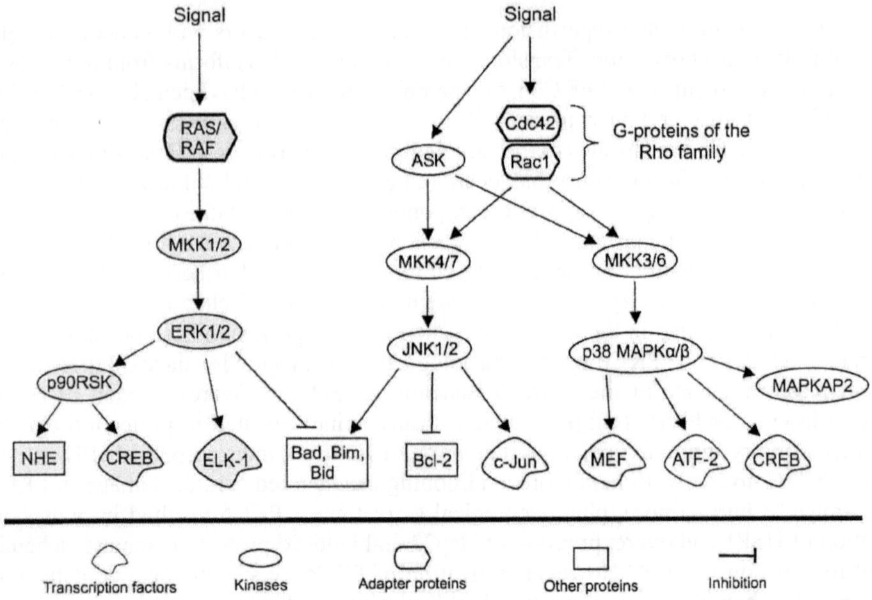

Figure 19. Schematic of Ras/Raf and Rho signaling. Growth, pro-death and pro-survival signals are tranduced through these cascades. Transcription factors are activated and link extracellular stimuli to RNA synthesis in the nucleus. Stimulation of ERK is pro-survival, JNK is pro-apoptotic and p38 MAPK can be either pro-survival or pro-apoptotic. See text for a more detailed explanation.

ing simulated ischemia decreased cell injury as measured by LDH release.[144] Similarly, inhibition of p38 MAPK activation reduced myocardial injury in isolated rabbit and rat heart models of ischemia and reperfusion.[145,146] Multiple cycle ischemic preconditioning attenuates ischemia and reperfusion induced p38 MAPK activation.[147, 148] However, transient activation of p38 MAPK during the brief episodes of ischemia and reperfusion seems to be an essential element of the preconditioning effect. In fact, treatment with SB203580 during preconditioning abrogated the protective effect.[149] Lastly, an isoform specific function is identified for the p38 MAPK with the isoform p38α exhibiting a pro-apoptotic effect, while p38β displaying an anti-apoptotic effect. Transgenic mice expressing dominant–negative mutants of p38α in the heart show reduced infarct size, TUNEL, and DNA laddering following ischemia and reperfusion.[150].

Increased JNKs activation in response to ischemia and reperfusion is observed in an adult rabbit cardiomyocytes model of simulated ischemia and reoxygenation. Attenuation of JNKs activity by transfection with a dominant negative mutant of the upstream activator of JNKs, JNK kinase–2 or JNK interacting protein–1, JIP-1, reduced cell death.[151] Furthermore, ischemia and reperfusion induced JNKs activation was decreased in perfused hearts subjected to ischemic preconditioning or heat stress treatment.[152]

2.3.4. The Ras/Raf signaling

This signaling pathway is activated by tyrosine kinase receptors, Gi receptors, or non receptor stimuli. Figure 10. Ras is a small GTP binding protein. When GTP is bound to Ras, activation of the downstream kinases occurs. The cascade includes the MAP-KKK (MAP kinase kinase kinase) known as Raf-1, the MAP-KK, known as MEK and the MAPK, known as ERK. Activation of this pathway leads to the phosphorylation of target proteins in both cytosol and nucleus. Such molecules are the p90RSK ribosomal S6 kinase and the transcription factors ELK-1 and CREB. p90RSK is involved in NHE regulation and can also be activated by ERK independent pathways. ERK1/2 facilitates cell survival through several downstream mediators and end-effectors. ERK1/2 forms a complex with PKCε in mitochondria, and increases the phosphorylation and inactivation of the pro-apoptotic Bcl-2 family member Bad. Similarly, inactivation of Bad occurs through the ERK/p90RSK ribosomal S6 kinase. ERK1/2 antagonizes the extrinsic apoptotic pathway through a mechanism involving inhibition of caspase–8 cleavage. Furthermore, ERK1/2 activation in cardiac myocytes may provide protection through direct transcription linkage with GATA4.[129] Ras/Raf signaling can interact with other signaling pathways (e.g JAK/STAT). Figure 19.

ERK is activated in response to ischemia and reperfusion and seems to be of cardioprotective nature. Inhibition of ERK activation by PD98059, an ERK inhibitor, increases apoptosis in neonatal cardiomyocytes exposed to simulated ischemia and re-oxygenation.[153] Similarly, in an isolated perfused rat heart model of ischemia and reperfusion, postischemic functional recovery was reduced after treatment with PD98059.[153] Furthermore, an interplay seems to exist between the ERK anti-apoptotic pathway and the p38 MAPK and JNKs pro-apoptotic pathways and cell fate is shown to depend on this balance. In fact, simultaneous inhibition of the p38 MAPK and JNKs pathways attenuated the increased ischemia and reoxygenation induced apoptosis that occurred by inhibition of the ERK pathway.[153] Activation of ERK1/2 occurs during preconditioning cycles and inhibition of its activity by PD98059, attenuated the preconditioning effect in an in vivo rat model.[135] However, similar effect was not observed in the perfused rat heart model of ischemia and reperfusion.[154]

2.3.5 The PI3K signaling

The PI3K signaling is mediated by receptors with intrinsic enzymatic activity (tyrosine kinase receptors) or non receptor stimuli. PI3K is activated by the receptor's association to Src-like tyrosine kinase or Ras kinase or to insulin receptor substrate-1 (IRS-1), an important docking site for several kinases and phosphatases. Figure 7. PI3K (α isoform) in turn activates PKD1/PKD2 and Akt while PI3K (γ isoform) negatively regulates c-AMP and hence GPCRs related signaling. The physiological role of PI3K kinase is now revealed by studies on transgenic animals showing that overexpression of PI3Kα can result in hypertrophy without the activation of the fetal program, while overexpression of dnPI3Kα blocks hypertrophy without depressing contractility, reviewed by Abel.[155] In contrast, deletion of PI3Kγ increases contractility without an increase in cardiac size. PI3K activation leads to the activation of the protein kinase B, known as Akt, through the phosphorylation of PDK1/PDK2. Transgenic animals lacking Akt1 isoform show a phenotype of generalized reduction in organ/body size, while deficiency of Akt2 results in type-2 diabetes. Overexpression of Akt induces hypertrophy and increases contractility both in vivo and in vitro.[155] This signaling is considered to facilitate cell survival through several targets. Bad, Bax, GSK-3β, caspace–9, eNOS and K_{ATP} channels are downstream to Akt. p70S6K is a S6 kinase activated by Akt and is critical for the hypertrophic effect mediated by Akt. This kinase can also be activated by PKC

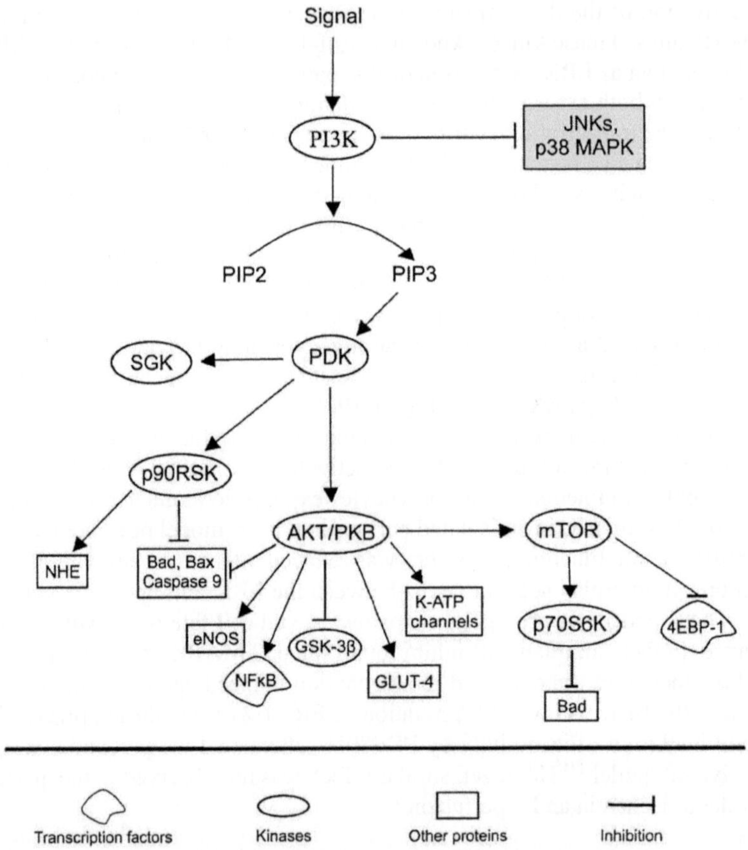

Figure 20. Schematic of the PI3K signaling pathway. PI3K mediates survival signaling. Activation of this pathway results in inactivation of caspase 9, inactivation of the pro-apoptotic proteins Bad and Bax, activation of eNOS, producing nitric oxide which may protect by inhibiting opening of the mitochondrial transition pore, and activation of p70S6K which inhibits Bad. A negative interaction between PI3K signaling and the pro-apoptotic JNK and p38 MAPK pathways also exists. Growth factors and G-protein coupled ligands induce cardioprotection by acting through the PI3K pathway.

in the absence of the PI3K activation.[156] An anti-apoptotic effect of P13K/Akt pathway may also be mediated through its modulatory interaction with the pro-apoptotic p38 MAPK and JNK pathways. This interplay seems to occur through the phosphorylation and inhibition of the apoptosis signal regulating kinase-1 (ASK1), the upstream activator of mitogen activated kinases.[157] Figure 19, 20.

PI3K/Akt activation occurs during reperfusion and interventions that further enhance its activation limited ischemia and reperfusion injury, indicating a cardioprotective role of the PI3K/Akt pathway. Activation of the PI3K/Akt by insulin, insulin like growth factor–1, TGFβ–1, cardiotrophin–1, urocortin, atorvastatin and bradykinin administration at reperfusion results in cardioprotection, reviewed by Hausenloy.[158] Activation of PI3K/Akt pathway is increased at the time of reperfusion in the ischemic preconditioned isolated rat hearts subjected to sustained ischemia and reperfusion. Furthermore, PI3K/Akt acts in parallel with ERK1/2 cascade and seems that they are both required for the ischemic preconditioning effect. Interestingly, these pathways are shown to interact in such a way that inhibiting one kinase cascade upregulates the activity of the other pathway, reviewed by Hausenloy.[158]

2.3.6 The JAK/STAT signaling

JAK/STAT pathway is activated by the IL-6 cytokine family through the gp130 receptor, G-protein coupled receptors and ischemia and reperfusion. Figure 8. JAK/STAT signaling has been recently linked to the cell response to ischemic stress. Simulated ischemia and reoxygenation in neonatal cardiomyocytes resulted in rapid induction and phosphorylation of STAT1 but not of the STAT3. Transfection of myocytes with STAT1 increased apoptosis following simulated ischemia, indicating a detrimental role of STAT1. On the contrary, transfection with STAT3 reduced ischemia induced apoptosis.[159] JAK/STAT signaling is shown to mediate the late preconditioning cardioprotective effect in a mouse model of coronary occlusion and reperfusion. This effect was associated with transcriptional upregulation of the inducible nitric oxide synthase (iNOS) and the cyclooxygenase-2 (COX-2).[160]

2.3.7 Calcineurin

Calcineurin (PP2B) is a calcium–calmodulin–activated, serine/threonine protein phosphatase that responds to sustained elevations of intracellular calcium. Calcineurin consists of a catalytic subunit (CnA), a calcium binding subunit (CnB) and calmodulin. Once activated, calcineurin directly dephosphorylates members of the NFAT transcription factor family in the cytoplasm promoting their nuclear translocation and the transcriptional induction of various genes. It is suggested that transient activation of calcineurin antagonizes myocyte apoptosis, whilst long standing activation induces cardiac hypertrophy and deleterious ventricular remodeling associated with heart failure, reviewed by Baines.[129]

A potential cardioprotective role for calcineurin is provided by studies in transgenic mice. Calcineurin A beta (-/-) gene targeted mice showed a greater loss of viable myocardium, enhanced DNA laddering and TUNEL and a greater loss of cardiac performance after ischemia and reperfusion compared with strain–matched wild–type control mice. This response was accompanied by reduced expression of the NFAT at baseline and after ischemia and reperfusion. Furthermore, expression of an activated NFAT mutant in cardiac myocytes resulted in protection while directed inhibition of NFAT augmented cell death.[161]

2.4. TRANSCRIPTION

A reprogramming of the expression of several genes can occur in the cell in response to stress contributing to cell defense and survival. Several regulators of transcription are implicated in this response.

NF–κB is a pleiotropic transcription factor that responds rapidly to a variety of stimuli including cytokines, endotoxin and oxidative stress. NF–κB controls both cell survival and cell death. Ligand binding to cell surface receptor leads to the phosphorylation of the inhibitor protein IkB and release of the sequestered NF–ϰB in the cytosol. Figure 21. NF-ϰB then translocates into the nucleus followed by phosphorylation and binds to the promoter region of the target gene. Figure 21. Genes regulated by this transcription factor include the inducible nitric oxide synthase (iNOS), cyclooxygenase-2 (COX-2), manganese–conjugated superoxide dismutase (MnSOD), anti-apoptotic proteins, such as Bcl-2, inhibitor of apoptosis factors (IAFs) and members of the cytokine family (e.g TNF-α), interleukins (e.g IL–1 and IL-6), cell adhesion molecules (ICAM, VCAM, selectins), Fas ligand and other transcription factors (p53).[162] Figure 21.

NF–ϰB activation occurs shortly after initiation of ischemia and is augmented by reperfusion in isolated heart models of ischemia and reperfusion. In in vivo models of coronary occlusion, NF–ϰB activation occurs at reperfusion in two phases; The first phase is at an early time of reperfusion due to oxidative stress and the second phase occurs later probably due to circulation of the de novo synthesized cytokines and interleukins. Studies with NF–kB decoys, blocking NF–ϰB activity, show a detrimental effect of NF–ϰB on the ischemic tolerance of the heart.[163] Furthermore, genetic blockade of NF–ϰB reduced infarct size in murine heart after ischemia and reperfusion. However, transient increased activity of the NF–ϰB has been linked to cardioprotection. Binding activity of NF–ϰB is significantly increased by brief episodes of ischemia and reperfusion (ischemic preconditioning) and is attenuated by perfusing the hearts with a NF–ϰB blocker (SN-50) with subsequent loss of the preconditioning effect.[164]

AP-1 is a transcription factor for a variety of genes and seems to play an important role in cellular responses to stress. The binding site of AP-1 is recognized by Jun family

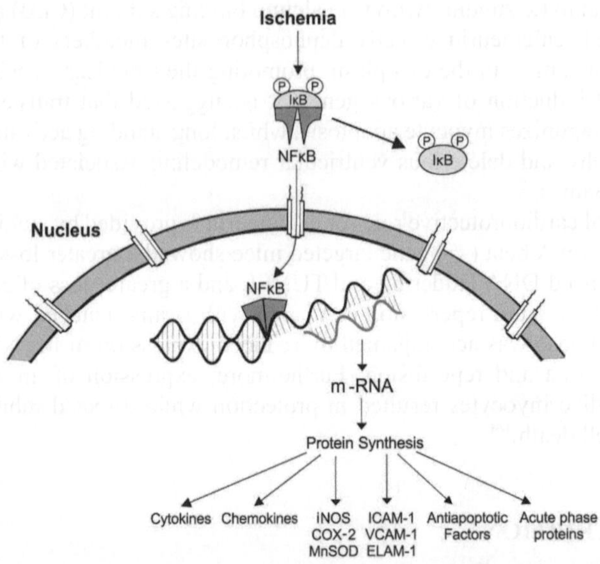

Figure 21. Schematic of activation of the NF–ϰB transcription factor. Phosphorylation of the inhibitor protein IkB results in release of the sequestered NF–ϰB to the cytosol. NF-ϰB then translocates into the nucleus followed by phosphorylation and binds to the promoter region of the target gene. NF–ϰB transcription factor can regulate the transcription of either survival or pro-death genes See text for more detailed explanation.

member homodimers and Jun/Fos family member heterodimers. The balance between Jun and Fos is critical for gene expression. Ischemia and reperfusion induces the activation of AP-1. When the heart is preconditioned to ischemic stress by short episodes of ischemia and reperfusion, AP-1 activation is reduced, reviewed by Das.[165]

p53 is a tumor suppressor protein and transcription factor that is activated by various stresses. p53 is known to promote apoptosis and this probably involves Bax and a series of p53 inducible genes signaling through Fas related pathways or caspases. Ischemia and reperfusion increases the activity of p53. Such an increase in p53 is prevented in ischemically adapted heart (ischemic preconditioning).[165]

GATA-4 is a member of the GATA family of zinc finger transcription factors which plays an important role in transducing nuclear events that modulate cell lineage differentiation during development. GATA-4 has been linked to cell survival and GATA-4 downregulation may be involved in the mechanism of the induction of cardiac myocyte apoptosis. In an isolated rat heart preparation, ischemia and reperfusion decrease GATA-4 DNA binding activity and GATA-4 mRNA. In contrast, in preconditioned hearts, GATA-4 DNA binding activity was increased in response to subsequent ischemia and reperfusion, indicating a cardioprotective role for GATA-4.[166]

2.4.1 Hypoxia inducible factor

Oxygen sensing and response to changes in the concentration of oxygen is a fundamental property of cell physiology. Lack of oxygen results in several adaptive responses in the cell, a process that is largely controlled by a transcription factor, known as hypoxia inducible factor (HIF-1). This factor consists of two subunits; the hypoxia regulated alpha subunit (HIF-1α) and the oxygen insensitive HIF-1β subunit. The activity of HIF-1 is predominantly regulated via stability of its α-subunit. Under normoxic conditions, HIF-1α protein turns over rapidly and steady state levels are often below the detection limit. HIF-1β is constitutively present. HIF-1α destruction is accomplished by a family of enzymes sensitive to oxygen (PHDs). Subsequently, a E3-ubiquitin ligase complex containing the von Hippel Lindau protein (pVHL) facilitates HIF-1α ubiquitination which is then recognized and degraded by the 26S proteasome. Figure 22. Oxygen deficiency attenuates PHD activity, prevents pVHL and proteosomal degradation and increases HIF-1α accumulation.[167] Figure 22. Non hypoxia stimuli also lead to the induction and activation of HIF-1α. Growth factors, cytokines, vascular hormones and viral proteins are shown to induce HIF-1. Contrary to hypoxia, stabilization of HIF-1α does not play a role in the non hypoxic induction of HIF-1α and the degradation of HIF-1α is not inhibited under non hypoxic activation of HIF-1α. This process leads to the increased translation rate of the HIF-1α protein and the PI3K pathway and its downstream effectors mTOR and p70S6K are involved.[168] HIF-1α activation leads to the transcription of genes encoding for erythropoietin (EPO), vascular endothelial growth factor (VEGF), insulin growth factor (IGF), glucose transporters (GLUT) and glycolytic enzymes. Figure 23. Such changes may favor cell survival under conditions of low oxygen tension. The impact of HIF-1α in respect to its pro- vs anti-apoptotic role remains elucive. HIF-1α can interact with the pro-apoptotic transcription factor p53 which is hypoxia inducible and the induction of HIF-1α transcriptional activity in the early phase of hypoxia serves a protective role. With time progressing, inhibition of HIF-1α and further induction of p53 may contribute to cell death.[169]

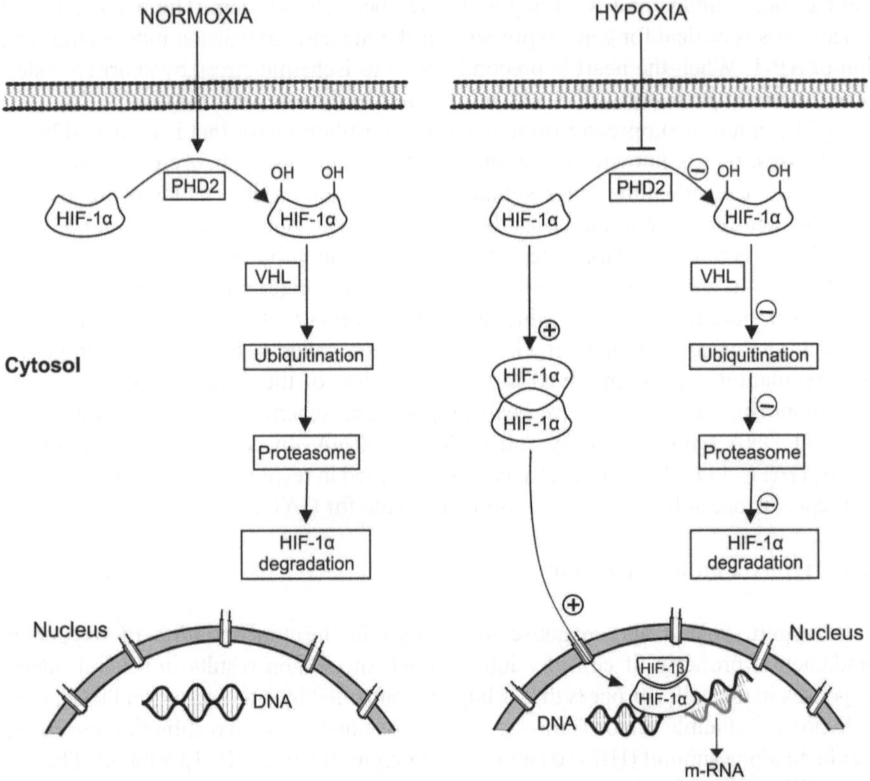

Figure 22. Schematic of proteasome dependent degradation of HIF-1α. Normoxia enhances HIF-1α degradation and hypoxia prevents it. Hydroxylation by oxygen sensing enzymes (PHD2) and ubiquitination by a E3-ubiquitin ligase complex containing the von Hippel Lindau protein (pVHL) are critical steps of HIF-1α degradation process. See text for a more detailed explanation.

A potential cardioprotective role of HIF-1α has been demonstrated in mice heterozygous for a knockout allele at the locus encoding HIF-1α (HIF1α+/-). Intermittent hypoxia resulted in protection of the isolated rat hearts against ischemia and reperfusion injury, in wild type and not in HIF1α+/- animals.[170]

2.4.2 Heat shock factor- Heat shock proteins

The heat shock response is a highly conserved defense mechanism against tissue and cell stress injury. This system represents an endogenous mechanism which antagonizes protein unfolding or misfolding that occurs during stress. It requires heat shock transcription factors (HSF) which phosphorylate and bind heat shock elements within the promoter regions of heat shock protein genes. Figure 24. HSF1 appears to be the primary mediator of the heat shock response system and is activated by ischemia and reperfusion. Activation is triggered by low energy levels, acidosis, alterations in redox state and by increased concentration of unfolded proteins, reviewed by Chi.[171]

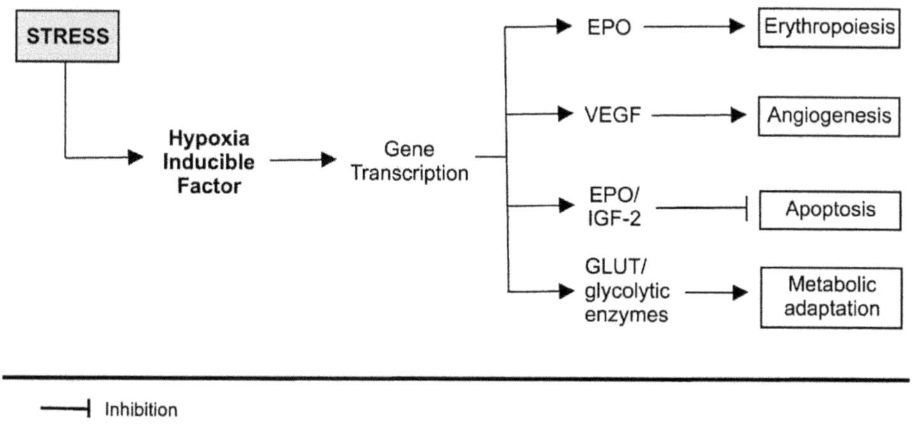

Figure 23. Schematic of HIF1 regulated gene program allowing cell to adjust to oxygen deficiency.

Heat shock proteins is a family of proteins which were identified in relation to heat stress response and they are categorized on the basis of their approximate molecular weights. Heat shock protein induction is a rapid response to altered redox state and closely corresponds to the activity of antioxidant enzymes such as catalase. Heat shock proteins are induced in response to a number of stresses, including sublethal heat, hypoxia, reoxygenation and ischemia and reperfusion.

Hsp70 is the most well studied protein in the context of ischemia and reperfusion injury. It is present in two forms; the constitutive Hsp70c and the inducible Hsp70i. Increased expression of Hsp70 is shown to confer tolerance of the cardiac cell to ischemic stress and Hsp70i seems to be the predominant isoform involved.[172-174] The beneficial effects of Hsp70 are mediated through different actions; Hsp70 inhibits apoptosis, attenuates activation of the pro-apoptotic JNK pathway induced by ischemia and reperfusion and decreases cytokine production. Furthermore, Hsp70 enhances mitochondrial function, restores redox balance and triggers NO induced protection.[175] Figure 24.

Heat shock proteins other than Hsp70 also provide added myocardial protection. These include the small heat shock proteins Hsp22, Hsp27, αβ-crystallin and Hsp32. Small heat shock proteins have anti-apoptotic effects and interfere with cytoskeletal stability. Hsp27 binds to cytochrome c and prevents its binding to Apaf-1.[176] Furthermore, overexpression of Hsp27 protects the integrity of the microtubules and the actin cytoskeleton in cardiac myocytes and endothelial cells exposed to ischemia.[177-178] Small heat shock proteins are induced by several stressful stimuli and phosphorylation is required for their function. This phosphorylation is mediated by p38 MAPK or PKCδ activation.[179, 180] Several studies provide evidence for a potential cardioprotective role of Hsp27 in the context of ischemia and reperfusion. Enhanced expression of Hsp27 in canine cardiac myocytes resulted in decreased susceptibility to simulated reperfusion injury.[181] Overexpression of Hsp27 or αB-crystallin protected adult cardiomyocytes against ischemic injury[182] and transgene overexpression of αB-crystallin confered simultaneous protection against cardiomyocyte apoptosis and necrosis during myocardial

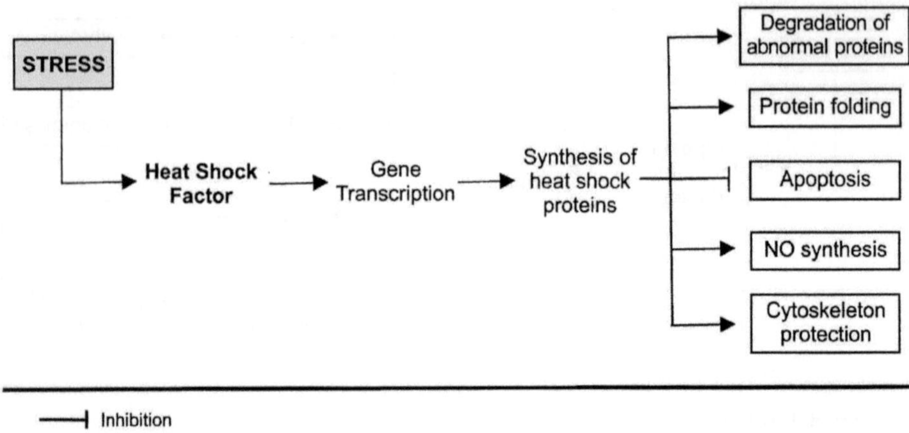

Figure 24. Heat shock proteins constitute an endogenous defense system antagonizing protein unfolding or misfolding that occurs upon stress. They enhance cytoskeletal stability, inhibit apoptosis and increase NO synthesis. Overexpession of heat shock proteins increases cellular tolerance to ischemia and reperfusion injury.

ischemia and reperfusion.[183] Ischemic preconditioning induced cardioprotection has been associated with accelerated αB-crystallin translocation and phosphorylation during the prolonged ischemia.[184] Similarly, ischemic and isoproterenol preconditioning resulted in activation of p38 MAPK with subsequent induction of Hsp27. However, during the index ischemia, Hsp27 phosphorylation remained increased while p38 MAPK activation was attenuated.[148] Accordingly, thyroxine induced cardioprotection was associated with increased Hsp27 expression and acceleration of Hsp27 phosphorylation and translocation to the cytoskeleton upon ischemia.[185]

Hsp60 and Hsp10 are located predominantly in the mitochondria. Accumulation of unfolded proteins within the mitochondrial matrix results in transcriptional upregulation of genes encoding these proteins. Their overexpression in rat neonatal cells leads to protection associated with increased ATP recovery and preservation of complex III and IV activities in the mitochondria.[186] A small amount of Hsp60 is also found in cytosol and forms a macromolecular complex with Bax and Bak but not with Bcl-2. Reduction of Hsp60 levels by antisense oligonucleotides increases the unbound Bax, indicating an important role of the cytosolic Hsp60 in the process of apoptosis.[187] Hypoxia results in dissociation of the Hsp60–Bax and translocation of Hsp60 to membrane and Bax to mitochondria, a process sufficient to trigger apoptosis.[188]

Hsp90 is an ATP dependent molecular chaperone involved in the folding and activation of various substrate proteins which include kinases and transcription factors such as HIF-1α and HSF1. Furthermore, Hsp90 has a regulatory effect on steroid receptors. Figure 12. Steroid hormones via the interaction of HSF1 and Hsp90 regulate heat shock protein expression in adult rat cardiomyocytes.[189] Disruption of Hsp90 by geldanamycin promotes HIF-1α degradation with marked reduction in both accumulation of the hypoxia–induced VEGF mRNA and hypoxia–dependent angiogenic activity.[190] Hsp90 acts also as anti-apoptotic in concert with Hsp70. Evidence for a cardioprotective role of Hsp90 is provided by studies in rat neonatal cardiomyocytes showing that urocortin induced cardioprotection is associated with increased expression of heat shock protein 90 in a MEK1/2 dependent pathway manner.[191]

Concluding remarks

Complex cell signaling pathways exist in the cell and are involved in growth, cell survival or cell death. Intracellular signaling is a transducer of adaptive and/or maladaptive responses of the cell to stress. Signals are transduced through kinase cascades to nucleus via transcription factors. Receptor and non receptor stimuli activate intracellular cascades. Several endogenous mediators such as catecholamines, acetylcholine, adenosine, angiotensin, endothelin, bradykinin or opioids released in myocardial ischemia and bound to G protein coupled receptors can mediate pro-survival or pro-death signaling. Non receptor stimuli such as nitric oxide (NO) and reactive oxygen species (ROS) also induce signaling which may be either beneficial or detrimental, depending on their amount. Protein kinase A and protein kinase C isoforms serve an important role in the adaptive response of the heart to ischemia and reperfusion. The role of PKA in ischemic tolerance remains elusive. Beneficial or detrimental effects are reported with PKA activation. PKCε and PKCδ have been mostly studied in relation to ischemia and reperfusion. PKCε has been linked to cardioprotection while PKCδ is shown to be either cardioprotective or detrimental. MAP kinases are activated during ischemia and/or reperfusion and their role in the adaptive response of the cell to ischemia has been intensively studied. ERK activation is associated with cardioprotection. JNK is pro-apoptotic and p38 MAPK can be either pro-survival or pro-apoptotic. Transient activation of p38 MAPK or JNK may be beneficial while sustained activation is detrimental. Activation of the PI3K/Akt pathway facilitates cell survival. Transcription factors, such as NF-kB, AP-1 or p53 are activated under ischemia and reperfusion and regulate the transcription of either survival or pro-death genes.

Lack of oxygen induces an adaptive response of the cell, a process that is largely controlled by a transcription factor known as hypoxia inducible factor (HIF-1). HIF-1α activation leads to the transcription of genes encoding for erythropoietin, vascular endothelial growth factor (VEGF), insulin growth factor, glucose transporters and glycolytic enzymes. This HIFα regulated gene program allows cell survival under conditions of low oxygen tension.

Heat shock proteins are involved in an endogenous defense mechanism which antagonizes protein unfolding or misfolding occuring upon stress. They enhance cytoskeletal stability, inhibit apoptosis and increase NO synthesis. Overexpression of heat shock proteins in the myocardium increases ischemic tolerance.

3. THE ADAPTED HEART

3.1. Ischemic preconditioning

In 1986 Murry, Jennings and Reimer made the observation that brief episodes of ischemia and reperfusion have the ability to adapt the heart to a subsequent prolonged episode of ischemia followed by reperfusion and this phenomenon is known as ischemic preconditioning.[192] This form of adaptation consists of an early transient phase lasting hours (classic or early preconditioning) and a late phase, lasting 1 to 3 days (delayed

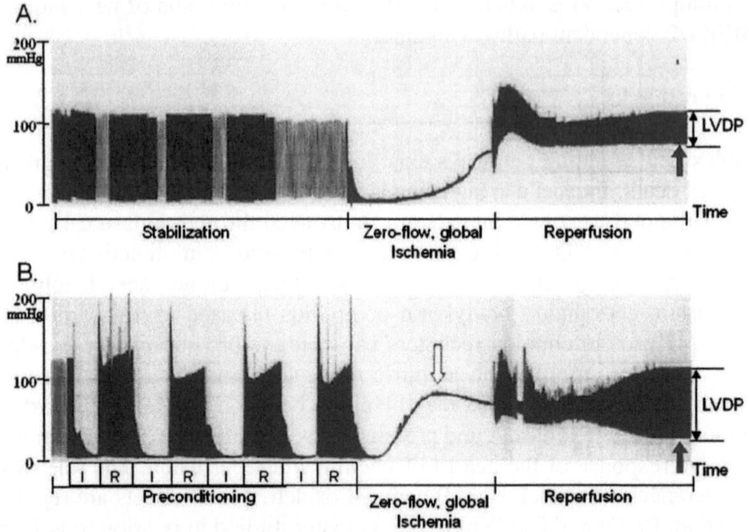

Figure 25. Left venricular developed pressure recordings from isolated rat hearts perfused with Krebs-Henseleit in Langendorff mode (LVDP is defined as the difference between systolic and diastolic left ventricular pressure). After stabilization, zero-flow global ischemia was induced by clamping the supply of the preheated perfusate to the heart followed by reperfusion. A. Note the high diastolic pressure (black arrow) and the low LVDP at reperfusion. B. The same protocol of ischemia and reperfusion was applied to a heart that had been subjected to four brief episodes of ischemia-reperfusion (preconditioning). Note the acceleration of ischemic contracture (white arrow), the lower diastolic pressure (black arrow) and the higher LVDP, indicating improved functional recovery (data from our laboratory).

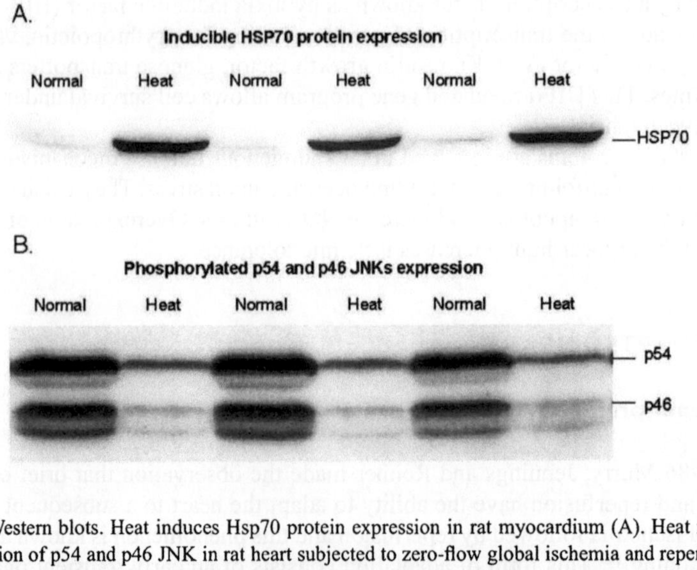

Figure 26. Western blots. Heat induces Hsp70 protein expression in rat myocardium (A). Heat reduces the phosphorylation of p54 and p46 JNK in rat heart subjected to zero-flow global ischemia and reperfusion (B). This is probably the effect of a negative interaction between Hsp70 and JNKs (modified by Pantos[152]). "Normal" stands for normal hearts and "Heat" stands for hearts subjected to heat stress.

preconditioning). Ischemic preconditioning limits infarct size, reduces reperfusion arrhythmias (not in pigs) and improves recovery of function in various experimental models. Figure 25. During the preconditioning episodes, intracellular triggering of the response may be due to the release of adenosine, bradykinin, opioids, prostacycline, nitric oxide, reactive oxygen species or TNF-α. The trigger substances also cause activation of kinase cascades either through G-protein coupled membrane receptors or directly. Protein kinase C, tyrosine kinase, as well as mitogen activated protein kinase families, are important mediators in different experimental models. The mitochondrial ATP dependent potassium channel has been implicated as a trigger or mediator, or even as end-effector, of the immediate cardioprotective effect. The early triggering response leads to the transcription of cardioprotective mediators, such iNOS, COX-2, antioxidant enzymes and heat shock proteins and their expression coincides with the late preconditioning effect, reviewed by Schulz[193] and Valen.[194] Ischemic preconditioning provides an important paradigm to unravel the cellular defense mechanisms against ischemic stress. (for a detailed description see chapter 3).

3.2 Heat stress induced 'cross tolerance' to myocardial ischemia

The phenomenon of ischemic preconditioning is mimicked by multiple environmental stresses. Prominent among them are heat stress and hypoxia. Transient hyperthermia is shown to induce delayed myocardial protection against reperfusion injury by preserving ventricular function, preventing arrhythmias and reducing myocardial necrosis. NO or ROS release by a sublethal hyperthermic stress triggers a complex cascade of signaling events that include activation of protein kinase C, and mitogen–activated protein kinases (MAPK) that ultimately lead to the expression of important cardioprotective proteins, such as the inducible nitric oxide synthase, cyclooxygenase-2, antioxidant enzymes and heat shock proteins.[195] Furthermore, in heat stress treated perfused hearts, ischemia and reperfusion induced activation of the pro-apoptotic JNKs is shown to be decreased due to its negative regulation by Hsp70.[152] Figure 26.

3.3 Chronic hypoxia

Clinical-epidemiological observations point out that the incidence of myocardial infarction is less in people living at high altitude, suggesting that hypoxia corresponds to a phenotype of increased ischemic tolerance. Subsequent experiments demonstrated that hearts exposed to chronic hypoxia are more tolerant to ischemic stress. In fact, coronary artery occlusion followed by reperfusion resulted in smaller infarctions in rats exposed to hypobaric hypoxia of 7000m for 8h/day, 5 days a week. This response was associated with overexpression of active PKCδ and the infarct size–limiting effect induced by chronic hypoxia was abolished by rottlerin, a specific inhibitor of PKCδ activation. K_{ATP} channels, ROS, NO, opioids and erythropoietin have also been implicated in the cardioprotection induced by chronic hypoxia.[196, 197] Furthermore, in animals with systemic hypoxia, downregulation of PPAR-α and PPAR-α regulated genes is observed[198] and this is accompanied by an isoform switch from α-MHC to β-MHC.[199]

Concluding remarks

Ischemic preconditioning is the phenomenon characterized by increased myocardial tolerance to ischemia and reperfusion injury induced by prior brief episodes of ischemia and reperfusion. There is an early phase lasting hours and a late phase lasting 1 to 3 days. The mechanisms of this phenomenon are not fully understood. It seems that substances released during the brief episodes of ischemia and reperfusion trigger a sequence of intracellular cascades and protective events. The phenomenon of ischemic preconditioning is mimicked by multiple environmental stresses. Prominent among them are heat stress and hypoxia.

4. THE DISEASED AND AGEING HEART

Ischemia and reperfusion injury has been extensively investigated in the laboratory using health tissues. However, in clinical settings, ischemic heart disease coexists with certain illnesses that could potentially influence the response of the myocardium to ischemia.

4.1 Cardiac hypertrophy

In general, the hypertrophied heart seems to be more susceptible to the deleterious effects of ischemia and reperfusion (reviewed by Friehs and Del Nido[200]). This may be attributed to alterations in myocardial energy metabolism and calcium handling or to anatomic and functional abnormalities of the coronary bed, such as reduced capillary density and coronary flow reserve.

Long chain fatty acid oxidation rate is lower in hypertrophied hearts while glucose uptake and glycolysis are accelerated without a concomitant increase in glucose oxidation. Stimulation of oxidative phosphorylation by activation of pyruvate dehydrogenase with dichloroacetate at reperfusion restores postischemic cardiac function. This pattern of energy substrate utilization resembles that of fetal hearts especially in hearts with pressure overload induced cardiac hypertrophy and in genetically induced hypertension in spontaneously hypertensive rats (see also introduction). Ion homeostasis is also altered in pathological hypertrophy due to the sodium–proton and sodium–calcium exchanger increased activity and sodium–potassium ATPase decreased activity. These changes in ion homeostasis together with the reduction of the sarcoplasmic reticulum calcium ATPase activity, might contribute to calcium overload and consequently to the impairment of postischemic recovery of function in hypertrophied hearts subjected to ischemia and reperfusion.[200, 201]

4.2 Heart failure

The response of the failing heart to ischemic stress appears to be variable. Increased incidence of ischemia and reperfusion arrhythmias is observed in hearts from rabbits with heart failure induced by pressure or volume overload.[202] Furthermore, hearts from rats with heart failure are shown to be more vulnerable to ischemic injury and acute blockade of RAS with ACE inhibitors improved postischemic recovery of function.[203] However, increased susceptibility to ischemia was not evident in specimens of right atrium from patients with impaired ventricular function.[204] A number of changes occur in heart failure that potentially could influence the response of the heart to ischemia. Oxidative stress is increased, sustained overexpression of pro-inflammatory mediators is observed, and the activity of the renin-angiotensin system is enhanced.

4.3. Diabetes

Much controversy seems to exist as to whether the diabetic heart is more or less sensitive to ischemic injury. A large number of studies using animal models of experimental diabetes (induced by streptozotocin or alloxan) report no change, increased or decreased sensitivity to ischemia and reperfusion. Differences in the experimental design in relation to metabolic and ion changes that occur in diabetic heart might be the basis of such discrepancies. Short-term diabetes is associated with decreased sensitivity to zero-flow ischemia and reperfusion injury. This beneficial effect disappears with increased duration or severity of diabetes. The diabetic heart appears to be more vulnerable in low-flow ischemia and in the presence of elevated fatty acids in the perfusate. Furthermore, hearts from Zucker diabetic fatty and lean Goto-Kakizaki Type-2 diabetic rats are resistant to reperfusion injury.[205]

Several mechanisms appear to underlie the response of the diabetic heart to ischemia and reperfusion. Reduction in glucose uptake and metabolism increases the sensitivity of the diabetic heart to an episode of hypoxia or mild ischemia (low-flow ischemia). In contrast, decrease in glycolytic product accumulation (lactate and protons) as well as alterations in the regulation of pH (decrease in Na^+/H^+ exchanger activity) make the diabetic heart less sensitive to an episode of severe ischemia (zero-flow ischemia).[205, 206] Studies demonstrating increased tolerance of the diabetic heart to ischemia and reperfusion implicate the involvement of cardioprotective intracellular signaling. In fact, ERK phosphorylation was increased at baseline and during ischemia, while inhibition of PKC activation abolished the enhanced tolerance of the diabetic heart to ischemia and reperfusion injury. Persistent translocation of PKCε during ischemia is also observed in the diabetic heart.[207] Furthermore, thyroid hormones decline in streptozotocin induced diabetes and this appears to contribute to the decreased incidence of reperfusion arrhythmias.[208]

4.4 Hypercholesterolemia

Hypercholesterolemia is a major risk factor for coronary artery disease and the investigation of the response of the myocardium to ischemia and reperfusion in the presence of hypercholesteremia is clinically relevant. This issue though is surrounded by much controversy and factors such as the component of diet, the presence of atherosclerosis, the experimental model of ischemia and reperfusion, and the duration of treatment may account for conflicting reports. The duration of high cholesterol levels appears to be an important determinant of the postischemic outcome. Hypercholesterolemia is associated with larger myocardial infarcts in rabbit hearts subjected to ischemia and reperfusion after short-term cholesterol treatment.[209] Similarly, in mice, short-term exposure (2 weeks) to high cholesterol levels does not alter the infarct size in the wild type animal but increases infarct size in animals deficient in the low-density lipoprotein receptor.[210] Prolonged exposure to elevated circulating cholesterol levels protects the myocardium from ischemia and reperfusion injury in rabbit and in wild type and in low density lipoprotein receptor deficient mice.[210, 211] However, several other studies show that prolonged hypercholesteremia increases susceptibility of the myocardium to ischemia and reperfusion injury.[212, 213] No change in the response of the heart to ischemic stress is also reported.[214]

Myocardial GSH levels are reduced within 2 weeks of cholesterol diet with a subsequent increase thereafter and this probably accounts for the different ischemic response in early and late stages of hypercholesterolemia.[210] Increased susceptibility of the hypercholesterolemic rabbit hearts to ischemia and reperfusion injury has been associated with increased caspase-1 and caspase-3 activity and apoptosis. Selective inhibition of caspase-1 reduced the detrimental effect conferred by hypercholesterolemia.[212]

4.5 Post-infarcted heart

Observations from our laboratory show that post-infarcted myocardium is more tolerant to ischemia and reperfusion injury. Increased postischemic recovery of function and decreased LDH release were found in perfused rat hearts after 8 weeks of an acute myocardial infarction. This response was associated with downregulation of TRα1 and TRβ1 thyroid hormone nuclear receptors. Thus, it is likely that tissue hypothyroidism (at the receptor level) might account for the increased tolerance of those hearts to ischemia and reperfusion injury.[215] See also chapter 2.

4.6 Ageing heart

Myocardial response to ischemia and reperfusion seems to vary with age. Immature rat hearts (14-21 days) are more tolerant to zero-flow global ischemia than hearts from adult animals (50 days).[216] Old age is associated with an increase in myocardial susceptibility to ischemia. In a model of low-flow global ischemia in perfused senescent hearts (24 months), severe coronary vasoconstriction and contractile dysfunction occurred with lower postischemic recovery of both coronary flow and contractility. This age associated decrease in ischemic tolerance was attributed to the accelerated accumulation of intracellular sodium and calcium due to the overactivity of sodium–proton exchanger (NHE). Administration of cariporide, a NHE inhibitor significantly improved postischemic contractile function and recovery of coronary function.[217] In experimental models of zero-flow global ischemia, susceptibility to ischemia and reperfusion is shown to increase with moderate ageing (16 months). In perfused hearts from 4 month (adults), 16 month (old) and 24 month (senescent) rats, susceptibility to ischemia and reperfusion injury increases from 4 to 16 months, while it decreases thereafter up to 24 months. Furthermore, postischemic arrhythmias are also increased at the age of 16 months. The enhanced susceptibility to ischemia at the moderate ageing was associated with decreased catalase activity and decreased ability of the cell to eliminate hydrogen peroxide.[218] Reduced antioxidative capacity rather increased reactive oxygen production was found in aged rat hearts with decreased tolerance to ischemic injury.[219] In addition, intermittent episodes of ischemia in aged hearts have been shown to promote the induction of hypertrophy and apoptosis related genes.[220]

Concluding remarks

Ischemic heart disease coexists with certain illnesses which may potentially influence the response of the myocardium to ischemia. Experimental evidence shows that the diseased myocardium may be either vulnerable or tolerant to ischemia and reperfusion injury. Much of the controversy could be attributed to differences in the experimental design, such as the duration and severity of the disease or the severity of the ischemic insult. The response of the myocardium to ischemia seems to vary with age.

5. EXPERIMENTAL MODELS

Differences in species, gender or experimental techniques may account for variable or conflicting reported results. The evolution of necrosis within an area of regional ischemia occurs extremely rapidly in animals that have little or no collateral flow such as rabbits or rats whilst it occurs slowly in animals with collateral circulation such as the canine model. In guinea pig, necrosis does not occur since this myocardium is richly supplied by collateral vessels. Several other species differences also exist including changes in myosin expression, ion homeostasis and inflammatory response. α-MHC is predominant in rodents, while β-MHC is predominant in larger animals. The action potential is short in rats compared to larger species. Ischemia and reperfusion induced arrhythmias in small animals such as rabbit and mouse are far less frequent than in canine or pig. Differences in postinfarction inflammatory response are also observed. In mice, unlike canine, infarcted hearts show only transient macrophage infiltration and no significant mast cell accumulation.[221] Calcium physiology is also species related (reviewed by Kim[67]). Rodent hearts contract and relax at physiological frequency that would be considered pathological tachycardia in large animals and therefore the required calcium for contraction is mainly provided by intracellular stores such as the sarcoplasmic reticulum. In contrast, in pigs and other large mammals with slower heart rate, a large amount of calcium is derived from extracellular calcium entry through the L-type calcium channel. Removal of calcium during diastole is also species–dependent. The sodium–calcium exchanger contributes more to calcium removal in large animals than in rodents.

Age matched adult females seem to be relatively protected against ischemia and reperfusion injury compared to males. TNF-alpha, IL-beta and IL-6 and activation of p38 MAPK are all decreased in hearts from female rats subjected to ischemia and reperfusion.[222] Furthermore, intracellular sodium after ischemia and reperfusion is higher in hearts from male than female rats.[223]

Different experimental techniques have been also used to investigate ischemia-reperfusion injury. Table 2. Experimental models of isolated hearts cannot consider the contribution of blood components or neurohormonal changes as this occurs in in vivo studies. However, these studies are able to dissect potential underlying mechanisms of the ischemic injury. The mode of perfusion (working heart vs Langendorff mode or constant flow vs constant pressure), the use of pacing, the composition of the perfusate and the end-points chosen to assess myocardial injury (arrhythmias, functional recovery

Table 2. Characteristics of various experimental models used to study ischemia-reperfusion injury.

Models	Characteristics
In vivo model of coronary occlusion	• Anesthesia, intubation, thoracotomy. • Induction of ischemia by coronary artery occlusion using a suture; no-flow regional ischemia. Reperfusion is possible. • ECG recording and study of arrhythmias. • Measurement of infarct size by TTC staining. • Assessment of contractile function by ultrasonography.

Models	Characteristics
	• Measurement of hemodynamic parameters by catheterization. • Acute or chronic effects of ischemia/reperfusion or ischemia alone can be studied. • The contribution of blood components and neurohormonal changes is considered. • Experimental model close to clinical conditions but many confounding factors may be involved when investigating mechanisms. • Arrthythmias, hypotension or pulmonary edema can occur during the experimental procedure.
Isolated perfused heart (Langendorff preparation)	• Cannulation of the aorta, retrograde perfusion of the heart ex vivo. (See figure 5). • No innervation, no circulating neurohormonal factors, confounding factors can be controlled. • Preload of left ventricle, flow or perfusion pressure can be adjusted. • Pacing can maintain constant rhythm. Heart rate can be set. • Perfusate composition can vary; bicarbonate Krebs-Henseleit buffer is the most common. Blood perfused model also exists.Various energy providing substrates in varying concentrations can be used in the perfusate; glucose with or without insulin, glucose and fatty acids, lactate etc. • Induction of ischemia by stopping (no-flow) or reducing (low-flow) coronary flow, using a peristaltic pump. • Assessment of contractility via intraventricular balloon. • Electrocardiographic recordings can be obtained. • Tissue necrosis can be evaluated by measurement of biochemical indexes such as LDH or CK release in the effluent. • Biochemical parameters and proteins can be determined in tissue samples. • NMR spectroscopy allows for continuous measurement of metabolites and intracellular ions. • Assessment of direct effects of various pharmacological agents. • Only acute effects of ischemia/reperfusion can be studied.
Isolated working heart preparation	• Perfusion of the heart ex vivo through the left atrium and ejection via the aorta resembling physiological conditions. • Measurement of cardiac output. • Preload and afterload can be adjusted. • Other characteristics similar to Langendorff preparation.

Models	Characteristics
Model of isolated heart muscle	• A thin myocardial strip dissected from atrium or ventricle is used. • Cardiac muscle strip is perfused in a chamber with oxygenated solution (Krebs or Tyrode). Preload is set by applying an initial stretching force. • The muscle is usually stimulated at 1 Hz. • Simulated ischemia is induced by decreasing pO2 and limiting or eliminating energy providing substrates in the perfusate. Simulated ischemia is also induced by decreasing pH and inhibiting glycolysis. • Contractility is assessed by tension measurement. • CK and LDH release in the effluent are used as biochemical indexes of tissue injury. • Tissue viability is assessed by MTT. • Action potential can be recorded using intracellular electrodes. Various parameters of the action potential can be measured.
Cell-based models	• Cells are cultured under controlled experimental conditions. • Pure population of cells can be obtained; embryonic myocytes, neonatal or adult cardiomyocytes. • Experiments are performed in unloading conditions. • Spontaneous rhythm, no innervation. • Ability to manipulate signalling proteins by the introduction of cDNAs, antisense RNA and interfering peptides. • Ability to induce efficient transfection of cardiomyocytes with certain genes. • Simulated ischemia is induced by decreasing pO2 and limiting or eliminating energy providing substrates in culture medium. Simulated ischemia is also induced by decreasing pH and inhibiting glycolysis. • Live-dead cells are detected by using specific staining (propidium iodine, trypan blue etc). • Metabolically active cells are detected by MTT measurement. • LDH and CK release in the medium are used as biochemical indexes of tissue injury. • Apoptotic cells are detected by using TUNEL. • Contractile function may be measured by cell shortening velocity.

or infarct size) may differentially influence the postischemic outcome. Furthermore, regional ischemia differs from global ischemia and low-flow ischemia from zero-flow ischemia in which metabolic end-products accumulate.[224, 225]

With transgenic and transfection approaches, intraspecies differences should be taken in account. For example, infarct size following 30 min of ischemia and 24 h of reperfusion is highly strain-dependent in rats.[226] Furthermore, overexpression of a certain protein with transfection might cause loss of its selectivity.[227]

Concluding remarks

Differences in species, gender and experimental design infuence various aspects of ischemia and reperfusion and ultimately the postischemic outcome despite the identical burden of ischemia. These factors should be considered in interpreting experimental data and translating basic research findings to clinical practice.

6. TREATMENT STRATEGIES

6.1. Pharmacological treatments

Treatment strategies aim at interventions targeting either the preischemic period mimicking the preconditioning effect or the reperfusion phase. Myocardial protection prior to ischemia is more difficult to institute than after ischemia. An example for the former is ischemic preconditioning. Ischemic preconditioning by brief aortic cross-clamping followed by reperfusion in controlled ischemia and reperfusion such as during cardiopulmonary bypass did not show any beneficial effect. However, in the off-pump bypass surgery, clamping of the individual coronary artery followed by reperfusion resulted in less troponin T enzyme release 48 h after surgery.[228] Concurrent medical treatments may prevent preconditioning effect. High doses of aspirin, which blocks both COX-1 and COX-2, prevented late preconditioning effect against myocardial stunning in conscious rabbits.[229] Furthermore, preconditioning response was abolished following oral treatment of propranolol or nipradilol in rats.[230] Preconditioning is now considered as a paradigm for the development of new pharmacological approaches. Drugs with preconditioning mimicking effect such as adenosine or K_{ATP} channel openers have already been tried in experimental and clinical studies.[231-234] Other pharmacological approaches include those aiming to reduce the detrimental effects of calcium overload,[235-240] the effects of reactive oxygen production[241] or modulators of the inflammatory response.[242, 243]

Newer treatments targeting stress related intracellular signaling, switching pro-death to survival signaling are now suggested as effective cardioprotective treatments. Inhibition of activation of pro-apoptotic p38 MAPK pathway by SB203580 during ischemia increases tolerance of the cardiac cell to ischemic stress.[244] Furthermore, activation of PI3K/Akt pathway by insulin or statins results in cardioprotection when administered at reperfusion.[158] PR39, a peptide that interacts with proteasome, inhibits HIF-1α degradation and increases peri-infarct vascularization in mouse cardiac tissue.[245] Similarly, the use of small molecule inhibitors of the HIF hydroxylases, which stabilize HIF, results in tissue preservation during myocardial infarction in rats. Furthermore, bomoclomol increases Hsp70 expression and reduces infarct size in rats.[246] The list of the pharmacological agents with cardioprotective properties continuous to grow but their efficacy still remains to be evaluated in clinical practice by conducting large clinical trials (see also chapter 7).

6.2. Gene and cell based therapies

Gene therapies are now considered as potential treatments for enhancing myocardial protection, reviewed by Melo.[247] The most common somatic gene therapy strategy for the myocardium involves the exogenous delivery and expression of genes whose endogenous activity may be either defective or attenuated due to mutation or pathological process. A full length or partial cDNA encoding the deficient gene is delivered to the target tissues using a vector system capable of expressing the therapeutic protein in the host cells. Furthermore, blockade of genes whose overactivity leads to disease can be achieved. Short–stranded deoxyoligonucleotides complementary to the target gene mRNA (antisense oligonucleotides) are delivered to the target cells or tissue by transfection with the aid of a vector. The antisense oligonucleotide binds to the target mRNA transcript and prevents it from being translated. The second strategy uses double–stranded deoxyoligonucleotides containing the consensus binding sequences (decoy oligonucleotides) for transcriptional factors involved in the activation of pathogenic genes. The decoy is usually delivered in molar excess, sequestering the target transcription factor and rendering incapable of binding to the promoter of the target gene.

The efficiency of gene transfer to the myocardium is highly dependent on the type of vector, route, dosage and the volume of delivery of the genetic material.[248] Recombinant viruses have become the preferred vectors for myocardial gene transfer. These are replication–deficient viral particles that retain their ability to penetrate target cells and deliver genetic material with much higher efficiency than non viral vectors. Some vectors are capable of sustained expression of the therapeutic gene which may be essential for the design of therapies for chronic myocardial disease. An immune reaction may be triggered by the host in response to the viral proteins and there is also a risk, although remote, that these vectors may revert to replication proficiency and be a cause for oncogenesis.[249]

Delivery of gene transfer systems of heat shock proteins (Hsp70),[250] antioxidant enzymes (catalase)[251] or survival genes (Akt)[252] has been associated with myocardial protection against ischemia and reperfusion. A vector gene therapy system has also been developed with a hypoxia response element–incorporated promoter to turn on the gene expression in response to hypoxic signal.[253]

Cardiac cell therapy consists of transplanting cells into the infarcted area of the myocardium to increase or preserve the number of cardiomyocytes, improve vascular supply and increase contractile function. There are different types of regenerating cells with the capacity to proliferate and differentiate into functional cardiomyocytes. These include embryonic stem cells and adult stem cells.

Studies using embryonic stem cells (ES) have shown cell maturation, successful engraftment, and an improvement of myocardial function. However, there are also certain drawbacks. ES are allogenic and immunosuppressive therapy might be needed, they are susceptible to ischemia and human ES may have the potential to form teratomas when injected into immunocompromized mouse, reviewed by Davani.[254]

Adult stem cells include skeletal myoblasts and bone marrow stem cells. Skeletal myoblasts are highly resistant to ischemia, they are harvested as autologous cells and differentiate efficiently into adult skeletal muscle after transplantation. Electromechanical coupling between mature skeletal grafts and cardiac muscle has yet to be demonstrated. Furthermore, arrhythmias are reported to occur with the use of skeletal myoblasts.[255]

Bone marrow contains several stem cell types including haematopoeitic stem cells (HSCs), endothelial stem/progenitor cells (EPCs), mesenchymal stem cells (MSCs), and multipotent adult progenitor cells (MAPCs). In injured heart, different bone marrow cells are shown to be able to form cardiomyocytes and /or vessels and result in functional improvement, reviewed by Davani.[254] A number of experimental and phase I non randomized clinical studies show the potential of bone marrow–derived stem cells fractions to regenerate the injured myocardium. Furthermore, in a large randomized controlled clinical trial, a significant increase in the ejection fraction was shown after six months in patients who underwent stent implantation for acute myocardial infarction and received autologous bone marrow mononuclear cells (BM-MNCs). However, the left ventricular diastolic volume was not different between groups, indicating lack of improvement of ventricular remodeling during follow up. No adverse effects were reported.[256] The major concern of using BM-MNCs may be the development of angiogenic neoplasias.[257] Furthermore, one trial which utilized peripheral blood stem cell mobilized by granulocyte–colony stimulating factor (G-CSF) has been stopped. In this study, an intracoronary infusion of stem cells after coronary stenting was performed. An improvement of myocardial function and angiogenesis was observed, but this was accompanied by an unacceptable rate of stent restenosis.[258]

It is now suggested that the adult heart may not be a terminally differentiated organ because it contains stem cells supporting its regeneration. Adult cardiac stem cells are multipotent, giving rise to endothelial cells, smooth muscle cells and functional cardiomyocytes. The existence of these cells opens new opportunities for myocardial repair.[259] See chapter 6.

Concluding remarks

Treatment strategies for protecting the myocardium aim at interventions before ischemia, mimicking the preconditioning effect or target the reperfusion phase. Myocardial protection prior to ischemia is more difficult to institute than after ischemia. Although several pharmacological agents have been tried in patients, there is a need for large randomized clinical trials. Newer treatments including gene and cell based therapies appear to be promising.

ACKNOWLEDGEMENTS

Prof. Taegtmeyer and Prof. Swynghedauw for reviewing this manuscript. Due to restrictions on the number of references, we have frequently cited reviews rather than original papers and apologise to the authors of the latter for not citing them directly.

REFERENCES

1. Z.Q. Zhao, D.A. Velez, N.P. Wang, K.O. Hewan-Lowe, M. Nakamura, R.A. Guyton and J. Vinten-Johansen, Progressively developed myocardial apoptotic cell death during late phase of reperfusion, *Apoptosis* **6(4)**, 279–90 (2001).

2. H. Yaoita, K. Ogawa, K. Maehara and Y. Maruyama, Attenuation of ischemia/reperfusion injury in rats by a caspase inhibitor, *Circulation* **97(3)**, 276–281 (1998).
3. Z.Q. Zhao, C.D. Morris, J.M. Budde, N.P. Wang, S. Muraki, H.Y. Sun and R.A. Guyton, Inhibition of myocardial apoptosis reduces infarct size and improves regional contractile dysfunction during reperfusion, *Cardiovasc Res.* **59(1)**, 132–142 (2003).
4. C. Ganote and S. Armstrong, Ischemia and the myocyte cytoskeleton: review and speculation, *Cardiovasc. Res.* **27**, 1387–1403 (1993).
5. V. Borutaite, A. Budriunaite, R. Morkuniene and G.C. Brown, Release of mitochondrial cytochrome c and activation of cytosolic caspases induced by myocardial ischemia, *Biochim. Biophys. Acta* **1537**, 101–109 (2001).
6. R.A. Gottlieb, K.O. Burleson, R.A. Kloner, B.M. Babior and R.L. Engler, Reperfusion injury induces apoptosis in rabbit cardiomyocytes, *J. Clin. Invest.* **94**, 1621–1628 (1994).
7. S. Nagata, Apoptosis by death factor, *Cell* **88**, 355–365 (1997).
8. M.Y. Heinke, M. Yao, D. Chang, R. Einstein and dos Remedios, Apoptosis of ventricular and atrial myocytes from pacing-induced canine heart failure, *Cardiovasc. Res.* **49**, 127–134 (2001).
9. P. Lee, M. Sata, D.J. Lefer, S.M. Factor, K. Walsh and R.N. Kitsis, Fas pathway is a critical mediator of cardiac myocyte death and MI dyring ischemia-reperfusion in vivo, *J. Physiol.* **284**, H456–463 (2003)
10. J. Yang, X. Liu, K. Bhala, C.N. Kim, A.M. Ibrado, J. Cai, T.I. Peng, D.P. Jones and X. Wang, Prevention of apoptosis by Bcl-2: release of cytochrome c from mitochondria blocked, *Science* **275**, 1129–1132 (1997).
11. N. Zamzani and G. Kroemer, The mitochondrion in apoptosis: how Pandora's box opens, *Nat. Rev. Mol. Cell. Biol.* **2**, 67–71 (2001).
12. A.P. Halestrap, S.J. Clarke and S.A. Javadov, Mitochondrial permeability transition pore opening during myocardial reperfusion–a target for cardioprotection, *Cardiovasc. Res.* **61**, 372–385 (2004).
13. A.M. Verhagen and D.L. Vaux, Cell death regulation by the mammalian IAP antagonist DIABLO/smac, *Apoptosis* **7**, 163–166 (2002).
14. C. Cande, I. Cohen, E. Daugas, L. Ravagnan, N. Larochette, N. Zamzami and G. Kroemer, Apoptosis-inducing factor (AIF): a novel caspase-independent death effector released from mitochondria, *Biochimie* **84(2-3)**, 215–222 (2002).
15. C. Adrain and S.J. Martin, The mitochondrial apoptosome: a killer unleashed by the cytochrome seas, *Trends Biochem. Sci.* **26**, 390–397 (2001).
16. A. Gross, J.M. McDonnell and S.J. Korsmeyer, Bcl-2 family members and the mitochondria in apoptosis, *Genes Dev.* **13**, 1899–1911 (1999).
17. M.P. Mattson and G. Kroemer, Mitochondria in cell death: novel targets for neuroprotection and cardioprotection, *Trends Mol. Med.* **9**, 196–205 (2003).
18. X.M. Yin, Signal transduction mediated by Bid, a pro-death Bcl-2 family protein, connects the death receptor and mitochondria apoptosis pathway. *Cell Res.* **10**, 161–167 (2000).
19. A. Bergmann, Survival signaling goes BAD, *Dev Cell.* **3(5)**, 607–8 (2002). Review.
20. R. Ley, K. Balmanno, K. Hadfield, C. Weston and S.J. Cook, Activation of the ERK1/2 signaling pathway promotes phosphorylation and proteasome-dependent degradation of the BH3-only protein, *Bim. J. Biol. Chem.* **278**, 18811–18816 (2003).
21. A.L. Harris, Emerging issues of connexin channels: biophysics fills the gap, *Q. Rev. Biophys.* **34**, 325–472 (2001).
22. D. Garcia-Dorado, A. Rodriguez-Sinovas and M. Ruiz-Meana, Gap junction–mediated spread of cell injury and death during myocardial ischemia-reperfusion, *Cardiovasc Res* **61**, 386–401 (2004).
23. W. Schlack, B. Preckel, H. Barthel, D. Obal and V. Thamer, Halothane reduces reperfusion injury after regional ischemia in the rabbit heart in vivo, *Br. J. Anaesth.* **79**, 88–96 (1997).
24. W. Schlack, B. Preckel, D. Stunneck, and V. Thamer, Effects of halothane, enflurane, isoflurane, sevoflurane and desflurane on myocardial reperfusion injury in the isolated rat heart, *Br. J. Anaesth.* **81**, 913–919 (1998).
25. R. Schulz, P. Gres and A. Skyschally, Ischemic preconditioning preserves connexin 43 phosphorylation during sustained ischemia in pig hearts in vivo, *FASEB. J.* **17**, 1355–1357 (2003).
26. K. Yasui, K. Kada, M. Hozo, J.K. Lee, K. Kamiya, J. Toyama, T. Opthof and I. Kodama, Cell-to-cell interaction prevents cell death in cultured neonatal rat ventricular myocytes, *Cardiovasc. Res.* **48**, 68–76 (2000).
27. N.G. Frangogiannis, Chemokines in the ischemic myocardium: from inflammation to fibrosis, *Inflamm Res.* **53(11)**, 585–95 (2004).

28. O. Dewald, N.G. Frangogiannis, M. Zoerlein, G.D. Duerr, C. Klemm, P. Knuefermann, G. Taffet, L.H. Michael, J.D. Crapo, A. Welz and M.L. Entman, Development of murine ischemic cardiomyopathy is associated with a transient inflammatory reaction and depends on reactive oxygen species, *Proc. Natl. Acad. Sci. USA.* **100(5)**, 2700–2705 (2003).
29. G. Ren, O. Dewald and N.G. Frangogiannis, Inflammatory mechanisms in myocardial infarction, *Curr Drug Targets Inflamm Allergy* **2**, 242–256 (2003).
30. M. La, A. Tailor, M. D'Amico, R.J. Flower and M. Perretti, Analysis of the protection afforded by annexin-1 in ischemia reperfusion injury: focus on neutrophil recruitment, *Eur. J. Pharmacol.* **429(1-3)**, 263–278 (2001).
31. G. Baxter, The neutrophil as a mediator of myocardial ischemia-reperfusion injury: time to move on, *Basic Res. Cardiol.* **97**, 268–275 (2002).
32. V. Stangl, G. Baumann, K. Stangl and S.B. Felix, Negative inotropic mediators released from the heart after myocardial ischemia-reperfusion, *Cardiovasc. Res.* **53**, 12–30 (2002).
33. S. Gilles, S. Zahler, U. Welsch, C.P. Sommerhoff and B.F. Becker, Release of TNF-α during myocardial reperfusion depends on oxidative stress and is prevented by mast cell stabilizers, *Cardiovasc. Res.* **60**, 608–616 (2003).
34. S. Lecour, P. Owira, C. Vergely, L. Rochette and L. Opie, TNF-alpha confers cardioprotection: A reactive oxygen species–mediated event, *Cardiovasc. J. S. Afr.*, **S8** (2004).
35. R. Schulz, E. Nava and S. Moncada, Induction and potential biological relevance of a Ca^{2+} - independent nitric oxide synthase in the myocardium, *Br. J. Pharmacol.* **105**, 575–580 (1992).
36. C.M. Thaik, A. Calderone, N. Takahashi and W.S. Colucci, Interleukin-1β modulates the growth and phenotype of neonatal rat cardiac myocytes, *J. Clin. Invest.* **96**, 1093–1099 (1995).
37. K. Yamauchi-Takihara, Y. Ihara, A. Ogata, K. Yoshizaki, J. Azuma and T. Kishimoto, Hypoxic stress induces cardiac myocyte-derived interleukin-6, *Circulation* **91(5)**, 1520–1524 (1995).
38. R.K. Chan, S.I. Ibrahim, N. Verna, M. Caroll, F.D. Moore Jr and H.B. Hechtman, Ischemia-reperfusion is an event triggered by immune complexes and complement, *British J Surgery* **90**, 1470–1478 (2003).
39. G. Montrucchio, G. Alloati and G. Camussi, Role of platelet-activating factor in cardiovascular pathophysiology, *Physiol. Rev.* **80**, 1669–1699 (2000).
40. B. Dawn, A.B. Stein, K. Urbanek, M. Rota, B. Whang, R. Rastaldo, D. Torella, X.L. Tang, A. Rezazadeh, J. Kajstura, A. Leri, G. Hunt, J. Varma, S.D. Prabhu, P. Anversa and R. Bolli, Cardiac stem cells delivered intravascularly traverse the vessel barrier, regenerate infarcted myocardium, and improve cardiac function, *Proc Natl Acad Sci USA.* **102(10)**, 3766–71 (2005).
41. C.L. Wainwright, Matrix metalloproteinases , oxidative stress and the acute response to acute myocardial ischemia-reperfusion, *Curr Opin Pharmacol* **4**, 132–138 (2004).
42. G. Sawicki, V. Menon and B.I. Jugdutt, Improved balance between TIMP-3 and MMP-9 after regional myocardial ischemia-reperfusion during AT1 receptor blockade, *J. Card. Fail.* **10(5)**, 442–449 (2004).
43. T. Reffemann and R.A. Kloner, Microvascular alterations after temporary coronary artery occlusion: the no-reflow phenomenon, *Cardiovasc. Pharmacol. Ther.* **9(3)**, 163–172 (2004).
44. R.R. Russell, J. Li, D.L. Coven, M. Pypaert, C. Zechner, M. Palmeri, F.J. Giordano, J. Mu, M.J. Birnbaum and L.H. Young, AMP-activated protein kinase mediates glucose uptake and prevents postischemic cardiac dysfunction, apoptosis and injury, *J Clin Invest* **114(4)**, 465–468 (2004).
45. L.H. Opie and M.N. Sack, Metabolic plasticity and the promotion of cardiac protection in ischemia and ischemic preconditioning, *J. Mol. Cell. Cardiol.* **34**, 1077–1089 (2002).
46. E.J. Lesnefsky, S. Moghaddas, B. Tandler, J. Kerner and C.L. Hoppel, Mitochondrial dysfunction in cardiac disease: ischemia-reperfusion , aging ,and heart failure, *J. Mol. Cell. Cardiol.* **33**, 1065–1089 (2001).
47. D.T. Lucas and L.I. Szweda, Declines in mitochondrial respiration during cardiac reperfusion: age-dependent inactivation of alpha-ketoglutarate dehydrogenase, *Proc. Natl. Acad. Sci. USA.* **96(12)**, 6689–6693 (1999).
48. H.A. Sadek, K.M. Humphries, P.A. Szweda and L.I. Szweda, Selective inactivation of redox-sensitive mitochondrial enzymes during cardiac reperfusion, *Arch. Biochem. Biophys*, **406(2)**, 222–228 (2002).
49. G.D. Lopaschuk, Alterations in fatty acid oxidation during reperfusion of the heart after myocardial ischemia, *Am J Cardiol* **80(3A)**, 11A–16A (1997). Review.
50. M. Avkiran and R. Haworth, Regulatory effects of G protein –coupled receptors on cardiac sarcolemmal Na^+/H^+ exchanger activity: signaling and significance, *Cardiovasc. Res.* **57**, 942–952 (2003).
51. T. Gan, C. Subrata and K. Morris, Modulation of Na^+/H^+ exchanger isoform 1 m-RNA expression in isolated rat hearts, *Am. J. Physiol.* **277**, H993–H998 (1999).

52. H.Y. Sun, N.P. Wang, M.E. Halkos, F. Kerendi, H. Kin, R.X. Wang, R.A. Guyton and Z.Q. Zhao, Involvement of Na^+/H^+ exchanger in hypoxia /re-oxygenation–induced neonatal rat cardiomyocyte apoptosis, *Eur. J. Pharmacol.* **486**, 121–131 (2004).
53. T. Shimohama, Y. Suzuki, C. Noda, H. Niwano, K. Sato, T. Masuda, K. Kawahara and T. Izumi, Decreased expression of Na^+/H^+ exchanger isoform 1 (NHE1) in non-infarcted myocardium after acute myocardial infarction, *Jpn. Heart J.* **43**, 273–282 (2002).
54. Y. Wang, J.W. Meyer, M. Ashraf and G.E. Shull, Mice with a null mutation in the NHE1 Na^+-H^+ exchanger are resistant to cardiac ischemia-reperfusion injury, *Circ Res* **93(8)**, 776–782 (2003).
55. E. Carmeliet, Cardiac ionic currents and acute ischemia: From channels to arrhythmias, *Physiol. Rev.* **79**, 917–1017 (1999).
56. K.D. Garlid, A.D. Kosta, M.V. Cohen, J.M. Downey and S.D. Critz, Cyclic GMP and PKG activate mito K(ATP) channels in isolated mitochondria, *Cardiovasc. J. S. Afr.* **15(4)**, S5 (2004).
57. R.J. Solaro, Integration of myofilament response to Ca^{2+} with cardiac pump regulation and pump dynamics, *Am J Physiol* **277(6 Pt 2)**, S155–63 (1999).
58. M.T. Stapleton and A.P. Allshire, Modulation of rigor and myosin ATPase activity in rat cardiomyocytes, *J. Mol. Cell. Cardiol.* **30**, 1349–1358 (1998).
59. M.L. Entman, M.A. Goldstein and A. Schwartz, The cardiac sarcoplasmic reticulum - glycogenolytic complex, an internal beta adrenergic receptor, *Life Sci* **19(11)**, 1623–30 (1976). Review.
60. C. Pantos, V. Malliopoulou, D. Varonos and D.V. Cokkinos, Thyroid hormone and phenotypes of cardioprotection, *Basic Res. Cardiol.* **99**, 101–120 (2004).
61. K.G. Kolocassides, M. Galinanes and D.J. Hearse, Dichotomy of ischemic preconditioning. Improved postischemic contractile function despite intensification of ischemic contracture, *Circulation* **93**, 1725–1733 (1996).
62. Piper HM, Abdallah Y, Schafer C. The first minutes of reperfusion: a window of opportunity for cardioprotection. *Cardiovasc. Res.* **61**, 365–371 (2004).
63. H Fujiwara, T. Onodera, M. Tanaka, S. Miyazaki, D.J. Wu, M. Matsuda, A. Kawamura, M. Ishida, G. Takemura, Y. Fujiwara, et al., Acceleration of cell necrosis following reperfusion after ischemia in the pig heart without collateral circulation, *Am J Cardiol* **63(10)**, 14E–18E (1989).
64. D. Garcia-Dorado, P. Theroux, J.M. Duran, J. Solares, J. Alonso, E. Sanz, R. Munoz, J. Elizaga, J. Botas, F. Fernandez-Aviles, et al., Selective inhibition of the contractile apparatus. A new approach to modification of infarct size, infarct composition, and infarct geometry during coronary artery occlusion and reperfusion, *Circulation* **85(3)**, 1160–1174 (1992).
65. J.A. Barrabes, D. Garcia-Dorado, M. Ruiz-Meana, H.M. Piper, J. Solares, M.A. Gonzalez, J. Oliveras, M.P. Herrejon and J. Soler Soler, Myocardial segment shrinkage during coronary reperfusion in situ. Relation to hypercontracture and myocardial necrosis, *Pflugers Arch.* **431(4)**, 519–526 (1996).
66. E. Braunwald and R.A. Kloner, Myocardial reperfusion: a double-edged sword? *J Clin Invest* **76**, 1713–1719 (1985).
67. S.J. Kim, C. Depre and S. Vatner, Novel mechanisms mediating stunned myocardium, *Heart Failure Reviews* **8**, 143–153 (2003).
68. R Bolli and E Marban, Molecular and cellular mechanisms of myocardial stunning. *Physiol. Rev.* **79**, 609–634 (1999).
69. R. Bolli, M. Zughaib, X.Y. Li, X.L. Tang, J.Z. Sun, J.F. Triana and P.B. McCay, Recurrent ischemia in the canine heart causes recurrent bursts of free radical production that have a cumulative effect on contractile function. A pathophysiological basis for chronic myocardial stunning. *J. Clin. Invest.* **96**, 1066–1084 (1995).
70. S. Sekili, P.B. McCay, X.Y. Li, M. Zughaib, J.Z. Sun, L. Tang, J.I. Thornby and R. Bolli, Direct evidence that the hydroxyl radical plays a pathogenetic role in myocardial "stunning" in the conscious dog and demonstration that stunning can be markedly attenuated without subsequent adverse effects, *Circ. Res.* **73(4)**, 705–723 (1993).
71. K. Przyklenk, P. Whittaker and R.A. Kloner, In vivo infusion of oxygen free radical substrates causes myocardial systolic but not diastolic dysfunction, *Am. Heart J.* **119**, 807–815 (1990).
72. M.C. Corretti, Y. Koretsune, H. Kusuoka, V.P. Chacko, J.L. Zweier and E. Marban, Glycolytic inhibition and calcium overload as consequences of exogenously generated free radicals in rabbit hearts, *J. Clin. Invest.* **88(3)**, 1014–1025 (1991).
73. P.M. Grinwald, Calcium uptake during post-ischemic reperfusion in the isolated rat heart: influence of extracellular sodium, *J Mol Cell Cardiol* **14(6)**, 359–365 (1982).

74. H. Kusuoka, J.K. Porterfield, H.F. Weisman, M.L. Weisfeldtand and E. Marban, Pathophysiology and pathogenesis of stunned myocardium. Depressed Ca^{2+} activation of contraction as a consequence of reperfusion-induced cellular calcium overload in ferret hearts, *J. Clin. Invest.* **79(3)**, 950–961 (1987).
75. W.D. Gao, D. Atar, Y. Liu, N.G. Perez, A.M. Murphy and E. Marban, Role of troponin I proteolysis in the pathogenesis of stunned myocardium, *Circ. Res.* **80(3)**, 393–399 (1997).
76. W.D. Gao, Y. Liu and E. Marban, Mechanism of decreased myofilament Ca^{2+} responsiveness in stunned rat ventricular myocardium: relative roles of soluble cytosolic factors versus structural alterations, *Circ. Res.* **78**, 455–465 (1996).
77. A. M. Murphy, H. Kogler, D. Georgakopoulos, J.L. McDonough, D.A Kass, J.E. Van Eyk and E. Marban, Transgenic mouse model of stunned myocardium, *Science* **287**, 488–491 (2000).
78. S.J. Kim, R.K. Kudej, A. Yatani, Y.K. Kim, G. Takagi, R. Honda, D.A. Colantonio, J.E. Van Eyk, D.E. Vatner, R.L. Rasmusson and S.F. Vatner, A novel mechanism for myocardial stunning involving impaired Ca(2+) handling, *Circ. Res.* **89**, 831–837 (2001).
79. C. Depre, J. Tomlinson, R.K. Kudej, V. Gaussin, E. Thompson, S.J. kim, D. Vatner, J. Topper and S. Vatner, Gene program for cardiac cell survival induced by transient ischemia in conscious pig, *Proc. Natl. Acad. Sci. USA.* **98**, 9336–9341 (2001).
80. G. Heusch, R. Schulz and S.H. Rahimtoola, Myocardial hibernation – a delicate balance, *Am. J. Physiol.* **288**, H984–H999 (2005).
81. J.A. Fallavollita and J.M. Canty Jr, Differential 18F-2-deoxyglucose uptake in viable dysfunctional myocardium with normal resting perfusion: evidence for chronic stunning in pigs, *Circulation* **99(21)**, 2798–2805 (1999).
82. C. Depre, J.L. Vanoverschelde, J.A. Melin, M. Borgers, A. Bol, J. Ausma, R. Dion and W. Wijns, Structural and metabolic correlates of the reversibility of chronic left ventricular ischemic dysfunction in humans, *Am J Physiol* **268**, H1265–1275 (1995).
83. G. Heusch, J. Rose, A. Skyschally, H. Post and R. Schulz, Calcium responsiveness in regional myocardial short-term hibernation and stunning in the in situ porcine heart. Inotropic responses to postextrasystolic potentiation and intracoronary calcium, *Circulation* **93(8)**, 1556–66 (1996).
84. C. Depre, S.J. Kim, A.S. John, Y. Huang, O.E. Rimoldi, J.R. Pepper, G.D. Dreyfus, V. Gaussin, D.J. Pennell, D.E. Vatner, P.G. Camici and S.F. Vatner, Program of cell survival underlying human and experimental hibernating myocardium, *Circ. Res.* **95(4)**, 433–440 (2004).
85. C.S. Baker, D.P. Dutka, D. Pagano, O. Rimoldi, M. Pitt, R.J. Hall, J.M. Polak, R.S. Bonser and P.G. Camici, Immunocytochemical evidence for inducible nitric oxide synthase and cyclooxygenase-2 expression with nitrotyrosine formation in human hibernating myocardium, *Basic Res Cardiol* **97(5)**, 409–415 (2002).
86. D.K. Kalra, X. Zhu, M.K. Ramchandani, G. Lawrie, M.J. Reardon, D. Lee-Jackson, W.L. Winters, N. Sivasubramanian, D.L. Mann and W.A. Zoghbi, Increased myocardial gene expression of tumor necrosis factor-alpha and nitric oxide synthase-2: a potential mechanism for depressed myocardial function in hibernating myocardium in humans, *Circulation* **105(13)**, 1537–1540 (2002).
87. M. Thielmann, H. Dorge, C. Martin, S. Belosjorow, U. Schwanke, A. van De Sand, I. Konietzka, A. Buchert, A. Kruger, R. Schulz and Heusch G, Myocardial dysfunction with coronary microembolization: signal transduction through a sequence of nitric oxide, tumor necrosis factor-alpha, and sphingosine, *Circ. Res.* **90(7)**, 807–813 (2002).
88. V. Bito, F.R. Heinzel, F. Weidemann, C. Dommke, J. van der Velden, E. Verbeken, P. Claus, B. Bijnens, I. De Scheerder, G.J. Stienen, G.R. Sutherland and K.R. Sipido, Cellular mechanisms of contractile dysfunction in hibernating myocardium, *Circ. Res.* **94(6)**, 794–801 (2004).
89. J.M. Canty, G. Suzuki Jr, M.D. Banas, F. Verheyen, M. Borgers J.A. Fallavollita, Hibernating myocardium chronically adapted to ischemia but vulnerable to sudden death, *Circ. Res.* **94**, 507–516 (2004).
90. G. Simonis, R. Marquetant, J. Rothele and R.H. Strasser, The cardiac adrenergic system in ischemia : differential role of acidosis and energy depletion, *Cardiovasc. Res.* **38**, 646–654 (1998).
91. C. Communal, K. Singh, D.B. Sawyer and W.S. Colucci, Opposing effects of β_1- and β_2-adrenergic receptors on cardiac myocyte apoptosis, *Circulation* **100**, 2210–2212 (1999).
92. C. Frances, P. Nazeyrollas, A. prevost, F. Moreau, J. Pisani, S. Davani, J.P. Kantelip and H. Millart, Role of β_1- and β_2-adrenoceptor subtypes in preconditioning against myocardial dysfunction after ischemia-reperfusion, *J. Cardiovasc. Pharmacol.* **41**, 396–405 (2003).
93. C. Pantos, I. Mourouzis, S. Tzeis, P. Moraitis, V. Malliopoulou, D.D. Cokkinos, H. Carageorgiou, D. Varonos, D.V. Cokkinos, Dobutamine administration exacerbates postischemic myocardial dysfunction in isolated rat hearts; An effect reversed by thyroxine pre-treatment, *Eur J Pharmacol* **460**, 155–161 (2003).

94. X. Meng, B.D. Shames, E.J. Pulido D.R. Meldrum, L. Ao, K.S. Joo, A.H. Harken and A. Banerjee, Adrenergic induction of bimodal myocardial protection: signal transduction and cardiac gene reprogramming, *Am. J. Physiol.* **276**, R1525– R1533 (1999).
95. O. Oldenburg, S.D. Critz, M.V. Cohen and J.M. Downey, Acetylcholine–induced production of reactive oxygen species in adult rabbit ventricular myocytes is dependent on phosphatidyl inositol 3 and Src–kinase activation and mitochondrial K_{ATP} channel opening, *J. Mol. Cell. Cardiol.* **35**, 653–660 (2003).
96. F.E. Rey, M.E. Cifuentes, A. Kiarash, M.T. Quinn and P.J. Pagano, Novel competitive inhibitor of NAPH oxidase assembly attenuates vascular O_2- and systolic blood pressure in mice, *Circ. Res.* **89**, 408–414 (2001).
97. M. Ushio-Fukai, R.W. Alexander, M. Akers, Q. Yin, Y. Fujio, K. Walsh and K.K. Griendling, Reactive oxygen species mediate the activation of Akt/protein kinase B by angiotensin II in vascular smooth muscle cells, *J. Biol. Chem.* **274(32)**, 22699–704 (1999).
98. W.R. Ford, A.S. Clanachan, C.R. Hiley and B.I. Jugdutt, Angiotensin II reduces infarct size and has no effect on post-ischemic contractile dysfunction in isolated rat hearts, *Br. J. Pharmacol.* **134**, 38–45 (2001).
99. G. Baxter and Z. Ebrahim, Role of bradykinin in preconditioning and protection of the ischemic myocardium, *Br. J. Pharmacol.* **135**, 843–854 (2002).
100. M. Yanagisawa, H. Kurihara, S. Kimura, Y. Tomobe, M. Kobayashi, Y. Mitsui, Y. Yazaki, K. Goto and T. Masaki, A novel potent vasoconstrictor peptide produced by vascular endothelial cells, *Nature* **332(6163)**: 411–415 (1988).
101. E. Bugge and K. Ytrehus, Endothelin-1 can reduce infarct size through protein kinase C and K_{ATP} channels in the isolated rat heart, *Cardiovasc. Res.* **32**, 920–929 (1996).
102. T. Kakita, K. Hasegawa, E. Iwai-Kanai, S. Adachi, T. Morimoto, H. Wada, T. Kawamura, T. Yanazume and S. Sasayama, Calcineurin pathway is required for endothelin-1-mediated protection against oxidant stress-induced apoptosis in cardiac myocytes, *Circ. Res.* **88(12)**, 1239–1246 (2001).
103. A.T. Gonon, A.V. Gourine, R.J.M. Middelveld, K. Alving and J. Pernow, Limitation of infarct size and attenuation of myeloperoxidase activity by an endothelin A receptor antagonist following ischemia and reperfusion, *Bas. Res. Cardiol.* **96**, 454–462 (2001).
104. G. Rossoni, M.N. Muscara, G. Cirino, J.L. Wallace, Inhibition of cyclo-oxygenase -2 exacerbates ischemia –induced acute myocardial dysfunction in the rabbit, *Br. J. Pharmacol.* **135**, 1540–1546 (2002).
105. M.A. Romano, E.M. Seymour, J.A. Berry, R.A. Mc Nish and S.F. Bolling, Relative contribution of endogenous opioids to myocardial ischemic tolerance, *J. Surg. Res.* **118**, 32–37 (2004).
106. S. Okubo, Y. Tanabe, K. Takeda, M. Kitayama, S. Kanemitsu, R.C. Kukreja and N. Takekoshi, Ischemic preconditioning and morphine attenuate apoptosis and infarction after ischemia-reperfusion in rabbits: role of delta-opioid receptor, *Am. J. Physiol.* **287(4)**, H1786–H1791 (2004).
107. D.A. Mei, K. Nithipatikom, R.D. Lasley and G.J. Gross, Myocardial preconditioning produced by ischemia, hypoxia and a K(ATP) channel opener: effects on intestitial adenosine in dogs, *J. Mol. Cell. Cardiol.* **30**, 1225–1236 (1998).
108. M. Kitakaze and M. Hori, It is time to ask what adenosine can do for cardioprotection, *Heart Vessels* **13(5)**, 211–228 (1998).
109. G.S. Liu, J. Thornton, D.M. Van Winkle, A.W. Stanley, R.A. Olsson and J.M. Downey, Protection against infarction afforded by preconditioning is mediated by A_1 adenosine receptors in rabbit heart, *Circulation* **84(1)**, 350–356 (1991).
110. G.S. Liu, S.C. Richards, R.A. Olsson, K. Mullane, R.S. Walsh and J.M. Downey, Evidence that the adenosine A_3 receptor may mediate the protection afforded by preconditioning in the isolated rabbit heart, *Cardiovasc Res.* **28(7)**, 1057–1061 (1994).
111. M. Koyama, P.M. Heerdt and R. Levi, Increased severity of reperfusion arrhythmias in mouse hearts lacking histamine H_3 receptors, *Biochem. Biophys. Res. Commun.* **306**, 792–796 (2003).
112. N. Haramaki, D.B. Stewart, S. Aggarwal, H. Ikeda, A.Z. Reznick and L. Packer, Networking antioxidants in the isolated rat heart are selectively depleted by ischemia-reperfusion, *Free Radic Biol Med* **25(3)**, 329–339 (1998).
113. L.B. Becker, New concepts in reactive oxygen species and cardiovascular reperfusion physiology, *Cardiovasc. Res.* **61**, 461–470 (2004).
114. T. Miura, J.M. Downey, D. Hotta and O. Iimura, Effect of superoxide dismutase plus catalase on myocardial infarct size in rabbits, *Can. J. Cardiol.* **4(8)**, 407–411 (1988).

115. G.K. Asimakis, S. Lick and C. Patterson, Postischemic recovery of contractile function is impaired in SOD2(+/-) but not SOD1(+/-) mouse hearts, *Circulation* **105(8)**, 981–986 (2002).
116. T. Miki, M.V. Cohen and J.M. Downey, Failure of N-2-mercaptopropionyl glycine to reduce myocardial infarction after 3 days of reperfusion in rabbits, *Basic Res. Cardiol.* **94(3)**, 180–187 (1999).
117. J. Sochman, N-acetylcysteine in acute cardiology: 10 years later: what do we know and what would we like to know? *J. Am. Coll. Cardiol.* **39(9)**, 1422–1428 (2002).
118. H. He, M. Chen, N.K. Scheffler, B.W. Gibson, L.L. Spremulli and R.A. Gottlieb, Phosphorylation of mitochondrial elongation factor Tu in ischemic myocardium: basis for chloramphenicol-mediated cardioprotection. *Circ. Res.* **89(5)**, 461–467 (2001).
119. D.K. Das and N. Maulik, Preconditioning potentiates redox signalling and converts death signal into survival signal, *Arch. Biochem. Biophys.* **420**, 305–311 (2003).
120. D.K. Das, N. Maulik, M. Sato and P. Ray, Reactive oxygen species function as second messengers during ischemic preconditioning of heart, *Mol. Cell. Biochem.* **196**, 59–67 (1999).
121. R. Schulz, M. Kelm and G. Heusch, Nitric oxide in myocardial ischemia/reperfusion injury, *Cardiovasc. Res.* **61**, 402–413 (2004).
122. Y. Shizukuda and P.M. Buttrick, Subtype specific roles of β-adrenergic receptors in apoptosis of adult rat ventricular myocytes, *J. Mol. Cell. Cardiol.* **34**, 823–831 (2002).
123. Y.J. Geng, Y. Ishikawa, D.E. Vatner, T.E. Wagner, S.P. Bishop, S.F. Vatner and C.J. Homcy, Apoptosis of cardiac myocytes in Gsalpha transgenic mice, *Circ. Res.* **84(1)**, 34–42 (1999).
124. C. Communal, K. Singh, D.R. Pimentel and W.S. Colucci, Norepinephrine stimulates apoptosis in adult rat ventricular myocytes by activation of the β-adrenergic pathway, *Circulation* **98**, 1329–1334 (1998).
125. D.M. Valks, S.A. Cook, F.H. Pham, P.R. Morrison, A. Clerk and P.H. Sugden, Phenylephrine promotes phosphorylation of Bad in cardiac myocytes through the extracellular signal regulated kinases 1/2 and protein kinase A, *J. Mol. Cell. Cardiol.* **34**, 749–763 (2002)
126. S. Sanada, H. Asanuma, O. Tsukamoto, T. Minamino, K. Node, S. Takashima, T. Fukushima, A. Ogai, Y. Shinozaki, M. Fujita, A. Hirata, H. Okuda, H. Shimokawa, H. Tomoike, M. Hori and Kitakaze M, Protein kinase A as another mediator of ischemic preconditioning independent of protein kinase C, *Circulation* **110(1)**, 51–7 (2004).
127. S. Makaula, A. Lochner, S. Genade, M.N. Sack, M.M. Awan and L.H. Opie, H-89, a non-specific inhibitor of protein kinase a, promotes post-ischemic cardiac contractile recovery and reduces infarct size, *J Cardiovasc Pharmacol* **45(4)**, 341–347 (2005).
128. K. Mackay and D. Mochly-Rosen, Localization, anchoring and functions of protein kinase C isozymes in the heart, *J. Mol. Cell. Cardiol.* **33**, 1301–1307 (2001).
129. C.P. Baines and J.D. Molkentin, Stress signaling pathways that modulate cardiac myocyte apoptosis, *J. Mol. Cell. Cardiol.* **38**, 47–62 (2005).
130. K. Yoshida, T. Hirata, Y. Akita, Y. Mizukami, K. Yamaguchi, Y. Sorimachi, T. Ishihara and S Kawashiama, Translocation of protein kinase C–α, δ and ε isoforms in ischemic rat heart, *Biochim. Biophys. Acta* **1317**, 36–44 (1996).
131. M.B. Mitchell, X. Meng, L. Ao, J.M. Brown, A.H. Harken and A. Banerjee, Preconditioning of isolated rat heart is mediated by protein kinase C, *Circ. Res.* **76(1)**, 73–81 (1995).
132. P. Ping, J. Zhang, Y. Qiu, X.L. Tang, S. Manchikalapudi, X. Cao and R. Bolli, Ischemic preconditioning induces selective translocation of protein kinase C isoforms epsilon and eta in the heart of conscious rabbits without subcellular redistribution of total protein kinase C activity, *Circ. Res.* **81(3)**, 404–14 (1997).
133. A.T. Saurin, D.J. Pennington, N.J. Raat, D.S. Latchman, M.J. Owen, M.S. Marber, Targeted disruption of protein kinase C epsilon gene abolishes the infarct size reduction that follows ischemic preconditioning of isolated buffer-perfused mouse hearts, *Cardiovasc. Res.* **55**, 672–680 (2002).
134. H.R. Cross, E. Murphy, R. Bolli, P. Ping and C. Steenbergen, Expression of activated PKC epsilon (PKC epsilon) protects the ischemic heart, without attenuating ischemic H(+) production, *J Mol Cell Cardiol* **34(3)**, 361–367 (2002).
135. R.M. Fryer, P.F. Pratt, A.K. Hsu and G.J. Gross, Differential activation of ERK isoforms in preconditioning and opioid-induced cardioprotection, *J. Pharmacol. Exp. Ther.* **296**, 642–649 (2001).
136. Y. Wang, K. Hirai and M. Ashraf, Activation of mitochondrial ATP-sensitive K(+) channel for cardiac protection against ischemic injury is dependent on protein kinase C activity, *Circ Res* **85(8)**, 731–741 (1999).
137. J. Zhao, O. Renner, L. Wightman, P.H. Sugden, L. Stewart, A.D. Miller, D.S. Latchman and M.S. Marber, The expression of constitutively active isotypes of protein kinase C to investigate preconditioning, *J. Biol. Chem.* **273**, 23072–23079 (1998).

138. C. Pantos, V. Malliopoulou, I. Mourouzis, E. Karamanoli, I. Paizis, N. Steimberg, D. Varonos and D.V. Cokkinos, Long-term Thyroxine Administration Protects the Heart in a Similar Pattern as Ischemic Preconditioning, *Thyroid* **12**, 325–329 (2002).
139. M. Mayr, B. Metzler, Y.L. Chung, E. mcGregor, U. Mayr, H. troy, Y. Hu, M. Leitges, O. Pachinger, J.R. Griffiths, M.J. Dunn and Q. Xu, Ischemic preconditioning exaggerates cardiac damage in PKC –δ null mice, *Am. J. Physiol.* **287**, H946–H956 (2004).
140. K. Yamanaka, N. Takahashi, T. Ooie, K. Kaneda, H. Yoshimatsu and T. Saikawa, Role of protein kinase C in geranylgeranylacetone-induced expression of heat-shock protein 72 and cardioprotection in the rat heart, *J. Mol. Cell. Cardiol.* **35(7)**, 785–794 (2003).
141. Chen L, Hahn H, Wu G, Chen C-H, Liron T, Schechtman D, Cavallaro G, Banci.L., Guo Y, Bolli R, Dorn GWI and D. Mochly-Rosen, Opposing cardioprotective actions and parallel hypertrophic effects of δPKC and εPKC, *Proc. Natl. Acad. Sci.* **98**, 11114–11119 (2001).
142. H.E. Hoover D.J. Thuerauf, J.J Martindale and C.C. Glembotski, αB-crystallin gene induction and phosphorylation by MKK6-activated p38. A potential role for αB-crystallin as a target of the p38 branch of the cardiac stress response, *J. Biol. Chem.* **275**, 23825–23833 (2000).
143. H. Aoki, P.M. Kang, J. Hampe, K. Yoshimura, T. Noma, M. Matzuzaki and S. Izumo, Direct activation of mitochondrial apoptosis machinery by c-Jun N– terminal kinase in adult cardiac myocytes, *J. Biol. Chem.* **277**, 10244–10250 (2002).
144. K. Mackay and D. Mochly-Rosen, An inhibitor of p38 MAPK protects neonatal cardiac myocytes from ischemia, *J. Biol. Chem.* **274**, 6272–6279 (1999)
145. X.L. Ma, S. Kumar, F. Gao, C.S. Louden, B.L. Lopez, T.A. Christopher, C. Wang, J.C. Lee, G.Z. Feuerstein and T.L. Yue, Inhibition of p38 mitogen-activated protein kinase decreases cardiomyocyte apoptosis and improves cardiac function after myocardial ischemia and reperfusion. *Circulation* **99(13)**, 1685–1691 (1999).
146. S. Schneider, W. Chen, J. Hou, C. Steenbergen and E. Murphy, Inhibition of p38 MAPK alpha/beta reduces ischemic injury and does not block protective effects of preconditioning, *Am. J. Physiol.* **280(2)**, H499–508 (2001).
147. C. Pantos, V. Malliopoulou, I. Paizis, P. Moraitis, I. Mourouzis, S. Tzeis, E. Karamanoli, D.D. Cokkinos, H. Carageorgiou, D. Varonos and D.V. Cokkinos, Thyroid hormone and cardioprotection; study of p38 MAPK and JNKs during ischemia and at reperfusion in isolated rat heart, *Mol. Cell Biochem.* **242**, 173–180 (2003).
148. E. Marais, S. Genade, R. Salie, B. Huisamen, S. Maritz, J.A. Moolman and A. Lochner, The temporal relationship between p38 MAPK and Hsp27 activation in ischemic and pharmacological preconditioning, *Basic Res. Cardiol.* **100(1)**, 35–47 (2005).
149. S. Sanada, M. Kitakaze, P.J. Papst, K. Hatanaka, H. Asanuma, T. Aki,Y. Shinizaki, H. Ogita, K. Node, S. Takashima, M. Asakura, T. Yamada, T. Fukushima, A. Ogai, T. Kuzuya, H. Mori, N. Terada, K. Yoshida and M. Hori, Role of phasic dynamism of p38 MAPK activation in ischemic preconditioning of canine heart, *Circ. Res.* **88**, 175–180 (2001).
150. R.A. Kaiser, O.F. Bueno, D.J. Lips, P.A. Doevendans, F. Jones, T.F. Kimball and J.D. Molkentin, Targeted inhibition of p38 mitogen-activated protein kinase antagonizes cardiac injury and cell death following ischemia-reperfusion in vivo, *J Biol Chem* **279(15)**, 15524–15530 (2004).
151. H. He, H.L. Li, A. Lin and R.A. Gottlieb, Activation of the JNK pathway is important for cardiomyocyte death in response to simulated ischemia, *Cell Death Differ.* **6**, 987–991 (1999).
152. C. Pantos, V. Malliopoulou, I. Mourouzis, P. Moraitis, S. Tzeis, A. Thempeyioti, I. Paizis, A.D. Cokkinos, H. Carageorgiou, D. Varonos, D.V. Cokkinos, Involvement of p38 MAPK and JNK in the heat stress induced cardioprotection, *Bas Res Cardiol* **98**, 158–164 (2003).
153. T.L. Yue, C. Yang, J.L. Gu, X.L. Ma, S. Kumar, J.C. Lee, G.Z. Feuerstein, H. Thomas, B. Maleeff and E.H. Ohlstein, Inhibition of extracellular signal-regulated kinase enhances ischemia/reoxygenation-induced apoptosis in cultured cardiac myocytes and exaggerates reperfusion injury in isolated perfused heart, *Circ. Res.* **86**, 692–699 (2000).
154. M.M. Mocanu, R.M. Bell and D.M. Yellon, PI3 Kinase and not p42/p44 appears to be implicated in the protection conferred by ischemic preconditioning. *J. Mol. Cell. Cardiol.* **34**, 661–668 (2002).
155. E.D. Abel, Insulin signaling in heart muscle: lessons from genetically engineered mouse models, *Curr. Hypertens. Rep.* **6**, 416–423 (2004).
156. M. Ceci, J. Ross and G. Condorelli, Molecular determinants of the physiological adaptation to stress in the cardiomyocyte : a focus on Akt, *J. Mol. Cell. Cardiol.* **37**, 905–912 (2004).

157. A.H. Kim, G. Khursigara, X. Sun, T.F. Franke and M.V. Chao, Akt phosphorylates and negatively regulates apoptosis signal-regulating kinase 1, *Mol. Cell. Biol.* **21(3)**, 893–901 (2001).
158. D.J. Hausenloy, M.M. Mocanu D.M. and Yellon, Cross talk between the survival kinases during early reperfusion: its contribution to ischemic preconditioning, *Cardiovasc. Res.* **63**, 305–312 (2004).
159. A. Stephanou, B.K. Brar, T.M. Scarabelli, A.K. Jonassen, D.M. Yellon, M.S. Marber, R.A. Knight and D.S. Latchman, Ischemia-induced STAT-1 expression and activation play a critical role in cardiomyocyte apoptosis, *J. Biol. Chem.* **275(14)**, 10002–10008 (2000).
160. R. Bolli, B. Dawn and Y.T. Xuan, Role of the JAK-STAT pathway in protection against myocardial ischemia/reperfusion injury, *Trends Cardiovasc. Med.* **13**, 72–79 (2003).
161. O.F. Bueno, D.J. Lips, R.A. Kaiser, B.J. Wilkins, Y.S. Dai, B.J. Glascock, R. Klevitsky, T.E. Hewett, T.R. Kimball, B.J. Aronow, P.A. Doevendans and J.D. Molkentin, Calcineurin Abeta gene targeting predisposes the myocardium to acute ischemia-induced apoptosis and dysfunction. *Circ. Res.* **94(1)**, 91–99 (2004).
162. G. Valen, Z. Yan and G.K. Hanson, Nuclear factor kappa –B and the heart, *J. Am. Coll. Cardiol.* **38**, 307–314 (2001).
163. Y. Sawa, R. Morishita, K. Suzuki, K. Kagisaki, Y. Kaneda, K. Maeda, K. Kadoba and H. Matsuda, A novel strategy for myocardial protection using in vivo transfection of cis element 'decoy' against NFkappaB binding site: evidence for a role of NFkappaB in ischemia-reperfusion injury, *Circulation* **96(9 Suppl)**, 280–284 (1997).
164. N. Maulik, M. Sato, B.D. Price and D.K. Das, An essential role of NfkappaB in tyrosine kinase signaling of p38 MAP kinase regulation of myocardial adaptation to ischemia, *FEBS Lett.* **429(3)**, 365–369 (1998).
165. D.K. Das, Redox regulation of cardiomyocyte survival and death, *Antioxid. Redox Signal.* **3**, 23–37 (2001).
166. Y.J. Suzuki, H. Nagase, R.M. Day and D.K. Das, GATA-4 regulation of myocardial survival in the preconditioned heart, *J. Mol. Cell. Cardiol.* **37**, 1195–1203 (2004).
167. G.L. Semenza, Hydroxylation of HIF-1: oxygen sensing at the molecular level, *Physiology* **19**, 176–182 (2004).
168. M.C. Dery, M.D. Michaud and D.E. Richard, Hypoxia-inducible factor 1: regulation by hypoxic and non-hypoxic activators, *Int. J. Biochem. Cell Biol.* **37**, 535–540 (2005).
169. T. Schmid, J. Zhou and B. Brune, HIF-1 and p53: communication of transcription factors under hypoxia, *J. Cell. Mol. Med.* **8(4)**, 423–431 (2004).
170. Z. Cai, D.J. Manalo, G. Wei, E.R. Rodriguez, K. Fox-Talbot, H. Lu, J.L. Zweier and G.L. Semenza, Hearts from rodents exposed to intermittent hypoxia or erythropoietin are protected against ischemia-reperfusion injury, *Circulation* **108**, 79–85 (2003).
171. N.C. Chi and J.S. Karliner, Molecular determinants of responses to myocardial ischemia/reperfusion injury: focus on hypoxia-inducible and heat shock factors, *Cardiovasc Res* **61(3)**, 437–447 (2004). Review.
172. M.S. Marber, J.M. Walker, D.S. Latchman and D.M. Yellon, Myocardial protection following whole body heat stress in the rabbit is dependent on metabolic substrate and is related to the amount of the inducible 70 kb Dalton heat shock protein, *J. Clin. Invest.* **93**, 1087–1094 (1994).
173. S. Okubo, O. Wildner, M.R. Shah, J.C. Chelliah, M.L. Hess and R.C. Kukreja, Gene transfer of heat-shock protein 70 reduces infarct size in vivo after ischemia/reperfusion in the rabbit heart, *Circulation.* **103(6)**, 877–881 (2001).
174. J.J. Zhou, J.M. Pei, G.Y. Wang, S. Wu, W.P. Wang, C.H. Cho and T.M. Wong, Inducible Hsp70 mediates delayed cardioprotection via U-50488H pretreatment in rat ventricular myocytes, *Am J Physiol* **281(1)**, H40–47 (2001).
175. D.S. Latchman, Heat shock proteins and cardiac protection, *Cardiovasc. Res.* **51**, 637–646 (2001).
176. J.M. Bruey, C. Ducasse, P. Bonniaud, L. Ravagnan, S.A. Susin, C. Diaz-Latoud, S. Gurbuxani, A.P. Arrigo, G. Kroemer, E. Solary and C. Garrido, Hsp27 negatively regulates cell death by interacting with cytochrome c, *Nat. Cell. Biol.* **2(9)**, 645–652 (2000).
177. W.F. Bluhm, J.L. Martin, R. Mestril and W.H. Dillmann, Specific heat shock proteins protect microtubules during simulated ischemia in cardiac myocytes, *Am. J. Physiol.* **275**, H2243–H2249 (1998).
178. S.A. Loktionova, O.P. Ilyinskaya and A.E. kabakov, Early and delayed tolerance to simulated ischemia in heat-preconditioned endothelial cells: a role for Hsp27, *Am. J. Physiol.* **275**, H2147–H2158 (1998).

179. A. Clerk, A. Michael and P.H. Sugden, Stimulation of multiple mitogen-activated protein kinase subfamilies by oxidative stress and phosphorylation of heat shock protein Hsp25/27, in neonatal ventricular myocytes, *Biochem. J.* **333**, 581–589 (1998).
180. E.T. Maizels, C.A. Peters, M. Kline, R.E. Cutler and M. Shanmugam, Heat-shock protein-25/27 phosphorylation by the delta isoform of protein kinase C, *Biochem. J.* **332**, 703–712 (1998).
181. R.S. Vander Heide, Increased expression of Hsp27 protects canine myocytes from simulated ischemia-reperfusion injury, *Am. J. Physiol.* **282**, H935–H941 (2002).
182. J.L. Martin, R. Mestril, R. Hilal-Dandan, L.L. Brunton and W.H. Dillmann, Small heat shock proteins and protection against ischemic injury in cardiac myocytes, *Circulation* **96(12),** 4343–4348 (1997).
183. P.S. Ray, J.L. Martin, E.A. Swanson, H. Otani, W.H. Dillmann and D.K. Das, Transgene overexpression of alphaB crystallin confers simultaneous protection against cardiomyocyte apoptosis and necrosis during myocardial ischemia and reperfusion, *FASEB J.* **15(2)**, 393–402 (2001).
184. P. Eaton, W. Fuller, J.R. Bell and M.J. Shattock, αB crystallin translocation and phosphorylation: signal transduction pathways and preconditioning in the isolated rat heart, *J. Mol. Cell. Cardiol.* **33**, 1659–1671 (2001).
185. C. Pantos, V. Malliopoulou, I. Mourouzis, E. Karamanoli, P. Moraitis, S. Tzeis, I. Paizis, H. Carageorgiou, D. Varonos and D.V. Cokkinos, Thyroxine pretreatment increases basal myocardial Hsp27 expression and accelerates translocation and phosphorylation of this protein upon ischemia, *Eur. J. Pharmacol.* **478**, 53–60 (2003).
186. K.M. Lin, B. Lin, I.Y. Lian, R. Mestril, I.E. Scheffler and W.H. Dillmann, Combined and individual mitochondrial Hsp60 and Hsp10 expression in cardiac myocytes protects mitochondrial function and prevents apoptotic cell deaths induced by simulated ischemia-reoxygenation, *Circulation* **103(13),** 1787–1792 (2001).
187. S.R. Kirchhoff, S. Gupta and A.A. Kwolton, Cytosolic heat shock protein 60, apoptosis and myocardial injury, *Circulation* **105**, 2899–2904 (2002).
188. A.A. Knowlton and S. Gupta, Hsp60, Bax, and cardiac apoptosis, *Cardiovasc Toxicol.* **3(3)**, 263–268 (2003). Review.
189. A.A. Knowlton and L. Sun, Heat shock factor-1, steroid hormones, and regulation of heat shock protein expression in the heart, *Am. J. Physiol.* **280(1)**, H455–H464 (2001).
190. J.S. Isaacs, Y.J. Jung, E.G. Mimnaugh, A. Martinez, F. Cuttitta and L.M. Neckers, Hsp90 regulates a von Hippel Lindau-independent hypoxia-inducible factor-1 alpha-degradative pathway, *Biol. Chem.* **277(33)**, 29936–29944 (2002).
191. B.K. Brar, J. Railson, A. Stephanou, R.A. Knight and D.S. Latchman, Urocortin increases the expression of heat shock protein 90 in rat cardiac myocytes in a MEK1/2-dependent manner, *J. Endocrinol.* **172(2)**, 283–93 (2002).
192. C.E. Murry, R.B. Jennings and K.A. Reimer, Preconditioning with ischemia: a delay of lethal cell injury in ischemic myocardium, *Circulation* **74(5)**, 1124–1136 (1986).
193. R.S. Schulz, M.V. Cohen, M. Behrends, J.M. Downey, G. Heusch, Signal transduction of ischemic preconditioning, *Cardiovasc. Res.* **52**, 181–198 (2001).
194. G. Valen, Cellular signaling mechanisms in adaptation to ischemia-induced myocardial damage, *Ann. Med.* **35**, 300–307 (2003).
195. M. Joyeux-Faure, C. Arnaud, D. Godin–Ribuot and C. Ribuot, Heat stress preconditioning and delayed myocardial protection : what is new? *Cardiovasc Res* **60**, 469–477 (2003).
196. F. Kolar and B. Ostadal, Molecular mechanisms of cardiac protection by adaptation to chronic hypoxia. *Physiol. Res.* **53**, S3–S13 (2004).
197. J. Neckar, I. Markova, F. Novak, O. Novakova, O. Szarszoi, B. Ostadal and F. Kolar, Increased expression and altered subcellular distribution of PKC isoform delta in chronically hypoxic rat myocardium: involvement in cardioprotection, *Am. J. Physiol.* **288(4)**, H1566–72 (2004)
198. P. Razeghi, M.E. Young, S. Abbasi and H. Taegtmeyer, Hypoxia in vivo decreases peroxisome proliferator-activated receptor alpha-regulated gene expression in rat heart, *Biochem Biophys Res Commun.* **287(1)**, 5–10 (2001).
199. P. Razeghi, M.F. Essop, J.M. Huss, S. Abbasi, N. Manga and H. Taegtmeyer, Hypoxia-induced switches of myosin heavy chain iso-gene expression in rat heart, *Biochem Biophys Res Commun.* **303(4)**, 1024–1027 (2003).
200. I. Friehs and P.J. del Nido, Increased susceptibility of hypertrophied hearts to ischemic injury, *Ann. Thorac. Surg.* **75**, S678–S684 (2003).

201. M.F. Allard, Energy substrate metabolism in cardiac hypertrophy, *Curr. Hyperten. Rep.* **6**, 430–435 (2004).
202. A. Bril, M.C. Forest and B. Gout, Ischemia and reperfusion induced arrhythmias in rabbits with chronic heart failure, *Am. J. Physiol.* **261**, H301–H307 (1991).
203. P.K. Podesser, J. Schirnhofer, O.Y. Bernecker, A. Kroner, M. Franz, S. Semsroth, B. Fellner, J. Neumuller, S. Hallstrom and E. Wolner, Optimizing ischemia/reperfusion in the failing rat heart: improved myocardial protection with acute ACE inhibition, *Circulation* **106(12 Suppl 1)**, I277–83 (2002).
204. S. Ghosh, N.B. Standen and M. Galinanes, Failure to precondition pathological myocardium, *J. Am. Coll. Cardiol.* **37**, 711–718 (2001).
205. D.J. Paulson, The diabetic heart is more sensitive to ischemic injury, *Cardiovasc. Res.* **34**, 104–112 (1997).
206. D. Feuvray and G.D. Lopaschuk, Controversies on the sensitivity of the diabetic heart to ischemic injury: the sensitivity of the diabetic heart to ischemic injury is decreased, *Cardiovasc. Res.* **34**, 113–120 (1997).
207. T. Ooie, N. Takahashi, T. Nawata, M. Arikawa, K. Yamanaka, M. Kajimoto, T. Shinohara, S. Shigematsu, M. Hara, H. Yoshimatsu and T. Saikawa, Ischemia-induced translocation of protein kinase C-epsilon mediates cardioprotection in the streptozotocin-induced diabetic rat, *Circ. J.* **67(11)**, 955–961 (2003).
208. L. Zhang, J.R. Parratt, G. H. Beastall, N. J. Pyne and B.L. Furman, Streptozotocin diabetes protects against arrhythmias in rat isolated hearts: role of hypothyroidism, *Eur. J. Pharmacol.* **435**, 269–276 (2002).
209. P. Golino, P.R. Maroko and T.E. Carew, The effect of acute hypercholesterolaemia on myocardial infarct size and the no-reflow phenomenon, during coronary occlusion-reperfusion, *Circulation* **75**, 292–298 (1987).
210. W.G. Girod, S.P. Jones, N. Sieber, T.Y. Aw and D.J. Lefer, Effect of hypercholesterolaemia on myocardial ischemia-reperfusion injury in LDL receptor-deficient mice, *Arterioscler. Thromb. Vasc. Biol.* **19**, 2776–2781 (1999).
211. B. Le Grand, B. Vie, P. Faure, A.D. Degryse, P. Mouillard and G.W. John, Increased resistance to ischemic injury in the isolated perfused atherosclerotic heart of the cholesterol-fed rabbit, *Cardiovasc Res* **30(5)**, 689–696 (1995).
212. T.D. Wang, W.J. Chen, T.J. Mau, J.W. Lin, W.W. Lin and Y.T. Lee, Attenuation of increased myocardial ischemia-reperfusion injury conferred by hypercholesterolemia through pharmacological inhibition of the caspase–1, *Br. J. Pharmacol.* **138**, 291–300 (2003).
213. O. Jung, W. Jung, T. Malinski, G. Wiemer, B.A. Schoelkens and W. Linz, Ischemic preconditioning and infarct mass: the effect of hypercholesterolemia and endothelial dysfunction Clin. *Exp. Hypertens.* **22(2)**, 165–79 (2000).
214. X.L. Tang, A.B. Stein, G. Shirk and R. Bolli, Hypercholesterolemia blunts NO donor-induced late preconditioning against myocardial infarction in conscious rabbits, *Basic Res Cardiol* **99(6)**, 395–403 (2004).
215. C. Pantos, I. Mourouzis, T. Saranteas, I. Paizis, C. Xinaris, V. Malliopoulou and D.V. Cokkinos, Thyroid hormone receptors α1 and β1 are downregulated in the post-infarcted rat heart: consequences on the response to ischaemia-reperfusion, *Basic Res Cardiol* (2005), in press.
216. W.I. Awad, M.J. Shattock and D.J. Chambers, Ischemic preconditioning in immature myocardium, *Circulation*, **98**, 206–213 (1998).
217. S. Besse, S. Tanguy, F. Boucher, C. Le Page, S. Rozenberg, B. Riou, J. Leiris and B. Swynghedauw, Cardioprotection with cariporide, a sodium-proton exchanger inhibitor, after prolonged ischemia and reperfusion in senescent rats, *Exp. Gerontol.* **39(9)**, 1307–14 (2004).
218. F. Boucher, S. Tanguy, S. Besse, N. Tresallet, A. Favier and J. de Leiris, Age dependent changes in myocardial susceptibility to zero flow ischemia and reperfusion in isolated perfused rat hearts: relation to antioxidant status, *Mechanisms Ageing Develop.* **103**, 301–316 (1998).
219. P. Liu, B. Xu, T.A. Cavalieru and C.E. Hock, Attenuation of Anti-oxidative capacity enhances reperfusion-injury in aged rat myocardium, *Am. J. Physiol* **9**, 287(6), H2719–2727 (2004)
220. B.Z. Simkhovich, P. Marjoram, C. Poizat, L. Kedes and R.A. Kloner, Age-related changes of cardiac gene expression following myocardial ischemia/reperfusion, *Arch Biochem Biophys.* **420(2)**, 268–278 (2003).
221. O. Dewald, G. Ren, G. Duerr, M. Zoerlein, C. Klemm, C. Gersch, S. Tinsey, L.H. Michael, M.L. Entman and N.G. Frangogiannis, Of mice and dogs: species-specific differences in the inflammatory response following myocardial infarction, *Am. J. Path.*, **164**, 665–677 (2004)

222. M. Wang, L. Baker, B.M. Tsai, K.K. Meldrum and D.R. Meldrum, Sex differences in the myocardial inflammatory response to ischemia/reperfusion injury, *J. Physiol. Endocrinol. Metab.* **288(2)**, E321–326 (2005).
223. K. Imahashi, R.E. London, C. Steenbergen and E. Murphy, Male/female differences in intracellular Na(+) regulation during ischemia/reperfusion in mouse heart, *J. Mol. Cell. Cardiol.* **37**, 747–753 (2004).
224. F.J. Sutherland and D. Hearse, The isolated blood and perfusion fluid perfused heart, *Pharmacol. Res.* **41**, 613–627 (2000).
225. D. Hearse and F.J. Sutherland, Experimental models for the the study of cardiovascular function and disease, *Pharmacol Res* **4**, 597–603 (2000).
226. J.E. Baker, E.A. Konorev, G.J. Gross, W.M. Chilian and H.J. Jacob, Resistance to myocardial ischemia in five rat strains: is there a genetic component of cardioprotection? *Am. J. Physiol.* **278**, H1395–H1400 (2000).
227. J.M. Pass, Y. Zheng, W.B. Wead, J. Zhang, R.C. Li, R. Bolli and P. Ping, PKCepsilon activation induces dichotomous cardiac phenotypes and modulates PKCepsilon-RACK interactions and RACK expression, *Am. J. Physiol.* **280(3)**, H946–H955 (2001).
228. S. Ghosh and M. Galinanes, Protection of the human heart with ischemic preconditioning during cardiac surgery: role of cardiopulmonary bypass, *J. Thorac Cardiovasc. Surg.* **126**, 133–142 (2003).
229. K. Shinmura, E. Kodani, Y.T. Xuan, B. Dawn, X.L. Tang and R. Bolli, Effect of aspirin on late preconditioning against myocardial stunning in conscious rabbits, *J. Am. Coll. Cardiol.* **41(7)**, 1183–1194 (2003).
230. Y. Suematsu, V. Anttila, S. Takamoto and P.J. del Nido, Cardioprotection afforded by ischemic preconditioning interferes with chronic beta-blocker treatment, *Scan. Cardiovasc. J.* **38**, 293–299, (2004).
231. S.L. Kopecky, R.J. Aviles, M.R. Bell, J.K. Lobl, D. Tipping, G. Frommell, K. Ramsey, A.E. Holland, M. Midei, A. Jain, M. Kellett and R.J. Gibbons, A randomized, double-blinded, placebo-controlled, dose-ranging study measuring the effect of an adenosine agonist on infarct size reduction in patients undergoing primary percutaneous transluminal coronary angioplasty: the ADMIRE (AmP579 Delivery for Myocardial Infarction REduction) study, *Am. Heart J.* **146(1)**, 146–152 (2003).
232. A. Ross, R. Gibbons, R.A. Kloner, V.J. Marder, G.W. Stone and R.W. Alexander, Acute myocardial infarction study of adenosine (AMISTAD II), *J. Am. Coll. Cardiol.* **39(Suppl A)**, 338A (2002).
233. IONA study group, Effect of nicorandil on coronary events in patients with stable angina: the impact of nicorandil in angina (IONA) randomized trial, *Lancet* **359**, 1269–1275 (2002).
234. T Miura and T. Miki, ATP-sensitive K^+ channel openers: old drugs with new clinical benefits for the heart, *Curr. Vasc. Pharmacol.* **1(3)**, 251–258 (2003).
235. P. Theroux, B.R. Chaitman, L. Erhardt, A. Jessel, T. Meinertz, W.U. Nickel, J.S. Schroeder, G. Tognoni, H. White and J.T. Willerson, Design of a trial evaluating myocardial cell protection with cariporide, an inhibitor of the transmembrane sodium-hydrogen exchanger: the Guard During Ischemia Against Necrosis (GUARDIAN) trial, *Curr Control Trials Cardiovasc Med.* **1(1)**, 59–67 (2000).
236. R.M. Mentzer Jr, Sodium-proton exchange inhibition to prevent coronary events in acute cardiac conditions trial, Paper presented at the American Heart Association Scientific Sessions. *November* **12**, (2003).
237. H. Tadokoro, A. Miyazaki, K. Satomura, L. Ryden, S. Kaul, S. Kar, E. Corday, and K. Drury, Infarct size reduction with coronary venous retroinfusion of diltiazem in the acute occlusion/reperfusion porcine heart model, *J Cardiovasc Pharmacol.* **28(1)**, 134–141 (1996).
238. P. Theroux, J. Gregoire, C. Chin, G. Pelletier, P. de Guise and M. Juneau, Intravenous diltiazem in acute myocardial infarction. Diltiazem as adjunctive therapy to activase (DATA) trial, *J Am Coll Cardiol.* **32(3)**, 620–628 (1998).
239. G. Pizzetti, A. Mailhac, L. Li Volsi, F. Di Marco, C. Lu, A. Margonato and S.L. Chierchia, Beneficial effects of diltiazem during myocardial reperfusion: a randomized trial in acute myocardial infarction, *Ital Heart J.* **2(10)**, 757–765 (2001).
240. V. Marangelli, C. Memmola, M.S. Brigiani, L. Boni, M.G. Biasco, D. Scrutinio, S. Iliceto and P. Rizzon, Early administration of verapamil after thrombolysis in acute anterior myocardial infarction. Effect on left ventricular remodeling and clinical outcome. VAMI Study Group. Verapamil Acute Myocardial Infarction, *Ital Heart J.* **1(5)**, 336–343 (2000).
241. J. Sochman, J. Vrbska, B. Musilova and M. Rocek, Infarct Size Limitation: acute N-acetylcysteine defense (ISLAND trial): preliminary analysis and report after the first 30 patients, *Clin Cardiol.* **19(2)**, 94–100 (1996).
242. C. de Zwaan, A.H. Kleine, J.H. Diris, J.F. Glatz, H.J. Wellens, P.F. Strengers, M. Tissing, C.E. Hack, M.P. van Dieijen-Visser and W.T. Hermens, Continuous 48-h C1-inhibitor treatment, following reperfusion therapy, in patients with acute myocardial infarction, *Eur. Heart J.* **23(21)**, 1670–1677 (2002).

243. J.C. Fitch, S. Rollins, L. Matis, B. Alford, S. Aranki, C.D. Collard, M. Dewar, J. Elefteriades, R. Hines, G. Kopf, P. Kraker, L. Li, R. O'Hara, C. Rinder, H. Rinder, R. Shaw, B. Smith, G. Stahl and S.K. Shernan, Pharmacology and biological efficacy of a recombinant, humanized, single-chain antibody C5 complement inhibitor in patients undergoing coronary artery bypass graft surgery with cardiopulmonary bypass, *Circulation* **100(25)**, 2499–2506 (1999).
244. T. Force, K. Kuida, M. Namchuk, K. Parang and J.M. Kyriakis, Inhibitors of protein kinase signaling pathways; Emerging therapies for cardiovascular disease, *Circulation* **109**, 1196–1205 (2004).
245. C. Willam, N. Masson, Y.M. Tian, S.A. Mahmood, M.I. Wilson, R. Bicknell, K.U. Eckardt, P.H. Maxwell, P.J. Ratcliffe and C.W. Pugh, Peptide blockade of HIFalpha degradation modulates cellular metabolism and angiogenesis. *Proc. Natl. Acad. Sci. USA.* **99(16)**, 10423–10428 (2002).
246. N.L. Lubbers, J.S. Polakowski, C.D. Wegner, S.E. Burke, G.J. Diaz, K.M. Daniell and B.F. Cox, Oral bimoclomol elevates heat shock protein 70 and reduces myocardial infarct size in rats, *Eur. J. Pharmacol.* **435(1)**, 79–83 (2002).
247. L.G. Melo, A.S. Pachori, D. Kong, M. Gnecchi, K. Wang, R.E. Pratt and V.J. Dzau, Gene and cell-based therapies for heart disease, *FASEB J.* **18(6)**, 648–663 (2004).
248. M.J. Wright, L.M. Wightman, D.S. Latchman and M.S. Marber, In vivo myocardial gene transfer: optimization and evaluation of intracoronary gene delivery in vivo, *Gene Ther.* **8(24)**, 1833–1839 (2001).
249. P.D. Robbins and S.C. Ghivizzani, Viral vectors for gene therapy, *Pharmacol Ther.* **80(1)**, 35–47 (1998). Review.
250. K. Suzuki, Y. Sawa, Y. Kaneda, H. Ichikawa, R. Shirakura and H. Matsuda, In vivo gene transfection with heat shock protein 70 enhances myocardial tolerance to ischemia-reperfusion injury in rat, *J Clin Invest.* **99(7)**, 1645–1650 (1997).
251. H.L. Zhu, A.S. Stewart, M.D. Taylor, C. Vijayasarathy, T.J. Gardner and H.L. Sweeney, Blocking free radical production via adenoviral gene transfer decreases cardiac ischemia-reperfusion injury, *Mol Ther.* **2(5)**, 470–475 (2000).
252. W. Miao, Z. Luo, R.N. Kitsis and K. Walsh, Intracoronary, adenovirus-mediated Akt gene transfer in heart limits infarct size following ischemia-reperfusion injury in vivo, *J Mol Cell Cardiol.* **32(12)**, 2397–2402 (2000).
253. Y. Tang, M. Jackson, K. Qian and M.I. Phillips, Hypoxia inducible double plasmid system for myocardial ischemia gene therapy, *Hypertension* **39(2)**, 695–698 (2002).
254. S. Davani, F. Deschaseaux, D. Chalmers, P. Tiberghien and J-P. Kantelip, Can stem cells mend a broken heart? *Cardiovasc Res* **65**, 305–316 (2005).
255. P. Menasche, Cell transplantation in myocardium, *Ann Thorac Surg.* **75(6 Suppl)**, S20–28 (2003). Review.
256. K.C. Wollert, G.P. Meyer, J. Lotz, S. Ringes-Lichtenberg, P. Lippolt, C. Breidenbach, S. Fichtner, T. Korte, B. Hornig, D. Messinger, L. Arseniev, B. Hertenstein, A. Ganser and H. Drexler, Intracoronary autologous bone-marrow cell transfer after myocardial infarction: the BOOST randomised controlled clinical trial, *Lancet* **364(9429)**, 141–148 (2004).
257. A.M. Davidoff, C.Y. Ng, P. Brown, M.A. Leary, W.W. Spurbeck, J. Zhou, E. Horwitz, E.F. Vanin and A.W. Nienhuis, Bone marrow-derived cells contribute to tumor neovasculature and, when modified to express an angiogenesis inhibitor, can restrict tumor growth in mice, *Clin Cancer Res.* **7(9)**, 2870–2879 (2001).
258. H.J. Kang, H.S. Kim, S.Y. Zhang, K.W. Park, H.J. Cho, B.K. Koo, Y.J. Kim, D. Soo Lee, D.W. Sohn, K.S. Han, B.H. Oh, M.M. Lee and Y.B. Park, Effects of intracoronary infusion of peripheral blood stem-cells mobilised with granulocyte-colony stimulating factor on left ventricular systolic function and restenosis after coronary stenting in myocardial infarction: the MAGIC cell randomised clinical trial, *Lancet Mar* **363(9411)**, 751–756 (2004).
259. A.P. Beltrami, L. Barlucchi, D. Torella, M. Baker, F. Limana, S. Chimenti, H. Kasahara, M. Rota, E. Musso, K. Urbanek, A. Leri, J. Kajstura, B. Nadal-Ginard and P. Anversa, Adult cardiac stem cells are multipotent and support myocardial regeneration, *Cell* **114(6)**, 763–776 (2003).

CHAPTER 2

HORMONES SIGNALING AND MYOCARDIAL ISCHEMIA

Constantinos Pantos*, Dennis V. Cokkinos**

Although hormones constitute an important component of the adaptive response of the living organism to various stresses, their role in myocardial ischemia has not been adequately explored. However, recent research reveals that hormone signaling is of physiological relevance in the context of ischemia and reperfusion. Furthermore, hormones or hormones' analogs are suggested as potential therapeutic agents for treating heart diseases.

1. ESTROGENS

Clinical observations have suggested a cardioprotective role for estrogens. Consistent with this notion are several experimental reports. Acute administration of 17β-estradiol before ischemia and at reperfusion is shown to increase functional recovery and reduce lactate dehydrogenase (LDH) release in perfused rat hearts from ovariectomized rats. This effect was associated with less intracellular Na^+ and Ca^{2+} and a blunted reduction in pH[1]. Similarly, acute pre-ischemic administration of 17β-estradiol and not 17α-estradiol limited infarct size in an in vivo model of coronary artery occlusion and reperfusion in ovariectomized rabbits. This response was abrogated by the administration of ICI 182,780, an estrogen receptor antagonist[2]. However, in a canine model of coronary occlusion and reperfusion, although 17β-estradiol reduced infarct size and arrhythmias, the administration of ICI 182,780 did not abolish these effects. Pretreatment with 5–hydroxydecanoate, a mitochondrial K_{ATP} channel blocker abrogated the estrogen infarct size limiting effect while blockade of sarcolemmal K_{ATP} channel abolished the effect of estrogen on reperfusion ventricular arrhythmias[3]. In open-chest dogs, infarct size and reperfusion ventricular arrhythmias were reduced by estrogen administration and this response was abrogated by inhibition of the NO synthase (NOS) or calcium-

* Department of Pharmacology, University of Athens, 75 Mikras Asias Ave. 11527 Goudi, Athens, Greece
**1st Cardiology Department, Onassis Cardiac Surgery Center, 356 Sygrou Ave. 176 74 Kallithea, Athens, Greece
Correspondence: Ass. Professor Constantinos Pantos, Department of Pharmacology, University of Athens, 75 Mikras Asias Ave. 11527 Goudi, Athens, Greece, Tel: (+30210) 7462560, Fax: (+30210) 7705185, Email: cpantos@cc.uoa.gr

activated potassium channels K (Ca^{2+})[4]. Furthermore, in humans, acute pretreatment with estrogens, in patients undergoing elective coronary angioplasty, limited myocardial ischemia while glibenclamide, a sarcolemmal K_{ATP} channel blocker abolished this effect. Post-angioplasty coronary vasoconstriction at the dilated and distal segments was attenuated while endothelin – 1 release was decreased.[5]

Chronic estrogens deficiency in overiectomized rats (3 weeks) resulted in impaired functional recovery in a perfused heart model of global ischemia and reperfusion while supplementation with estrogens improved the postischemic outcome[6]. However, estrogens replacement in ovariectomized female rats decreased the recovery of function in hearts perfused with palmitate.[7] In aged overiectomized female rats, chronic estrogens replacement increased postischemic functional recovery in isolated rat hearts.[8]

A modulatory effect of estrogens on heat stress response has also been observed. The cardioprotective effect induced by heat stress was pronounced in ovariectomized rats and not in those replaced by estrogens. In addition, male responded better than female hearts from intact animals while the induction of heat shock protein 72 in response to heat stress was less in female hearts.[9]

Additional evidence for the cardioprotective role of estrogens is derived from cell models of simulated ischemia. Treatment with 17β-estradiol enhanced cell survival after hypoxia–reoxygenation in cardiomyocytes from adult female rats. In addition, estrogens activated NF-kB and HSF1 and increased the expression of heat shock protein 72. Decoy–mediated blockade of nuclear HSF1 binding preserved the cardioprotective effect of 17β-estradiol while transfection with NFkB decoy prevented the increase in heat shock protein 72 and abolished protection.[10]

Estrogens induced cardioprotection seems to involve the ERα receptor. In fact, hearts from estrogens receptor–alpha knock out mice were sensitive to ischemia and reperfusion injury[11]. Furthermore, estrogens receptor modulators which lack some of the estrogens side effects are shown to be cardioprotective; raloxifene limited infarct size and incidence of ventricular fibrillation in an in vivo canine model of coronary occlusion and reperfusion. This effect was attenuated by the inhibition of NO synthase (NOS) or calcium activated potassium channels and completely abolished by both blocking NOS and Ca^{2+}-activated K^+ channels. Ischemia and reperfusion induced p38 MAPK activation was also attenuated in raloxifene treated hearts.[12]

2. ANDROGENS

Although the anabolic androgenic steroids have been associated with myocardial infarction and sudden cardiac death, a cardioprotective role for androgens is also suggested. In a cellular model of simulated ischemia, testosterone significantly decreased the percentage of cell death and this could be prevented by 5-hydroxydecainoic acid (a mitochondrial K_{ATP} channel blocker) but it was unaffected by the sarcoplasmic K_{ATP} blocker, HMR1098, and the testosterone receptor antagonist flutamide.[13] Accordingly, long-term (2 weeks) treatment with supraphysiological doses of 5α–dihydrotestosterone resulted in increased postischemic recovery of function in perfused rat hearts subjected to zero-flow global ischemia and reperfusion. This response was associated with less intracellular calcium at the end of the ischemic period and early phase of reperfusion without any change in the expression of genes related to calcium handling (phospholamban, sodium-calcium exchanger, ryanodine–receptor and SERCA expression was unchanged), indicating a possible increase in the activity of those regulatory proteins. Furthermore, hearts from orchectomized rats were susceptible to ischemia and reperfusion injury.[14]

A detrimental effect caused by androgens is also reported. Blockade of the endogenous testosterone by flutamide or depletion of testosterone (castration) improved myocardial function of the perfused rat hearts subjected to ischemia and reperfusion. This response was associated with decreased caspase–1, caspase-3, caspase–11, decreased TNF-alpha, IL-1 beta, IL-6, decreased ischemia and reperfusion induced p38 MAPK activation and increased Bcl-2 expression in castrated and flutamide treated males.[15] Accordingly, supraphysiological doses of nandrolone taken during exercise or under sedentary conditions increased myocardial susceptibility to ischemia and reperfusion injury in perfused rat hearts. Pre-ischemic c-AMP concentrations and pre-ischemic and reperfusion TNF-alpha concentrations were found to be increased in those hearts.[16]

3. GROWTH HORMONE

Experimental studies have suggested a cardioprotective role for growth hormone. Administration of anti-GH releasing hormone serum in rats exacerbated ventricular dysfunction induced by low-flow ischemia in perfused rat hearts. This effect was accompanied by increased responsiveness of the coronary vasculature to angiotensin II and decreased rate of formation of 6-keto-prostaglandin F1 alpha, a metabolite of prostacyclin. Hexarelin, a synthetic growth hormone secretagogue, restored postischemic recovery of function.[17] Administration of growth hormone in senescent rats also increased postischemic recovery of function in the perfused rat heart model of ischemia and reperfusion.[18] Furthermore, long-term treatment (2 weeks) with GHRP-2, a growth hormone releasing peptide, attenuated postischemic diastolic dysfunction in an isolated blood perfused rabbit heart model of ischemia and reperfusion without altering the circulating GH and IGF-1 levels, indicating a direct effect of this peptide on the myocardium.[19]

4. GHRELIN

Ghrelin, is a 28 amino acid peptide predominantly produced by the stomach and displays strong GH releasing activity mediated by the activation of GHSR–1α, a Gq protein–coupled GH secretagogue receptor. Ghrelin and its receptor are found in the myocardium. Acute pretreatment with ghrelin or hexarelin, the synthetic secretagogue, attenuated tissue necrosis in isolated rat hearts subjected to ischemia and reperfusion. Furthermore, the effect of hexarelin was abolished by chelerythrine, suggesting a possible role of the PKC in this response.[20] Administration of ghrelin at the time of reperfusion also increased postischemic recovery of function in the perfused rat heart model of ischemia and reperfusion with decreased myocardial MDA (an index of oxidative stress) and increased ATP myocardial content. This effect was independent from the release of GH and involved binding of ghrelin to cardiovascular ghrelin receptors, a process that was upregulated during ischemia and reperfusion.[21] Ghrelin is shown to prevent doxorubicin or serum starvation induced apoptosis in primary cultures of adult cardiomyocytes or embryonic H9c2 cardiomyocytes, an effect associated with increased activation of the extracellular signal–regulated kinases (ERK1/2) and Akt.[22]

5. GLUCOCORTICOIDS

Glucocorticoids are known for their anti-inflammatory action and as such have been used to limit the inflammatory response following ischemia and reperfusion. Glucocorticoids prevent leukocytes recruitment, suppress pro-inflammatory cytokines and leukocyte adhesion molecules and increase the induction of antioxidants. Glucocorticoid treatment before cardiopulmonary bypass reduces the inflammatory reaction during and after surgery.[23] However, glucocorticoids increase the incidence of left ventricular free wall rapture by delaying myocardial scar formation.[24] Glucocorticoids can induce cardioprotection independently of their antinflammatory effect. In fact, methylprednisolone treatment (1-5 days) reduced tissue necrosis and improved postischemic functional recovery in perfused rat hearts subjected to global ischemia and reperfusion. Hsp70 content in the myocardium was increased due to the post-transcriptional regulation of Hsp70 by glucocorticoids since concomitant increase in Hsp70 m-RNA was not observed.[25] Similarly, dexamethasone treatment significantly increased postischemic recovery of aortic flow and left ventricular developed pressure in a working rat heart model of ischemia and reperfusion. This response was abolished by actinomycin D.[26] (See also figure 12 in chapter 1 for glucocorticoid action on the cell).

6. UROCORTIN

Urocortin is a peptide related to hypothalamic corticotrophin–releasing factor and binds with a high affinity to the CRF-R2 beta receptor which is expressed in the heart. Urocortin is released from myocytes in response to stressful stimuli such as ischemia. Its cardioprotective role is demonstrated by several studies. In neonatal rat cardiomyocytes, the presence of urocortin at the time of reoxygenation following simulated ischemia limited cell death.[27] Accordingly, urocortin, given at reperfusion reduced infarct size in perfused rat hearts and in in vivo models of ischemia and reperfusion. Urocortin increases ERK phosphorylation at levels above that observed with reperfusion alone. Furthermore, the urocortin infarct size limiting effect was abrogated in the presence of PD098059, a MEK1/2 inhibitor, while phosphorylation of ERK1/2 was reduced. In addition, in rat cardiomyocytes, urocortin mediated cardioprotection was abolished by the specific PI3K inhibitors, wortmannin or LY294002. Similar response was observed in cardiomyocytes possessing dominant negative mutation of PI3K-Akt.[28]

7. MELANOCORTIN PEPTIDES

Melanocortin peptides display anti-oxidant and anti-inflammatory properties and may be beneficial in the context of ischemia and reperfusion. Administration of ACTH–1-24, a melanocyte–stimulating hormone before ischemia prevented reperfusion arrhythmias in an in vivo model of regional ischemia and reperfusion. Furthermore, administration of long acting melanocortin peptide NDP MSH resulted in infarct size reduction in rats subjected to permanent coronary occlusion.[29] Work in this area is not very extensive and awaits further exploration.

8. MELATONIN

The cardioprotective effect of melatonin is demonstrated in several studies in in vivo and ex vivo experimental rat models or cardiomyocytes, as reviewed by Reiter.[30] Melatonin administration in perfused rat hearts subjected to ischemia and reperfusion increased postischemic recovery of function, reduced the duration of ventricular tachycardia and ventricular fibrillation and this was associated with decreased lipid peroxidation products and OH radical formation, indicating an antioxidant effect of melatonin.[31] Furthermore, in pinealectomized rats, occlusion of the left coronary artery followed by reperfusion resulted in significant increase in infarct size than in intact animals.[32] Melatonin acts as scavenger of oxygen or nitrogen based reactants, stimulates antioxidant enzymes, stabilizes cellular membrane, increases the efficiency of oxidative phosphorylation, reduces leukocyte recruitment and adhesion molecule expression and reduces homocysteine induced damage (reviewed by Duncker[33]).

9. ERYTHROPOIETIN

The hematopoeitic cytokine erythropoietin (EPO) and its receptor have been shown to be present in various tissues including the myocardium, suggesting potential roles of erythropoietin signaling beyond haematopoiesis. EPO is produced by the kidney in response to hypoxia and stimulates erythroid progenitor cells, thereby increasing oxygen carrying capacity. EPO receptors are found in endothelial cells and fibroblasts as well as in cardiomyocytes.[34] EPO has a direct cardioprotective effect against ischemia and reperfusion. In fact, exposure of neonatal rat ventricular myocytes to hypoxia with recombinant EPO was associated with decreased apoptosis as measured by TUNEL staining, flow cytometry and caspase 3/7 like activity. The antiapoptotic effect of EPO was abrogated by LY 294002, a PI3K blocker.[35] Similarly, H9c2 embryonic cells pretreated with EPO were resistant to simulated ischemia. This effect was abrogated by wortmannin, a PI3K inhibitor and not by an ERK inhibitor. EPO is shown to increase the activation of ERK, Akt, JAK1 and STAT-3.[36] (See also chapter 1).

The cardioprotective effect of EPO has also been demonstrated in animal models. EPO administration at the time of reperfusion significantly reduced infarct size and apoptosis (assessed by TUNEL staining) in a rabbit model of acute coronary occlusion and reperfusion.[36] This effect was accompanied by increased activation of ERK and Akt in the unstressed myocardium.[36] Similarly, EPO administration throughout the period of low-flow ischemia reduced apoptosis and improved recovery of left ventricular pressure in perfused rat hearts.[34]

10. NATRIURETIC PEPTIDES

Natriuretic peptides (ANP, BNP, CNP) were first described by Genest and are now recognized to have several autocrine and paracrine effects within the myocardium and coronary circulation. Natriuretic peptide receptor A (NPR-A) and B (NPR- B) are widely expressed in the cardiovascular system. The natriuretic peptides produce cellular responses through the elevation of intracellular c-GMP concentration that in turn regulates

PKG and cyclic nucleotide phosphodiesterases (PDEs) (reviewed by Baxter[37]). A rapid release of natriuretic peptides and induction of their de novo synthesis occurs in myocardial ischemia. Natriuretic peptides may have a cardioprotective role. BNP–32 administration in perfused rat hearts prior to left main coronary artery occlusion and until 30 min of reperfusion resulted in limitation of infarct size in a concentration dependent manner. Furthermore, this effect was abolished by 5-hydroxydecanoate (presumed to be a selective blocker of mitochondrial K_{ATP} channels), L-NAME, an inhibitor of NOS and ODQ, a specific soluble guanyl cyclase inhibitor.[38] Similarly, human recombinant ANP limited infarct size and reperfusion arrhythmias in a canine model of coronary occlusion and reperfusion.[39]

A beneficial role of the natriuretic peptides on postischemic myocardial remodeling has also been suggested. Upregulation of the expression of these peptides in the heart following myocardial infarction results in suppression of growth and proliferative responses in myocytes and fibroblasts. This may be a negative regulatory mechanism to counteract the hypertrophy and pro-fibrotic response induced by angiotensin II and catecholamines after myocardial infarction (reviewed by Baxter[37]).

11. PTH - PARATHYROID HORMONE RELATED PEPTIDE (PTHrP)

PTHrP is structurally related to parathyroid hormone (PTH). In contrast to PTH, which is exclusively expressed in and secreted by the parathyroid gland, PTHrP is expressed and released by vascular smooth muscle cells and endothelial cells but not by ventricular myocytes. PTH and PTHrP are potent dilators and exert positive chronotropic and inotropic effects (reviewed by Halapas[40]). PTHrP activates adenyl cyclase and increases c-AMP levels with subsequent activation of PKA/PKC dependent pathways.[41,42]

The release of biologically active PTHrP is increased during hypoxic perfusion of isolated rat hearts with possible physiological consequences.[43] In fact, blockade of endogenous PTHrP at the receptor level significantly decreased the left ventricular pressure in the postischemic reperfused isolated rat hearts, in an in vivo model of stunning in pigs. Furthermore, exogenous PTHrP improved postischemic functional recovery.[44]

12. ALDOSTERONE

Evidence of the role of aldosterone in the response of the myocardium to ischemia is derived indirectly from studies in which the renin-angiotensin system was inhibited or directly from studies using spironolactone to inhibit the aldosterone effects. Long-term (30 days) treatment with lisinopril (an ACE inhibitor) in normal or infarcted rats increased postischemic contractile function in perfused rat hearts subjected to low-flow global ischemia and reperfusion. Furthermore, similar effects were obtained with spironolactone. The combined administration of the two agents (at a lower dose of spironolactone) resulted in synergistic effect both in normal and infarcted rats. However, in the case of high doses of spironolactone, a synergistic effect was evident only in the infarcted hearts.[45]

13. LEPTIN

Although leptin is being derived primarily from adipocytes, it is now shown that non adipocyte tissues can be a source of leptin. In fact, gene expression of leptin and its receptors OB-Ra, OB –Rb and OB-Re have been identified in rat heart.[46] It is likely that leptin serves an autocrine/paracrine role in regulating cardiac function. Leptin is shown to have a negative inotropic effect and promotes hypertrophy.[47, 48] The physiological role of leptin in myocardial ischemia remains unknown. Leptin activates cardiac fatty acid oxidation independent of changes in the AMP-activated protein kinase–acetyl–CoA carboxylase-malonyl-CoA axis.[49]

Plasma leptin levels are increased in patients with acute myocardial infarction and this has been suggested to be detrimental.[50] In an experimental model of ischemia and reperfusion, the expression of leptin and its receptors were decreased after ischemia while no change in the leptin efflux in the perfusate was detected. This was suggested to be an adaptive mechanism for increasing clearance of leptin from cardiac tissue.[46]

14. INSULIN

Insulin signaling regulates important metabolic and cardioprotective pathways with potential physiological consequences on cellular response to ischemic stress (reviewed by Abel[51] and Hue[52]).

Insulin by binding to insulin receptor (IR) activates the tyrosine kinase activity of IR leading to IR autophosphorylation and to the subsequent phosphorylation of IR substrates (IRS), Figure 1. Insulin signaling downstream to IRS is mediated by at least two pathways ; the first involves the activation of ERK cascade and the second pathway the activation of PI3K, Figure 1. PI3K (phosphatidylinositol-3 kinase, α isoform) leads to the activation of PDK1/2 (phosphoinositide dependent protein kinase). Downstream kinases to PDK1/2 include the protein kinase C (zeta and lambda), the insulin stimulated kinase (WISK), the serum and glucocorticoid regulated protein kinase (SGK) and Akt. The glycogen synthase kinase-3 beta (GSK-3β) and the mammalian target of rapamycin (mTOR) are shown to be downstream to Akt. mTOR regulates protein synthesis by activating p70 ribosomal S6 kinase (p70S6K), and inhibiting the eukaryotic initiator factor 4E-binding protein (4EBP1), Figure 1. Akt mediates short term effects of insulin such as the stimulation of glycogen synthesis by phosphorylation and inactivation of GSK-3β and the activation of phosphodiesterase (PDE), the enzyme responsible for the anti-cyclic AMP effects of insulin. Insulin stimulates glycolysis by a concomitant recruitment of GLUT4 and an increase in 6-phospho-fructo-2-kinase (PFK-2) activity. Insulin's effect on glucose uptake is mediated through activation of Akt and atypical PKCs with subsequent recruitment of GLUT4 transporter (reviewed by Hue[52]). However, glucose uptake is also increased by insulin through a PI3K–independent pathway involving the proto-oncogene Cbl, which translocates to lipid rafts in the plasma membrane and together with caveolae, results in the activation of the G protein TC10, which participates in the recruitment of GLUT4. (Figure 1, reviewed by Hue[52]). The effect of insulin on the 6-phospho-fructo-2-kinase (PFK-2) activity is mediated in PI3K/WISK pathway dependent manner.[53]

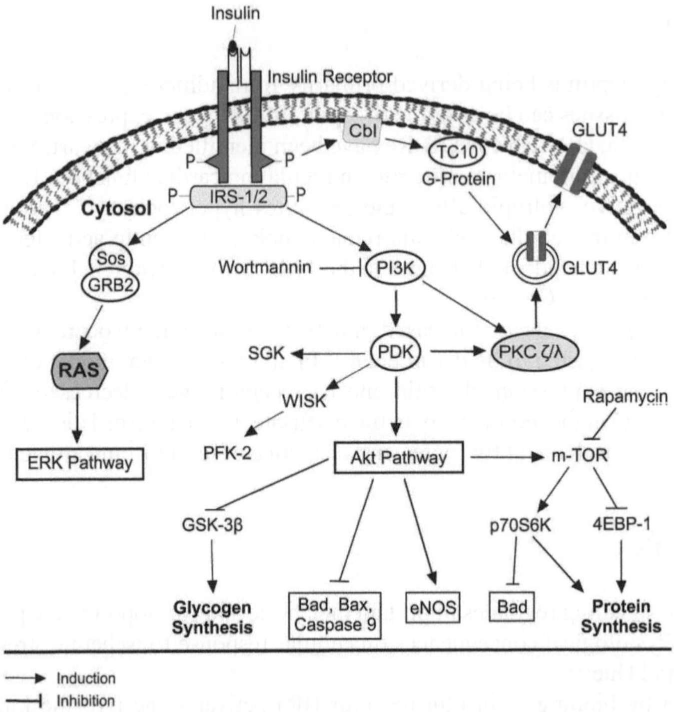

Figure 1. Schematic of insulin's intracellular signaling. Insulin induced cardioprotection is dependent on PI3K signaling. Blockade with wortmannin or rapamycin abrogates the protective effect of insulin. Signaling through PI3K results in inactivation of caspace –9, phosphorylation and inactivation of the proapoptotic proteins Bad and Bax and activation of eNOS producing nitric oxide which may protect by inhibiting opening of the mitochondrial permeability transition pore. Note also the involvement of PI3K signalling pathway in mediating insulin's effect on metabolism (e.g GLUT4 recruitment, activation of PFK-2, inactivation of GSK-3β and activation of m-TOR). See text for a more detailed explanation.
"P"=Phosphorylation

Insulin has also a regulatory role on cell metabolism under ischemic conditions by interacting with AMPK. AMPK is activated during ischemia in response to changes in AMP/ATP ratio causing an increase in glycolysis and fatty acid oxidation, Figure 2, chapter 1. Insulin inhibits the AMPK activation in a wortmannin sensitive manner.[54] However, in order insulin to exert this effect has to be administered before ischemia. Ischemic acidosis inhibits the IR tyrosine activity, thereby prevents the activation of downstream components of the insulin signaling pathway.[55]

Important cardioprotective targets are now recognized to be regulated by the insulin induced intracellular signaling. In fact, insulin induces phosphorylation and inactivation of the proapoptotic protein Bad and activation of the endothelial nitric oxide synthase (eNOS). [56, 57] Figure 1. Furthermore, a cardioprotective role for insulin is shown in a number of clinical and experimental studies. Glucose–insulin–potassium (GIK) administration in patients with acute myocardial infarction reduced in-hospital mortality.[58] In addition, GIK was effective in the treatment of refractory left ventricular failure after aortocoronary by-pass grafting.[59] (See also chapter 7 Table). Accordingly, experimental studies on animal and cell-based models of ischemia and reperfusion documented a cardioprotective role for GIK or insulin itself (reviewed by Sack[60]). GIK administration at the time of reperfusion or during the entire experimental period reduced infarct size in an in-vivo rat model of coronary occlusion and reperfusion. Furthermore, administration of GIK at reperfusion also improved postischemic recovery of function.[61] In a rabbit model of coronary occlusion and reperfusion, GIK or insulin administration throughout the experimental period resulted in increased postischemic recovery of function, infarct size limitation and a decrease in DNA fragmentation and apoptosis index.[62] Furthermore, early reperfusion with insulin (15min) limited infarct size, while delaying insulin administration 15 min after the onset of reperfusion was not protective in a perfused rat heart model of ischemia and reperfusion. Similarly, in cell-based models of hypoxia-reoxygenation, insulin administration at reoxygenation attenuated the apoptotic and necrotic components of cell death.[56, 63]

The promotion of cardiac glycolysis with concomitant reduction of fatty acid metabolism were initialy proposed as possible underlying mechanisms of insulin mediated cardioprotection.[64] However, GIK administration at reperfusion exerts cardioprotective effects without changes in FFA and glucose levels at early reperfusion, indicating an independent cardioprotective effect of insulin, in its own right. In fact, the infarct size limiting effect of insulin was abrogated by wortmannin (a PI3K inhibitor) or rapamycin (a mTOR-p70S6K inhibitor) in a perfused rat heart model of ischemia and reperfusion, indicating that PI3K signaling is an important component of the insulin induced cardioprotection.[56]

15. INSULIN LIKE GROWTH FACTOR (IGF-1)

IGF-1 is a serum factor implicated in cellular survival and growth and has been shown to protect the heart in a manner that is dependent on the PI3K-Akt and ERK1/2 signaling pathways.[65, 66] Furthermore, isolated rat hearts from transgenic mice overexpressing IGF-1 are shown to be resistant to ischemia and reperfusion. This response has been associated with an increase in basal activation of Akt with further activation at reperfusion shifting the balance between the antiapoptotic Akt and the proapoptotic p38 MAPK. In fact, SB 203580 administration reduced apoptosis in the wild type but increased apoptosis in transgenic hearts by inhibiting both p38 MAPK and Akt activation.[67]

16. PEROXISOME PROLIFERATED –ACTIVATED RECEPTORS (PPARS)

Peroxisome proliferator–activated receptors (PPARs) are members of the nuclear hormone receptors superfamily of ligand–activated transcription factors that are related to retinoid, steroid and thyroid receptors. All members of this superfamily have a similar structure: the amino-terminal region allows ligand–independent activation, confers constitutive activity on the receptor and is negatively regulated by phosphorylation. This region is followed by a DNA binding domain and the carboxyl–terminal ligand binding domain. PPARs regulate gene expression by binding as heterodimers with retinoid X receptors (RXRs, activated by 9-cis-retinoic acid) to specific PPARs response elements in the promoter regions of specific target genes. The PPAR subfamily is composed of three members; PPAR-α, PPAR-β, PPAR-γ. Transcriptional coactivators have also been identified. An important PPAR-γ transcriptional coactivator (PGC-1), has been recently discovered. PGC-1, serves as pleiotropic regulator of multiple pathways involved in cellular energy metabolism within and outside the mitochondria. Interestingly, PGC-1 activates the trancription of mitochondrial uncoupling protein–1 (UCP-1) through interactions with the nuclear hormone receptors PPAR-γ and thyroid hormone receptor. p38 MAPK, NO, β-adrenergic /c-AMP signaling, and calcineurin A have been identified as upstream regulators of PGC-1.[68] PPARs have been pharmacologically targeted by compounds displaying a selective action on PPARs. These include PPAR-γ activators, such as the thiazolidinediones, (TZDs) rosiglitazone, pioglitazone and ciglitazone and PPAR-α activators, such as clofibrate.

A cardioprotective role for PPARs has been recently suggested. Preischemic administration of rosiglitazone, ciglitazone or pioglitazone resulted in reduced infarct size in an in vivo rat model of ischemia and reperfusion.[69] Furthermore, a beneficial effect of rosiglitazone on postischemic recovery of function was observed in a model of coronary occlusion in rabbits with hypercholesterolemia. This response was associated with significant reduction in apoptosis and ischemia-induced activation of p38 MAPK.[70] However, rosiglitazone had no effect on contractile function in a pig model of low-flow regional ischemia and reperfusion. In contrast, in the same model, troglitazone resulted in cardioprotection due to its alpha-tocopherol moiety.[71] These findings, in conjuction with prior rat studies, suggest interspecies differences in the response of PPAR-γ activation in the heart. PPAR-α activation with clofibrate resulted also in infarct size limitation in a rat model of coronary occlusion and reperfusion.[69] However, reactivation of PPAR-α has been associated with resting contractile dysfunction in the hypertrophied rat heart.[72]

17. THYROID HORMONE

Thyroid hormone has multiple effects on the cardiovascular system with various physiological consequences. Several genes that encode important regulatory and structural proteins in the heart have been shown to be thyroid hormone responsive. Thyroid hormone increases cardiac contractility, induces vasorelaxation and angiogenesis, prevents fibrosis and has favorable effects on lipid metabolism (reviewed by Pantos[73]).

The role of thyroid hormone in the response of the heart to ischemia and reperfusion has not been extensively investigated due to the fact that thyroid hormone accelerates heart rhythm and increases oxygen consumption, effects which could be detrimental in the setting of ischemia and reperfusion. However, accumulating experimental evidence shows that either acute or chronic pretreatment with thyroid hormone can lead to cardioprotection. In an isolated working rat heart model, cardiac work and cardiac efficiency were increased after no-flow global ischemia and reperfusion in hearts acutely pretreated with T_3.[74] Furthermore, thyroxine pretreatment for two weeks resulted in increased recovery of function in isolated rat hearts subjected to zero-flow global ischemia followed by reperfusion.[75, 76] This functional improvement occurred despite ischemic contracture was accelerated and intensified in those hearts.[77] A similar pattern of contracture has also been observed in ischemicaly preconditioned hearts and has been attributed to the reduced content of preischemic myocardial glycogen due to thyroxine treatment and ischemic preconditioning.[77, 78]

Thyroid hormone pretreatment has not been consistently resulted in cardioprotection. Postischemic recovery of function has been reported to be reduced in hyperthyroid hearts subjected to no-flow global ischemia.[79-81] However, this discrepancy is due to differences in the experimental design (reviewed by Pantos[73]).

Thyroid hormone administration at the time of reperfusion has also been associated with improved postischemic recovery. Acute T_3 supplementation at reperfusion improved postischemic contractile recovery in isolated rat hearts.[82-84] Furthermore, in large animal models, a significant improvement of postischemic left ventricular contractility was observed after T_3 administration.[85, 86] Similar results were obtained in patients undergoing CABG.[87, 88]

A beneficial effect of thyroid hormone on left ventricular remodeling is also reported. In an experimental model of acute myocardial infarction in rats, a decline in serum T_3 was observed associated with left ventricular dysfunction and changes in T_3 responsive genes. Treatment with high doses of T_3 for three weeks resulted in improved cardiac function with normalization of most of the changes in gene expression.[89] Similarly, administration of DITPA (a thyroid analogue) after myocardial infarction in rabbits was associated with improved cardiac function.[90]

The mechanisms through which thyroid hormone can exert its cardioprotective effect are now under intense investigation. Chronic thyroid treatment has been associated with changes in the expression of important cardioprotective molecules. In fact, PKCδ is found to be overexpressed in hyperthyroid hearts while PKCε expression decreases. The cardioprotective role of PKCδ has been documented in several studies (see also chapter 1). PKCδ overexpression in cells results in cardioprotection through a negative regulation of the ischemia-induced p38 MAPK activation.[91] Furthermore, PKCδ can phosphorylate cardioprotective molecules such as Hsp27.[92] Interestingly, expression and phosphorylation of Hsp27, particularly in the cytoskeletal fraction was shown to be increased in the hyperthyroid hearts.[93] Figure 2. Furthermore, upon ischemia, phosphorylation and translocation of Hsp27 to cytoskeletal fraction was accelerated in thyroxine treated hearts with concomitant decrease in the ischemia induced activation of the pro-apoptotic p38 MAPK.[93, 94] Figure 2. Similar findings have been reported for the ischemic preconditioning and the isoproterenol induced cardioprotection.[95, 96] Based on this evidence, it has been suggested that thyroid hormone protects the heart against ischemia and reperfusion through a preconditioning like effect.[94] In fact, recent data from our labaratory, show that thyroxine administration induces mild oxidative stress (probably due to mitochondrial uncoupling) with subsequent expression of redox regulated cardioprotective molecules, such as Hsp70 and Hsp27 (unpublished data).

Enhanced tolerance of the heart to ischemia and reperfusion has also been observed in the case of low thyroid hormone levels. Several important changes in metabolism or energy utilization occur in hypothyroid hearts that could potentially alter the response of those hearts to ischemic stress. Hypothyroid hearts consume less oxygen in doing mechanical work due to the predominance of V3 myosin isoform. Myocardial glycogen is increased while the expression of the sodium-proton exchanger is decreased. ATP levels are shown to decline more slowly during ischemia and are higher at reperfusion.

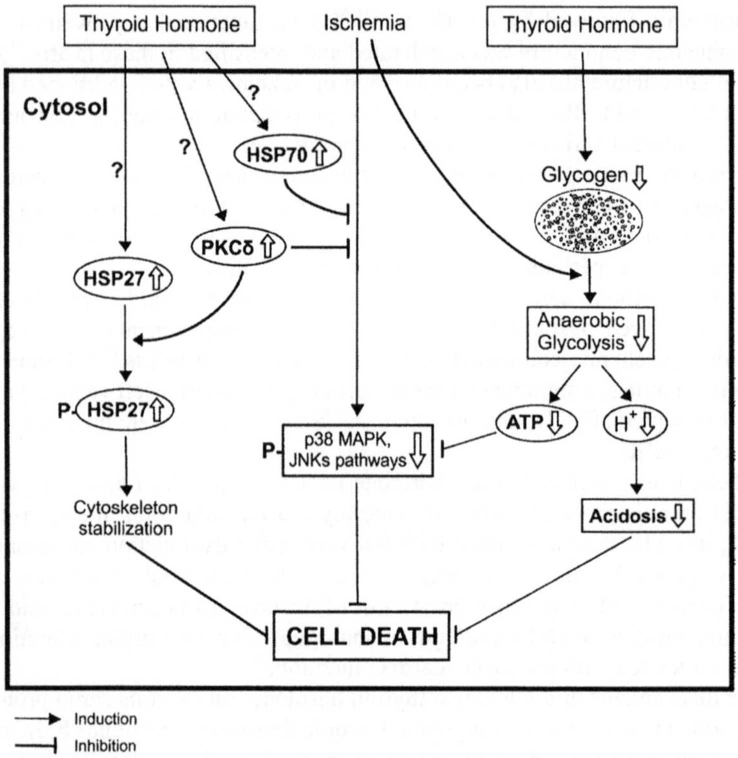

Figure 2. Proposed mechanisms for thyroid hormone mediated cardioprotection. Thyroid hormone results in glycogen depletion with less ATP formation and acidosis during ischemia. A critical balance between ATP production and H^+ formation is attained and cell injury is prevented. Activation of the pro-apoptotic p38 MAPK induced by ischemia and/or reperfusion is attenuated due either to negative regulation of PKCδ or to decreased phosphorylation because of reduced ATP availability. Thyroid hormone increases the expression of heart shock proteins. Hsp70 negatively regulates ischemia–reperfusion induced JNKs activation (similar mechanism as in heat stress mediated cardioprotection, see chapter 2). Phosphorylation of Hsp27 has a protective effect by stabilizing cytoskeleton and/or inhibiting apoptosis. The mechanism that leads to overexpression of heat shock proteins is elusive. Recent data from our laboratory show that these redox regulated proteins are overexpressed in response to mild oxidative stress induced by thyroid hormone (reviewed by Pantos[73]).
"P"=Phosphorylation, ⬆= Increase, ⬇= decrease

(reviewed by Pantos[73]). Furthermore, hypothyroidism results in increased expression of PKCε accompanied by decreased activation of the pro-apoptotic JNKs during ischemia and reperfusion.[97] Due to these characteristics, hypothyroid hearts are shown to withstand ischemia and reperfusion better than normal hearts. Postischemic recovery of function was enhanced while ischemic contracture was suppressed in isolated hypothyroid rat hearts subjected to zero-flow global ischemia and reperfusion.[97-100] Furthermore, hypothyroid hearts were protected against ischemia and reperfusion induced arrhythmias.[101] Accordingly, clinical data provide evidence that patients with long standing angina and decreased thyroid hormone levels develop smaller infarctions.[102]

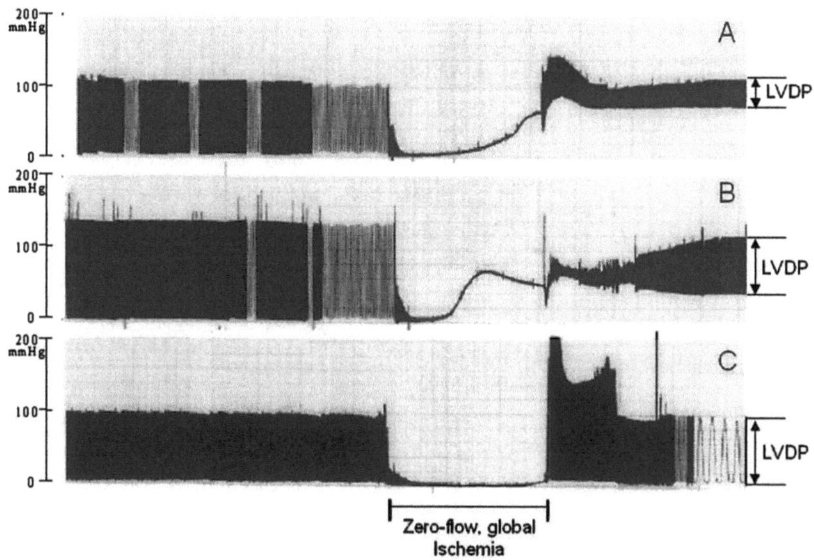

Figure 3. Left ventricular pressure recordings obtained from isolated rat hearts subjected to zero-flow global ischemia and reperfusion. Ischemic contracture is exacerbated in thyroxine treated hearts (B) and is suppressed in the hypothyroid hearts (C) as compared to normal hearts (A). Recovery of left ventricular developed pressure is increased in both hypothyroid and hyperthyroid as compared to normal hearts. LVDP is defined as the difference between systolic and diastolic left ventricular pressure (data from our laboratory).

On the basis of this experimental evidence, it seems likely that in the setting of the ischemic heart disease and hypothyroidism, thyroid hormone replacement may have adverse effects probably due to the loss of the cardioprotection conferred by hypothyroidism and not to the effects of thyroid hormone per se. In support to this notion are clinical observations showing that angina is not uncommon after thyroid hormone replacement in hypothyroid patients.

17.1 Thyroid hormone receptors

Thyroid hormone's genomic action is mediated by its binding to thyroid hormone nuclear receptors (TRs). TRs are ligand-activated transcription factors. Two genes encode the thyroid hormone receptors (TRs), and in mammalian heart, two splice variants of the TRα gene, TRα1 and TRα2 and two splice variants of the TRβ gene, TRβ1 and TRβ2 are expressed. All these receptors apart from the TRα2 receptor can bind thyroid hormone and transactivate thyroid hormone responsive elements on target genes. TRα2 negatively regulates TRα1 producing a hypothyroid like effect. Thyroid hormone receptor isoforms couple to the trancription of different genes and ultimately mediate different physiological functions. Studies on rats or rat cardiomyocytes demonstrate that TRβ1 is coupled to the trancription of genes encoding β-MHC, SERCA and TRβ1 itself while TRα1 regulates the transcription of α-MHC and potassium channels responsible for the heart rate. Thyroid hormone receptor isoform expression is altered in tissue

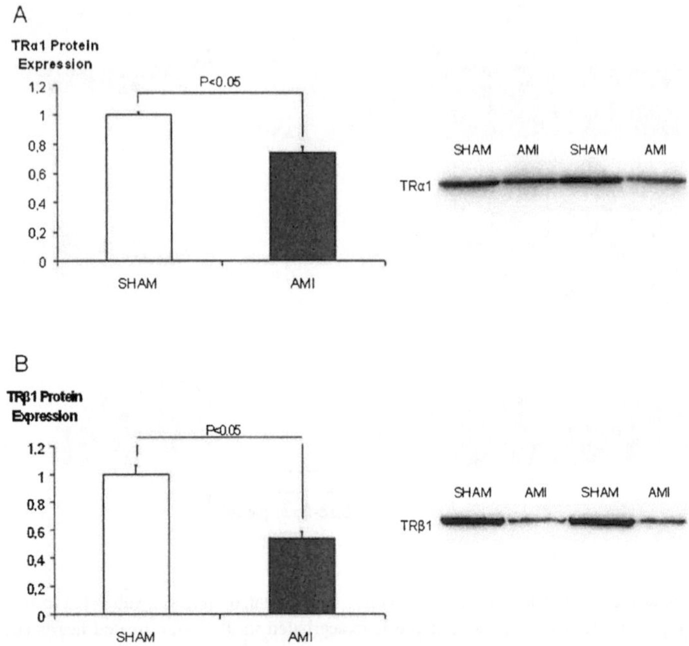

Figure 4. Densitometric assessment in arbitrary units and representative western blots of thyroid hormone receptor α1 (TRα1) expression (A) and thyroid hormone receptor β1 (TRβ1) expression (B) in sham-operated (SHAM) and post-infarcted (AMI) rat hearts (data from our labaratory).

specific manner and in various pathological conditions. Maturation of the myocardium depends on increasing thyroid hormone signaling after birth, which induces growth and the transcriptional programming that leads to the characteristic gene expression profile of the adult heart. It is now realized that gene expression profile of fetal heart (where thyroid hormone stimulation is relatively low) is recapitulated in the hypertrophic or failing heart and altered TR expression seems to be contributory to reactivation of the fetal transcriptional profile.[103] Phenylephrine or pressure-overload induced cardiac hypertrophy is also accompanied by a decreased expression of the TRs (TRβ1, TRα1 and TRα2). Overexpression of either TRα1 or TRβ1 was shown to counteract the phenotype effects of phenylephrine treatment upon α-MHC promoter activity or β-MHC and SERCA promoter activity, respectively.[103] Furthermore, TRα1 and TRβ1 receptors are found to be downregulated in the non-infarcted myocardium 8 weeks after acute myocardial infarction in rats, whereas thyroid hormone levels were unchanged. This tissue hypothyroidism is associated with increased tolerance of those hearts to ischemia and reperfusion. Hypothyroid like changes may constitute a part of an adaptive response aiming to protect the post-infarcted heart from recurrent ischemic insults, by reducing energy requirements.[104] Figure 4.

TRs can pharmacologically be regulated at the transcription level. In fact, amiodarone resulted in downregulation of the TRα1, TRβ1, TRβ2 mRNA but not TRα2 mRNA while co-administration of T_3 and amiodarone in upregulation of TRα2 and

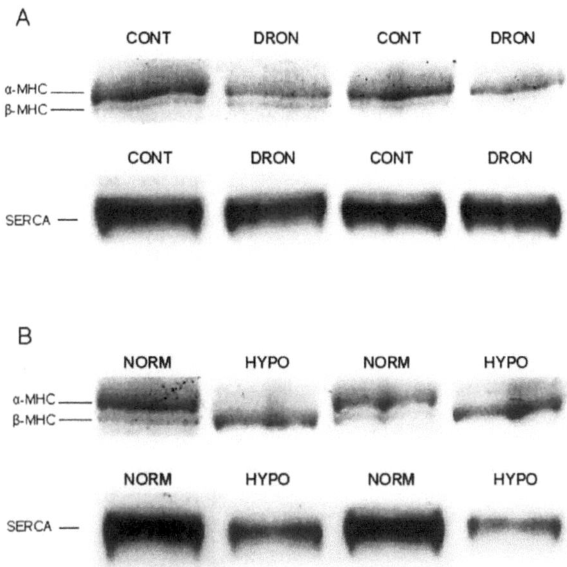

Figure 5. Images of SDS-PAGE for myosin heavy chain (MHC) α and β isoforms expression and immunoblots for sarcoplasmic reticulum Ca^{2+}-ATPase (SERCA) expression in normal hearts (CONT or NORM) and after A) TRα1 blockade with dronedarone treatment (DRON) and B) propylthiouracil induced hypothyroidism (HYPO). TRβ1-regulated β-MHC and SERCA are not altered with dronedarone treatment (data from our laboratory). Selective manipulation of thyroid hormone signaling may be of therapeutic importance.

TRβ1 mRNA.[105] Furthermore, pharmacological agents can specifically activate or antagonize thyroid hormone nuclear receptors or influence their binding to their coregulators. Thus, amiodarone or its metabolite desethyl-amiodarone (DEA) is reported to be a non competitive inhibitor of TRβ1 and a competitive inhibitor of TRα1. Interestingly, in the presence of thyroxine excess, DEA has a synagonistic action on TRβ1,[106] while it exhibits an antagonistic effect on TRα1.[107] This effect has been suggested to be due to the stabilizing action of DEA on the binding of TRβ1 with its coactivator. A non iodinated amiodarone like agent, dronedarone and particularly its metabolite is shown to be a selective TRα1 antagonist.[108, 109] Furthermore, a TRβ1 agonist, GC-1, has also been developed.[110]

Selective targeting of thyroid hormone receptors can elicit cardioprotection. Blockade of TRα1 with dronedarone, suppressed ischemic contracture, increased postischemic functional recovery and reduced tissue injury in a perfused rat model of zero-flow global ischemia and reperfusion. This response was associated with decreased expression of α-MHC without any change in the expression of β-MHC and SERCA, indicating a selective inhibitory effect of dronedarone on TRα1.[109] Figure 5. Furthermore, resting heart rate and contractility were reduced but not to the same extent as in hypothyroidism, while preischemic myocardial glycogen content was also increased.[109]

Non cardiac effects with important consequences on the course of the ischemic heart disease are elicited in a thyroid hormone receptor isoform manner. In fact, TRα1 blockade by dronedarone prevented body weight gain by reducing food intake, an ef-

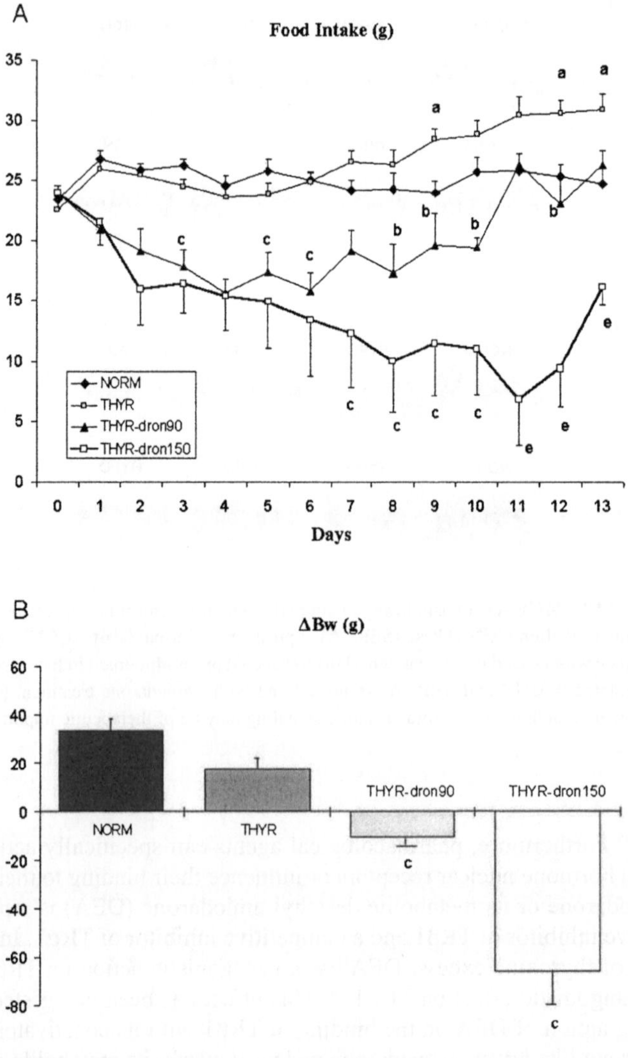

Figure 6. Non cardiac effects of thyroid hormone treatment (THYR) on food intake and body weight gain (ΔBw). A) Thyroid hormone increases food intake as compared to normal rats (NORM), an effect which is prevented by blockade of TRα1 by 90mg/Kg dronedarone administration (THYR-dron90) or 150 mg/Kg (THYR-dron150). B) Thyroid hormone has a weak effect on body weight reduction because of the concomitant increase in food intake. With dronedarone treatment, this effect is potentiated (data from our labaratory). a $p<0.05$ vs NORM, b $p<0.05$ vs THYR, c $p<0.05$ vs NORM and THYR, e $p<0.05$ vs NORM, THYR and THYR-dron90

fect which was further potentiated in the presence of increased doses of thyroxine.[109, 111] Figure 6. Furthermore, activation of TRβ1 by GC-1, a TRβ1 agonist, is shown to reduce cholesterol levels and body weight without accelerating heart rate.[110] It appears that thyroid hormone responsive signaling can be selectively manipulated at the level of thyroid hormone nuclear receptors and the beneficial effects of thyroid hormone could be therapeutically exploited in the treatment of heart diseases. Thyroid analogs have been synthesized and are tested in patients.[112]

Concluding remarks

Hormones signaling appears to be of physiological relevance in the context of ischemia and reperfusion. A cardioprotective effect can be elicited by hormones through their genomic or non genomic actions. This response resembles that of ischemic preconditioning and to some extent involves similar intracellular signaling pathways. Hormones signaling can be selectively manipulated and hormone analogs may have a place in the management of the ischemic heart disease.

ACKNOWLEDGEMENTS

Prof. Taegtmeyer and Prof. Swynghedauw for reviewing this manuscript.

REFERENCES

1. S.E. Anderson, D.M. Kirkland, A. Beyschau and P.M. Cala, Acute effects of beta–estradiol on myocardial pH, Na and Ca and ischemia and reperfusion, *Am. J. Physiol.* **288(1)**, C57-64 (2005)
2. E.R. Booth, M. Marchesi, E.J. Kilbourne and B.R. Lucchesi, 17β estradiol as a receptor-mediated cardioprotective agent, *J. Pharmacol. Exper. Ther.* **307**, 395–401 (2003).
3. C.H. Tsai, S.F. Su, T.F. Chou and T.M. Lee, Differential effects of sarcolemmal and mitochondrial K(ATP) channels activated by 17 beta estradiol on reperfusion arrhythmias and infarct sizes in canine hearts, *J. Pharmacol. Exp. Ther.* **301**, 234–240 (2002).
4. K. Node, M. Kitakaze, H Kosaka, T. Minamino, H. Funaya and M. Hori, Amelioration of ischemia and reperfusion-induced myocardial injury by 17beta-estradiol: role of nitric oxide and calcium activated potassium channels, *Circulation* **96(6)**, 1953–1963 (1997).
5. T.M. Lee, T.F. Chou and C.H. Tsai, Differential role of K_{ATP} channels activated by conjugated estrogens in the regulation of myocardial and coronary protective effects, *Circulation* **107**, 49–54 (2003).
6. S. Beer, M. Reincke, M. Kral, S.Z. Lie, S. Steinhauer, H.H. Schmidt, B. Allolio and S. Neubauer, Susceptibility to cardiac ischemia /reprfusion injury is modulated by chronic estrogen status, *J. Cardiovasc. Pharmacol.* **40**, 420–428 (2002).
7. M. Grist, R.B. Wambolt, G.P. Bondy, D.R. English and M.F. Allard, Estrogen replacement stimulates fatty acid oxidation and impairs postischemic recovery of hearts from ovariectomized female rats, *Can. J. Physiol. Pharmacol.* **80**, 1001–1007 (2002).
8. Y. Xu, S.J. Armstrong, I.A. Arenas, D.J. Pehowich, S.T. Davidge, Cardioprotection by chronic estrogen or superoxide dismutase mimetic treatment in the aged female rat, *Am. J. Physiol.* **287**, H165–H171 (2004).
9. T. Shinohara, N. Takahashi, T. Ooie, M. Ishinose, M. Hara, H. Yonemoshi, T. Saikawa and H. Yoshimatsu, Estrogen inhibits hyperthermia –induced expression of heat shock protein 72 and cardioprotection against ischemia/reperfusion injury in female rat heart, *J. Mol. Cell. Cardiol.* **37**, 1053–1061 (2004).
10. K.L. Hamilton, S. Gupta, A.A. Knowlton, Estrogen and regulation of heat shock protein expression in female cardiomyocytes: cross –talk with NFkB signaling, *J. Mol. Cell. Cardiol.* **36**, 577–584 (2004).
11. P. Zhai, T.E. Eurell, P.S. Cooke, D.B. Lubahn and D.R. Gross, Myocardial ischemia and reperfusion injury in estrogen receptor-alpha knockout and wild-type mice, *Am. J. Physiol.* **278(5)**, H1640–H1647 (2000).

12. H. Ogita, K. Node, H. Asanuma, S. Sanada, Y. Liao, S. Takashima, M. Asakura, H. Mori, Y. Shinozaki, M. Hori and M. Kitakaze, Amelioration of ischemia and reperfusion induced myocardial injury by the selective estrogen receptor modulator, raloxifene, in the canine heart, *J. Am. Coll. Cardiol.* **40**, 998–1005 (2002).
13. F. Er, G. Michels, N. Gassanov, F. Rivero and U.C. Hoppe, Testosterone induces cytoprotection by activating ATP-sensitive K^+ channels in the cardiac mitochondrial inner membrane, *Circulation* **110(19)**, 3100–3107 (2004).
14. F. Callies, H. Stromer, R. Schwinger, B. Bolck, K. Hu, S. Frantz, A. Leupold, S. Beer, B. Allolio and A.W. Bonz, Administration of testosterone is associated with a reduced susceptibility to myocardial ischemia, *Endocrinology* **144**, 4478–4483 (2004).
15. M. Wang, B.M. Tsai, A. Kher, L.B. Baker, G.M. Wairiuko, D.R. Meldrum, The role of endogenous testosterone in myocardial proinflammatory and proapoptotic signaling after acute ischemia and reperfusion, *Am. J. Physiol.* **288(1)**, H221–226 (2005).
16. E.F. Du Toit, E. Rossouw, J. Van Rooyen and A. Lochner, Proposed mechanism for the anabolic steroid induced increase in myocardial susceptibility to ischemia/reperfusion injury, *Cardiovasc. J. S. Afr.* **16(1)**, 21–28 (2005).
17. V. De Gennaro Colonna, G. Rossoni, M. Bernareggi, E.E. Muller and F. Berti, Cardiac ischemia and impairment of vascular endothelium function in hearts from growth hormone-deficient rats: protection by hexarelin, *Eur, J, Pharmacol.* **334(2–3)**, 201–207 (1997).
18. G. Rossoni, V. De Gennaro Colonna, M. Bernareggi, G.L. Polvani, E.E. Muller and F. Berti, Protectant activity of hexarelin or growth hormone against postischemic ventricular dysfunction in hearts from aged rats, *J. Cardiovasc. Pharmacol.* **32(2)**, 260–265 (1998).
19. F. Weekers, E. van Herck, J. Isgaard and G. van den Berghe, Pretreatment with growth hormone releasing peptide-2 directly protects against the diastolic dysfunction of myocardial stunning in an isolated, blood–perfused rabbit heart model, *Endocrinology* **141**, 3993–3999 (2000).
20. S. Frascarelli, S. Ghelardoni, S. Ronca-Testoni and R. Zucchi, Effect of ghrelin and synthetic growth hormone secretagogues in normal and ischemic rat heart, *Basic Res. Cardiol.* **98**, 401–405 (2003).
21. L. Chang, Y. Ren, X. Liu W.G. Li, J. Yang, B. Geng, N.L. Weintraub and C. Tang, Protective effects of ghrelin on ischemia/reperfusion injury in the isolated rat heart, *J. Cardiovasc. Pharmacol.* **43**, 165–170 (2004).
22. G. Baldanzi, N. Filigheddu, S. Cutrupi, F. Catapano, S. Bonissoni, A. Fubini, D. Malan, G. Baj, R. Granata, F. Broglio, M. Papotti, N. Surico, F. Bussolino, J. Isgaard, R. Deghenghi, F. Sinigaglia, M. Prat, G. Muccioli, E. Ghigo and A. Graziani, Ghrelin and des-acyl ghrelin inhibit cell death in cardiomyocytes and endothelial cells through ERK1/2 and PI3-kinase/Akt, *J. Cell. Biol.* **159(6)**, 1029–1037 (2002).
23. A. Bourbon, M. Vionnet, P. Leprince, E. Vaissier, J Copeland, P. McDonagh, P. Debre and I. Gandjbakhch, The effect of methylprednisolone treatment on the cardiopulmonary bypass-induced systemic inflammatory response, *Eur. J. Cardiothorac. Surg.* **26(5)**, 932–938 (2004).
24. D.E. Sholter and P.W. Armstrong, Adverse effects of corticosteroids on the cardiovascular system, *Can. J. Cardiol.* **16(4)**, 505–511 (2000).
25. G. Valen, T. Kawakami, Tahepold, A. Dumitrescu, C. Lowbeer and J. Vaage, Clucocorticoid pretreatment protects cardiac function and induces cardiac heat shock protein 72, *Am. J. Physiol.* **279**, H836–H843 (2000).
26. E. Varga, N. Nagy, J. Lazar, G. Czifra, I. Bak, T. Biro and A.Tosaki, Inhibition of ischemia/reperfusion–induced damage by dexamethasone in isolated working rat hearts: the role of cytochrome c release, *Life Sci.* **75**, 2411–2423 (2004).
27. B.K. Brar, A.K. Jonassen, A. Stephanou, G. Santilli, J. Railson, R.A. Knight, D.M. Yellon and D.S. Latchman, Urocortin protects against ischemic and reperfusion injury via a MAPK-dependent pathway, *J. Biol. Chem.* **275(12)**, 8508–8514 (2000).
28. D.J. Hausenloy and D.M. Yellon, New directions for protecting the heart against ischemia and reperfusion injury: targeting the Reperfusion Injury Salvage Kinase (RISK)-pathway, *Cardiovasc. Res.* **61**, 448–460 (2004).
29. C. Bazzani, S. Guarini, A. Botticelli, D. Zaffe, A. Tomasi, A. Bini, M.C. Cainazzo, G. Ferrazza, C. Mioni and A. Bertolini, Protective effect of melanocortin peptides in rat myocardial ischemia. *J. Pharmacol. Experimental. Therapeutics* **297**, 1082–1087 (2001).
30. R.J. Reiter and D.X. Tan, Melatonin: a novel protective agent against oxidative injury of the ischemic/reperfused heart, *Cardiovasc. Res.* **58**, 10–19 (2003).

31. S. Kaneko, K. Okumura, Y. Numaguchi, H. Matsui, K. Murase, S. Mokuno, I. Morishima, K. Hira, Y. Toki, T. Ito and T. Hayakawa, Melatonin scavenges hydroxyl radical and protects isolated rat hearts from ischemic reperfusion injury, *Life Sci.* **67(2)**, 101–112 (2000).
32. E. Sahna, A. Acet, M.K. Ozer and E. Olmez, Myocardial ischemia and reperfusion in rats: reduction of infarct size by either supplemental physiological or pharmacological doses of melatonin, *J. Pineal Res.* **33(4),** 234–238 (2002).
33. D.J. Duncker and P.D. Verdouw, Has melatonin a future as a cardioprotective agent? *Cardiovasc. Drugs Ther.* **15**, 205–207, (2001).
34. P. Van der Meer, E. Lipsic, R.H. Henning, R.A. de Boer, A.J.H. Suurmeijer, D.J. van Veldhuisen and W.H. van Gilst, Erythropoietin improves left ventricular function and coronary flow in an experimental model of ischemia and reperfusion injury, *Eur. J. Heart Fail.* **6**, 853–859 (2004).
35. A.F. Tramontano, R. Muniyappa, A.D. Black, M.C. Blendea, I. Cohen, L. Deng, J.R. Sowers, M.V. Cutaia and N. El-Sherif, Erythropoietin protects cardiac myocytes from hypoxia–induced apoptosis through an Akt–dependent pathway *Biochem. Biophys. Res. Commun.* **308**, 990–994 (2003).
36. C.J. Parsa, A. Matsumoto, J. Kim, R.U. Reil, L.S. Pascal, G.B. Walton, R.B. Thompson, J.A. Petrofski, B.H. Annex, J.S. Stamler and W.J. Koch, A novel protective effect of erythropoietin in the infracted heart, *J. Clin. Invest.* **112**, 999–1007 (2003).
37. G. Baxter, Natriuretic peptides and myocardial ischemia, *Basic Res. Cardiol.* **99**, 90–93 (2004).
38. S.P. D'Souza, M. Davis and G.F. Baxter, Autocrine and paracrine actions of natriuretic peptides in the heart, *Pharmacol, Ther.* **101(2)**, 113–129 (2004).
39. M.A. Rastegar, A. Vegh, J.G. Papp and J.R. Paratt, Atrial natriuretic peptide reduces the severe consequences of coronary artery occlusion in anaesthetized dogs, *Cardiovasc. Drugs Ther.* **14(5)**, 471–479 (2000).
40. A. Halapas, R. Tenta, C. Pantos, D.V. Cokkinos and M. Koutsilieris, Parathyroid hormone-related peptide and cardiovascular system, *In Vivo.* **17(5),** 425–32 (2003).
41. K.L. Laugwitz, H.J. Weig, A. Moretti, E. Hoffmann, P. Ueblacker, I. Pragst, K. Rosport, A. Schomig and M. Ungerer, Gene transfer of heterologous G protein-coupled receptors to cardiomyocytes: differential effects on contractility, *Circ Res.* **88(7)**, 688–95 (2001).
42. K.D. Schluter, M. Weber and H.M. Piper, Effects of PTH-rP(107–111) and PTH-rP(7–34) on adult cardiomyocytes, *J. Mol. Cell. Cardiol.* **29(11)**, 3057–65 (1997).
43. K. Schluter, C. Katzer, K. Frischkopf, S. Wenzel, G. Taimor and H.M. Piper, Expression, release, and biological activity of parathyroid hormone-related peptide from coronary endothelial cells, *Circ Res.* **86(9)**, 946–51 (2000).
44. J. Jansen, P. Gres, C. Umschlag, F.R. Heinzel, H. Degenhardt, K.D. Schluter, G. Heusch and R. Schulz, Parathyroid hormone–related peptide improves contractile function of stunned myocardium in rats and pigs, *Am. J. Physiol.* **284**, H49–H55 (2003).
45. A. Rochetaing, C. Chapon, L. Marescaux, A. Le Bouil, A. Furber, P. Kreher. Potential beneficial as well as detrimental effects of chronic treatment with lisinopril and (or) spironolactone on isolated hearts following low-flow ischemia in normal and infarcted rats, *Can. J. Physiol. Pharmacol.* **81**, 864–872 (2003).
46. D.M. Purdham, M.X. Zou, V. Rajapurohitam and M. Karmazyn, Rat heart is a site of leptin production and action. *Am. J. Physiol. Heart* **287(6)**, H2877–84 (2004).
47. M.W. Nickola, L.E. Wold, P.B. Colligan, G.J. Wang, W.K. Samson and J. Ren, Leptin attenuates cardiac contraction in rat ventricular myocytes. Role of NO, *Hypertension* **36(4)**, 501–5 (2000).
48. V. Rajapurohitam, X.T. Gan, L.A. Kirshenbaum and M. Karmazyn, The obesity-associated peptide leptin induces hypertrophy in neonatal rat ventricular myocytes, *Circ Res.* **93(4)**, 277–279 (2003).
49. L.L. Atkinson, M.A. Fischer and G.D. Lopaschuk, Leptin activates cardiac fatty acid oxidation independent of changes in the AMP-activated protein kinase-acetyl-CoA carboxylase-malonyl-CoA axis, *J. Biol. Chem.* **277(33)**, 29424–29430 (2002).
50. S.R. Meisel, M. Ellis, C. Pariente, H. Pauzner, M. Liebowitz, D. David and I. Shimon, Serum leptin levels increase following acute myocardial infarction, *Cardiology* **95(4),** 206–11 (2001).
51. E.D. Abel, Insulin signaling in heart muscle: lessons from genetically engineered mouse models, *Curr. Hypertens. Rep.* **6**, 416–423 (2004).
52. L. Hue, C. Beauloye, A.S. Marsin, L. Bertrand, S. Horman and M.H. Rider, Insulin and ischemia stimulate glycolysis by acting on the same targets through different and opposing signaling pathways, *J. Mol. Cell Cardiol.* **34**, 1091–1097 (2002).

53. J. Deprez, L. Bertrand, D.R. Alessi, U. Krause, L. Hue and M.H. Rider, Partial purification and characterization of a wortmannin-sensitive and insulin-stimulated protein kinase that activates heart 6-phosphofructo-2-kinase, *Biochem. J.* **347**, 305–312 (2000).
54. C. Beauloye, A.S. Marsin, L. Bertrand, U. Krause, D.G. Hardie, J.L. Vanoverschelde and L. Hue, Insulin antagonizes AMP-activated protein kinase activation by ischemia or anoxia in rat hearts, without affecting total adenine nucleotides, *FEBS Lett.* **505(3)**, 348–352 (2001).
55. C. Beauloye, L. Bertrand, U. Krause, A.S. Marsin, T. Dresselaers, F. Vanstapel, Vanoverschelde and L. Hue, No-flow ischemia inhibits insulin signalling in heart by decreasing intracellular pH, *Circ. Res.* **88(5)**, 513–519 (2001).
56. A.K. Jonassen, M.N. Sack, O.D. Mjos and D.M. Yellon, Myocardial protection by insulin at reperfusion requires early administration and is mediated via Akt and p70s6 kinase cell-survival signaling. *Circ. Res.* **89**, 1191–1198 (2001).
57. F. Gao, E. Gao, T.L. Yue, E.H. Ohlstein, B.L. Lopez, T.A. Christopher and X.L. Ma, Nitric oxide mediates the antiapoptotic effect of insulin in myocardial ischemia and reperfusion: the roles of PI3-kinase, Akt, and endothelial nitric oxide synthase phosphorylation, *Circulation* **105(12)**, 1497–502 (2002).
58. F. Fath-Ordoubadi and K.J. Beatt, Glucose-insulin-potassium therapy for treatment of acute myocardial infarction: an overview of randomized placebo-controlled trials, *Circulation* **96(4)**, 1152–1156 (1997).
59. S. Gradinac, G.M. Coleman, H. Taegtmeyer, M.S. Sweeney and O.H. Frazier, Improved cardiac function with glucose-insulin-potassium after aortocoronary bypass grafting, *Ann. Thorac. Surg.* **48(4)**, 484–489 (1989).
60. M.N. Sack and D. Yellon, Insulin therapy as an adjunct to reperfusion after acute coronary ischemia, *J. Am. Coll. Cardiol.* **41**, 1404–1407 (2003).
61. A.K. Jonassen, E. Aasum, R.A. Riemersma, O.D. Mjos and T.S. Larsen, Glucose–insulin–potassium reduces infarct size when administered during reperfusion, *Cardiovasc. Drugs Ther.* **14**, 615–623 (2000).
62. H.F. Zhang, Q. Fan, X.X. Qian, B.L. Lopez, T.A. Christopher, X.L. Ma and F. Gao, Role of insulin in the antiapoptotic effect of glucose–insulin–potassium in rabbits with acute myocardial ischemia and reperfusion. *Apoptosis* **9**, 777–783 (2004).
63. A.K. Jonassen, B.K. bar, O.D. Mjos, M.N. Sack, D.S. Latchman and D.M. Yellon, Insulin administered at reoxygenation exerts a cardioprotective effect in myocytes by a possible anti-apoptotic mechanism, *J. Moll. Cel. Cardiol.* **32(5)**, 757–764 (2000).
64. L.H. Opie, The glucose hypothesis: relation to acute myocardial ischemia, *J. Mol. Cell Cardiol.* **1**, 107–114 (1970).
65. Y. Fujio, T. Nguyen, D. Wencker, R.N. Kitsis and K. Walsh, Akt promotes survival of cardiomyocytes in vitro and protects against ischemia and reperfusion injury in mouse heart, *Circulation* **101(6)**, 660–667 (2000).
66. M. Parrizas, A.R. Saltiel and D. LeRoith, Insulin-like growth factor-1 inhibition of apoptosis is associated with increased expression of the bcl-xL gene product. *Endocrinology* **138(3)**, 1355–1358 (1997).
67. K. Yamashita, J. Kajstura, D.J. Discher, B.J. Wasserlauf, N.H. Bishopric, P. Anversa and K.A. Webster, Reperfusion-activated Akt kinase prevents apoptosis in transgenic mouse hearts overexpressing insulin-like growth factor-1, *Circ. Res.* **88**, 609–614 (2001).
68. D.P. Kelly and R.C. Scarpulla, Transcriptional regulatory circuits controlling mitochondrial biogenesis and function, *Genes Dev.* **18**, 357–368 (2004).
69. N.S. Wayman, Y. Hattori, M.C. Mc Donald, H. Mota-Filipe, S. Cuzzocrea, B. Pisano, P.K. Chatterjee and C. Thiemermann, Ligands of the peroxisome proliferator activated receptors (PPAR-γ and PPAR-α) reduce myocardial infarct size, *FASEB J.* **16**, 1027–1040 (2002).
70. H.R. Liu, L. Tao, E. Gao, B.L. Lopez, T.A. Christopher, R.N. Willette, E.H. Ohlstein, T.L. Yue and X.L. Ma, Antiapoptotic effects of rosiglitazone in hypercholesterolemic rabbits subjected to myocardial ischaemia and reperfusion, *Cardiovasc. Res.* **62**, 135–144 (2004).
71. Y. Xu, M. Gen, J. Fox, S.O. Weiss, R.D. Brown, D. Perlov, H. Ahmad, P. Zhu, C. Greyson, C.S. Long and G.G. Schwartz, PPAR-gamma activation fails to provide myocardial protection in ischemia and reperfusion in pigs, *Am. J. Physiol.* **288(30)**, H1314–H1323, 2005.
72. M.E. Young, F.A. Laws, G.W. Goodwin and H. Taegtmeyer, Reactivation of PPAR-alpha is associated with contractile dysfunction in hypertrophied rat heart, *Biol. Chem.* **276(48)**, 44390–44395 (2001).
73. C. Pantos, V. Malliopoulou, D. Varonos and D.V. Cokkinos, Thyroid hormone and phenotypes of cardioprotection, *Basic Res. Cardiol.* **99**, 101–120 (2004).

74. Q. Liu, A.S. Clanachan and G.D. Lopaschuk, Acute effects of tri-iodothyronine on glucose and fatty acid metabolism during reperfusion of ischemic rat hearts, *Am. J. Physiol.* **275(3)**, E392–399 (1998).
75. P.T. Buser, J. Wikman-Coffelt, S.T. Wu, N. Derugin, W.W. Parmley and C.B. Higgins, Postischemic recovery of mechanical performance and energy metabolism in the presence of left ventricular hypertrophy. A 31P-MRS study, *Circ. Res.* **66(3)**, 735–746 (1990).
76. C. Pantos, V. Malliopoulou, I. Mourouzis, E. Karamanoli, S.M. Tzeis, H. Carageorgiou, D. Varonos and D.V. Cokkinos, Long-term thyroxine administration increases Hsp70 mRNA expression and attenuates p38 MAP kinase activity in response to ischemia, *J. Endocrinol.* **170**, 207–215 (2001).
77. C. Pantos, D.D. Cokkinos, S. Tzeis, V. Malliopoulou, I. Mourouzis, H. Carageorgiou, C. Limas, D. Varonos and D.V. Cokkinos, Hyperthyroidism is associated with preserved preconditioning capacity but intensified and accelerated ischemic contracture in rat heart, *Basic Res. Cardiol.* **94**, 254–260 (1999).
78. K.G. Kolocassides, M. Galinanes and D.J. Hearse, Dichotomy of ischemic preconditioning. Improved postischemic contractile function despite intensification of ischemic contracture, *Circulation* **93**, 1725–1733 (1996).
79. T. Asahi, M. Shimabukuro, Y. Oshiro, H. Yoshida and N. Takasu, Cilazapril prevents cardiac hypertrophy and postischemic myocardial dysfunction in hyperthyroid rats, *Thyroid* **11(11)**, 1009–1015 (2001).
80. J.A. Lahorra, D.F. Torchiana, C. Hahn, C.A. Bashour, A.G. Denenberg, J.S. Titus, W.M. Daggett and G.A. Geffin, Recovery after cardioplegia in the hypertrophic rat heart, *J. Surg. Res.* **88(2)**, 88–96 (2000)
81. P. Venditti, C. Agnisola and S. Di Meo, Effect of ischemia and reperfusion on heart mitochondria from hyperthyroid rats, *Cardiovasc. Res.* **56(1)**, 76–85 (2002).
82. C.M. Dyke, T. Yeh Jr, J.D. Lehman, A. Abd-Elfattah, M. Ding, A.S. Wechsler and D.R. Salter, Tri-iodothyronine-enhanced left ventricular function after ischemic injury, *Ann. Thorac. Surg.* **52(1)**, 14–19 (1991).
83. F.W. Holland 2nd, P.S. Brown Jr and R.E. Clark, Acute severe postischemic myocardial depression reversed by tri-iodothyronine, *Ann. Thorac. Surg.* **54(2)**, 301–305 (1992).
84. M. Kadletz, P.G. Mullen, M. Ding, L.G. Wolfe and A.S. Wechsler, Effect of tri-iodothyronine on postischemic myocardial function in the isolated heart, *Ann. Thorac. Surg.* **57(3)**, 657–662 (1994).
85. C.M. Dyke, M. Ding, A.S. Abd-Elfattah, K. Loesser, R.J. Dignan, A.S. Wechsler and D.R. Salter, Effects of tri-iodothyronine supplementation after myocardial ischemia, *Ann. Thorac. Surg.* **56(2)**, 215–222 (1993).
86. D. Novitzky, N. Matthews, D. Shawley, D.K. Cooper and N. Zuhdi, Tri-iodothyronine in the recovery of stunned myocardium in dogs, *Ann. Thorac. Surg.* **51(1)**, 10–16 (1991).
87. J.D. Klemperer, I. Klein, M. Gomez, R.E. Helm, K. Ojamaa, S.J. Thomas, O.W. Isom and K. Krieger, Thyroid hormone treatment after coronary-artery bypass surgery, *N. Engl. J. Med.* **333(23)**, 1522–1527 (1995).
88. D. Novitzky, D.K. Cooper and A. Swanepoel, Inotropic effect of tri-iodothyronine (T_3) in low cardiac output following cardioplegic arrest and cardiopulmonary bypass: an initial experience in patients undergoing open heart surgery, *Eur. J. Cardiothorac. Surg.* **3(2)**, 140–145 (1989).
89. K. Ojamaa, A. Kenessey, R. Shenoy and I. Klein, Thyroid hormone metabolism and cardiac gene expression after acute myocardial infarction in the rat, *Am. J. Physiol.* **279**, E1319–E1324 (2000).
90. K.W. Mahaffey, T.E. Raya, G.D. Pennock, E. Morkin and S. Goldman, Left ventricular performance and remodeling in rabbits after myocardial infarction: effects of a thyroid hormone analogue, *Circulation* **91(3)**, 794–801 (1995).
91. A.T. Saurin, J.L. Martin, R.J. Heads, C. Foley, J.W. Mockridge, M.J. Wright, Y. Wang and M.S. Marber, The role of differential activation of p38-mitogen-activated protein kinase in preconditioned ventricular myocytes, *FASEB J.* **14(14)**, 2237–2246 (2000).
92. E.T. Maizels, C.A. Peters, M. Kline, R.E. Cutler and M. Shanmugam, Heat-shock protein–25/27 phosphorylation by the δ isoform of protein kinase C, *Biochem. J.* **332**, 703–712 (1998)
93. C. Pantos, V. Malliopoulou, I. Mourouzis, E. Karamanoli, P. Moraitis, S. Tzeis, I. Paizis, H. Carageorgiou, D. Varonos and D.V. Cokkinos, Thyroxine pretreatment increases basal myocardial Hsp27 expression and accelerates translocation and phosphorylation of this protein upon ischemia, *Eur. J. Pharmacol.* **478**, 53–60 (2003).
94. C. Pantos, V. Malliopoulou, I. Mourouzis, E. Karamanoli, I. Paizis, N. Steimberg, D. Varonos and D.V. Cokkinos, Long-term Thyroxine Administration Protects the Heart in a Similar Pattern as Ischemic Preconditioning, *Thyroid* **12**, 325–329 (2002).
95. C. Pantos, V. Malliopoulou, I. Paizis, P. Moraitis, I. Mourouzis, S. Tzeis, E. Karamanoli, D.D. Cokkinos, H. Carageorgiou, D. Varonos and D.V. Cokkinos, Thyroid hormone and cardioprotection; study of

p38 MAPK and JNKs during ischemia and at reperfusion in isolated rat heart, *Mol. Cell Biochem.* **242**, 173–180 (2003).

96. E. Marais, S. Genade, R. Salie, B. Huisamen, S. Maritz, J.A. Moolman and A. Lochner, The temporal relationship between p38 MAPK and Hsp27 activation in ischemic and pharmacological preconditioning, *Basic Res. Cardiol.* **100(1)**, 35–47 (2005).
97. C. Pantos, V. Malliopoulou, I. Mourouzis, K. Sfakianoudis, S. Tzeis, P. Doumba, C. Xinaris, A.D. Cokkinos, H. Carageorgiou, D. Varonos and D.V. Cokkinos, Propylthiouracil induced hypothyroidism is associated with increased tolerance of the isolated rat heart to ischemia and reperfusion. *J. Endocrinol.* **178(3)**, 427–435 (2003).
98. M. Abe, H. Obata and H. Tanaka, Functional and metabolic responses to ischemia in the isolated perfused hypothyroid rat heart, *Jpn. Circ. J.* **56(7)**, 671–680 (1992).
99. L.S. Carter, R.A. Mueller, E.A. Norfleet, F.B. Payne and L.S. Saltzman, Hypothyroidism delays ischemia-induced contracture and adenine nucleotide depletion in rat myocardium, *Circ. Res.* **60(5)**, 649–652 (1987).
100. M. Eynan, T. Knubuvetz, U. Meiri, G. Navon, G. Gerstenblith, Z. Bromberg, Y. Hasin and M. Horowitz, Heat acclimation-induced elevated glycogen, glycolysis, and low thyroxine improve heart ischemic tolerance, *J. Appl. Physiol.* **93(6)**, 2095–2104 (2002).
101. L. Zhang, J.R. Parratt, G.H. Beastall, N.J. Pyne and B.L. Furman, Streptozotocin diabetes protects against arrhythmias in rat isolated hearts: role of hypothyroidism, *Eur. J. Pharmacol.* **435(2–3)**, 269–276 (2002).
102. L. Friberg, S. Werner, G. Eggertsen and S. Ahnve, Rapid down-regulation of thyroid hormones in acute myocardial infarction: is it cardioprotective in patients with angina? *Arch. Intern. Med.* **162(12)**, 1388–1394 (2002).
103. K. Kinugawa, K. Yonekura, R.C. Ribeiro, Y. Eto, T. Aoyagi, J.D. Baxter, S.A. Camacho, M.R. Bristow, C.S. Long and P.C. Simpson, Regulation of thyroid hormone receptor isoforms in physiological and pathological cardiac hypertrophy, *Circ. Res.* **89(7)**, 591–598 (2001).
104. C. Pantos, I. Mourouzis, T. Saranteas, I. Paizis, C. Xinaris, V. Malliopoulou and D.V. Cokkinos, Thyroid hormone receptors α1 and β1 are downregulated in the post-infarcted rat heart: consequences on the response to ischaemia-reperfusion, *Bas. Res. Cardiol.* (2005), in press.
105. V. Drvota, M. Bronnegard, J. Hagglad, T. Barkhem and C. Sylven, Downregulation of thyroid hormone receptor subtype mRNA levels by amiodarone during catecholamine stress in vitro, *Biochem. Biophys. Res. Commun.* **211(3)**, 991–996 (1995).
106. O. Bakker, H.C. van Beeren and W.M. Wiersinga, Desethylamiodarone is a noncompetitive inhibitor of the binding of thyroid hormone to the thyroid hormone beta 1-receptor protein, *Endocrinology* **134(4)**, 1665–1670 (1994).
107. H.C. Van Beeren, O. Bakker and W.M. Wiersinga, Desethylamiodarone is a competitive inhibitor of the binding of thyroid hormone to the thyroid hormone alpha 1-receptor protein, *Mol. Cell Endocrinol.* **112(1)**, 15–19 (1995).
108. H.C. Van Beeren, W.M. Jong, E. Kaptein, T.J. Visser, O. Bakker and W.M. Wiersinga, Dronerarone acts as a selective inhibitor of 3,5,3'-tri-iodothyronine binding to thyroid hormone receptor-alpha1: in vitro and in vivo evidence. *Endocrinology* **144(2)**, 552–558 (2003).
109. C. Pantos, I. Mourouzis, V. Malliopoulou, I. Paizis, S. Tzeis, P. Moraitis, K. Sfakianoudis, D. Varonos and D.V. Cokkinos, Dronedarone administration prevents body weight gain and increases tolerance of the heart to ischemic stress: a possible involvement of thyroid hormone receptor α1, *Thyroid* **15**, 16–23 (2005).
110. S.U. Trost, E. Swanson, B. Gloss, D.B. Wang-Iverson, H. Zhang, T. Volodarsky, G.J. Grover, J.D. Baxter, G. Chiellini, T.S. Scanlan and W.H. Dillmann, The thyroid hormone receptor-beta-selective agonist GC-1 differentially affects plasma lipids and cardiac activity, *Endocrinology* **141(9)**, 3057–3064 (2000).
111. C. Pantos, I. Mourouzis, I. Paizis, P. Moraitis, A.D. Cokkinos and D.V. Cokkinos, Blockade of thyroid hormone receptor alpha 1: a new strategy for body weight reduction? *Obes. Rev.* **6(1)**, P146 (2005).
112. J.D. Baxter, D.H. Dillman, B.L. West, R. Huber, J.D. Furlow, R.J. Fletterick, P. Webb, J.W. Apriletti and T.S. Scanlan, Selective modulation of thyroid hormone receptor action, *J. Ster. Biochem. Mol. Biol.* **76**, 31–42 (2001).

CHAPTER 3

ISCHEMIC PRECONDITIONING

James M. Downey, Ph.D*. and Michael V. Cohen, M.D*.

1. INTRODUCTION

Acute myocardial infarction often results in a poorly functioning left ventricle and heart failure. In general these complications are a direct result of the loss of contractile mass of the ventricle. Loss of more than 1/3 of the ventricle through infarction will overtax the remaining viable myocardium and result in remodeling and subsequent heart failure. In 1971 Braunwald and associates proposed that treatment for acute myocardial infarction should be directed at reducing the size of the resulting infarct.[1] At that time there was a poor understanding of the determinants of infarction and in retrospect the proposed strategies for limiting necrosis were clearly flawed as they were based on attempts to improve the supply/demand relationship in the face of unrestored blood flow. Nevertheless it put cardiology on a path that was to eventually lead to reperfusion therapy, and the impact of timely reperfusion of the ischemic myocardium has been enormous. The pioneering work of Jennings and colleagues revealed that myocardium dies in a progressive wave-front with the first subendocardial cells dying after only 20 minutes of ischemia but with the last cells not dying until nearly 6 hours after the onset of the occlusion.[2] Reperfusion stops this progression and salvages myocardium that would have otherwise died in the absence of reflow. Nevertheless, few patients are reperfused before an appreciable amount of muscle has been lost. Thus heart failure has not been eliminated in patients following acute myocardial infarction and there is a clear need for additional treatment to further reduce cell death in the setting of reperfusion therapy.

In the 1980s there was much interest in free radical scavengers and the use of anti-inflammatory treatment as strategies for salvaging myocardium. The hypothesis was that free radicals generated at the time of reperfusion were killing cells resulting in "reperfusion" injury. A variation on that theme was that neutrophils which were clearly concentrated in the infarct were the source of free radicals and were attacking viable myocardium. While several glowing reports using animal models appeared in the lit-

Departments of Physiology* and Medicine*, College of Medicine, University of South Alabama, Mobile Alabama, USA. Correspondence to Professor James Downey, MSB 3024, University of South Alabama, Mobile, AL 36688, USA, FAX 251 460 6818, jdowney@usouthal.edu

erature it soon became clear that these strategies were not equally effective in the hands of all investigators.[3, 4] As the animal model became more refined, the effectiveness of these interventions seemed to diminish. Today most of the evidence indicates that free radicals primarily stun the heart but do not actually kill it. Furthermore neutrophils appear to enter the infarct only after myocardial cells have died and they may play an active role in debriding the necrotic tissue and in scar formation. Investigators in the mid 1980s wondered if it would ever be possible to make the ischemic heart less vulnerable to infarction.

2. ISCHEMIC PRECONDITIONING

In 1986 our outlook changed dramatically. Charles Murry working in Robert Jennings's laboratory at Duke University described the phenomenon of ischemic preconditioning.[5] Figure 1 summarizes the results of this landmark study. Dogs exposed to 40 min of coronary arterial branch occlusion followed by reperfusion suffered infarction of about 25% of the region of the ventricle that was rendered ischemic (often termed the region at risk). However, if the 40-minute index ischemia was preceded by 4 cycles of 5-min coronary arterial occlusion, each followed by 5 min of reperfusion, infarct size was reduced to less than 10% of the risk region. The brief periods of sublethal ischemia had actually caused the heart to quickly adapt itself to a phenotype that was very resistant to infarction and other sequelae of ischemia. This was termed ischemic preconditioning (IPC). The importance of this observation was soon to be appreciated by the entire scientific community. It meant that it was indeed possible to make the heart resistant to infarction. All that remained was to determine the mechanism and design a drug that would instill this same protection in the patient with acute myocardial infarction.

Unraveling the preconditioning puzzle has been amazingly elusive. Now almost 20 years after Murry's initial observation we still do not completely understand it. That search has been hampered by the fact that we do not know what the lethal event is when ischemia kills myocardium. We assume that IPC prevents that event. Nevertheless, we have made great strides over the past 2 decades and many details of this process have been elucidated in amazing detail even if the overall scheme remains unclear. More importantly these studies are beginning to bear fruit as a new generation of powerful agents based on modification of signal transduction pathways is emerging from the preclinical studies and should soon find their way into clinical trials.

3. ISCHEMIC PRECONDITIONING IS RECEPTOR-MEDIATED

IPC was first described by Murry and colleagues in dog hearts and has since been observed in virtually all mammalian species tested including rabbits, rats, and mice, and the evidence is strong that it also occurs in man [see[6] for an extensive review of the evidence that IPC does occur in man]. The first part of IPC's mechanism to be identified involved the release of adenosine from the myocardium during the preconditioning ischemia.[7] As the ischemic heart goes into negative energy balance adenosine triphosphate (ATP) is rapidly broken down to adenosine monophosphate (AMP). Some of the AMP that accumulates within the ischemic cell is dephosphorylated to adenosine which is free to leave the cell. During the preconditioning ischemia adenosine that moves

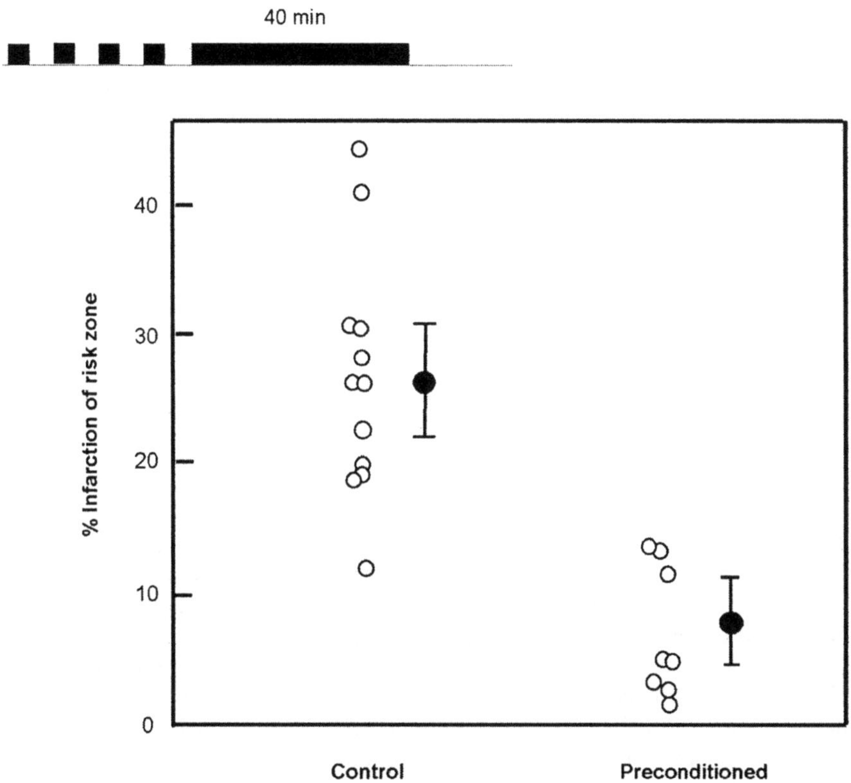

Figure 1. The original demonstration of preconditioning in open-chest dogs. Control dogs received 40 min of coronary artery occlusion plus 4 days reperfusion. In preconditioned animals the 40 min index ischemia was preceded by 4 cycles of 5-min coronary occlusion/5-min reperfusion. This caused a dramatic reduction in the percent of the ischemic tissue that infarcted. Open symbols represent individual hearts while the solid symbol shows the group mean and SEM. Adapted from Cohen.[40]

into the interstitial space populates adenosine receptors on cardiomyocytes. Adenosine receptor occupancy puts the heart into a preconditioned state that persists for approximately an hour even if the adenosine is washed away during the subsequent reperfusion cycle. It was also noted that IPC's protection was dependent on activation of an enzyme called protein kinase C (PKC).[8,9] A kinase is a signaling protein that modulates its target protein's function by phosphorylating it on a specific amino acid. Many kinases exist in the cell, each with its own specific targets. In IPC PKC was activated as a result of adenosine receptor occupation.

While the critical time for adenosine receptor activation is prior to the onset of the lethal ischemic insult (often called the index ischemia), the critical time for PKC activation is during the index ischemia and beyond.[10] Therefore, we classify receptor occupancy as a "trigger" of preconditioning while PKC activation serves as a "mediator". There are 4 known adenosine receptor subtypes. The A_{2a} and A_{2b} receptors are Gs-coupled causing an increase in cAMP within the cell. The A_1 and A_3 receptors are

Gi-coupled and act to lower cAMP. Evidence indicates that both A_1 and A_3 adenosine receptors act in parallel to trigger the preconditioned state.[11, 7]

It was subsequently shown that other Gi-coupled receptors on the cardiomyocyte, including α-1 adrenergic,[12, 13] angiotensin AT_1,[14] endothelin ET_1,[15] bradykinin B_2,[16] and δ opioid[17] receptors, were also able to trigger the preconditioned state in the heart. The protective effects of all of these receptors are dependent on PKC, and the latter two, the opioid[18] and bradykinin[19] receptors, were shown to be physiologically important in IPC. It would appear that adenosine, bradykinin, and opioid agonists are all released during the brief preconditioning ischemia and their receptors have couplings that act to activate PKC. If one of the receptor types is blocked, then a longer duration of ischemia will be required to release enough of the agonists of the other functioning receptors to cause sufficient PKC stimulation to precondition the heart. Thus blocking a single receptor does not actually prevent the ability to precondition the heart but rather simply raises the ischemic threshold needed to put the heart into a preconditioned state. This redundancy assures that the heart can be preconditioned in most circumstances.

There are six isoforms of PKC found in the myocardium and most data indicate that activation of the ε isoform is responsible for protection by IPC.[20, 21, 22] Some data suggest that PKCδ may be responsible for the protection,[23] but other data suggest that PKCδ may actually be detrimental and cause an apoptotic effect (programmed cell death) in cardiomyocytes.[24, 25] The substrate protein phosphorylated by PKCε, a potential candidate for the 'end-effector' of IPC, has not yet been identified. Many studies are focusing on the possibility that regulatory proteins associated with mitochondria are targets for PKCε.[26, 27, 28] As we will see later in this chapter the signal transduction pathways are extremely complex and PKC may well simply phosphorylate another signal transduction element and still be far upstream from the end-effector.

4. ATP-SENSITIVE POTASSIUM CHANNELS

In 1992 Garrett Gross discovered that IPC was dependent on the opening of ATP-sensitive potassium channels (K_{ATP}). These channels open when ATP levels fall in the cell. Opening of K_{ATP} channels exerts a powerful protective effect against infarction, whereas channel blockers abrogate IPC's protection.[29] These observations led to the hypothesis that preconditioning acted to open K_{ATP} channels in the heart. It was initially assumed that the target of preconditioning was the sarcolemmal K_{ATP} channel. The focus changed to the mitochondrial channel (mK_{ATP}) after Garlid et al.[30] observed that diazoxide which selectively opened this channel (EC50 ~30 μM) improved post-ischemic ventricular function by an amount similar to that of IPC. Liu et al.[31] showed that diazoxide opened mK_{ATP} in cardiomyocytes, and the drug mimicked IPC in a myocyte model of osmotic fragility. Finally, diazoxide also mimicked IPC by diminishing infarction in an intact heart, and the mK_{ATP} blocker 5-hydroxydecanoate (5HD) aborted IPC's protection.[32] These critical observations led to the proposal that it was the opening of mK_{ATP} rather than the sarcolemmal channel that was causing the cardioprotection.

The structure of mK_{ATP} is not known but it is assumed that it incorporates elements of the two known inward rectifier ATP-sensitive K^+ channel proteins, Kv6.1 or Kv6.2. All known sarcolemmal K_{ATP} channels contain 4 pore-forming channel proteins and 4 sulfonylurea-binding receptor (SUR) proteins. The SUR has the ATP binding site and, as the name implies, binds sulfonylurea compounds like glibenclamide. Sulfonylurea binding blocks the channel and thus glibenclamide has been a useful tool for testing for K_{ATP} involvement.[33] While agents like cromakalim open both sarcolemmal and mitochondrial channels, diazoxide is highly selective for the latter. Similarly 5HD blocks only the mitochondrial channels. Virtually all of our knowledge concerning mK_{ATP} in IPC is based on this pharmacology.

The mitochondria normally exclude potassium, thus creating a steep transmembrane potassium gradient. This gradient is required to maintain osmotic balance between the mitochondrial matrix and the cytosol. Opening mK_{ATP} will allow potassium to enter the matrix making it more osmotically active causing the mitochondria to swell and to be slightly uncoupled thanks to a potassium-hydrogen ion exchanger. It was originally not clear why either mitochondrial swelling or uncoupling would benefit the ischemic heart.

5. MITOCHONDRIAL K_{ATP} OPENING TRIGGERS ENTRANCE INTO THE PRECONDITIONED STATE

Opening mK_{ATP} was originally assumed to be a mediator rather than a trigger of IPC,[29] and mK_{ATP} has even been proposed to be the end-effector of protection.[34] More recently, it was shown that mK_{ATP} opening actually acts as a trigger of preconditioning. Forbes et al.[35] were the first to show that protection from the mK_{ATP} opener diazoxide is dependent on production of reactive oxygen species. Wang et al.[34] also found that a pulse of diazoxide preconditioned the rat heart although the diazoxide had been washed out prior to the index ischemia. That led Pain et al.[36] to test whether the critical time for opening of mK_{ATP} in IPC is prior to the index ischemia (and therefore acting as a trigger) or during it (and therefore acting as a mediator). They used the selective mK_{ATP} blocker 5HD and found that mK_{ATP} opening acted as a trigger rather than a mediator. Having 5HD present during the brief preconditioning ischemia and then washing it out prior to the index ischemia completely blocked IPC's protection, while starting the 5HD infusion just prior to the index ischemia had no effect on IPC's protection. They concluded that mK_{ATP} opening was acting as a trigger rather than mediator. When they repeated the experiment with a free radical scavenger they found the same behavior. Moreover, as Forbes et al.[35] had seen, the scavenger could block protection from the mK_{ATP} opener diazoxide indicating that radical generation was downstream of channel opening. They proposed that potassium entering the mitochondria caused them to produce reactive oxygen species (ROS). These ROS would then act as second messengers to activate PKC which then becomes a mediator of protection. It has been known for some time that ROS can directly activate PKC. Since the appearance of the report by Pain et al.[36] there has been widespread confirmation of the trigger roles of mK_{ATP} and ROS in preconditioning.

mK_{ATP} channels may also play a role as mediators. Wang et al.[37] found that a mK_{ATP} blocker could abort protection when given just prior to the onset of the index ischemia but that a much higher dose was required to block protection than when the drug was given during the preconditioning cycles of ischemia/reperfusion. In addition, Juhaszova et al.[38] found evidence that mK_{ATP} were both upstream and downstream of PKC in their cell model. As will be discussed below mK_{ATP} may modulate formation and/or opening of the mitochondrial permeability transition pore.

The involvement of K_{ATP} has been a matter of concern for clinicians because it is likely that some patients are actually preconditioned prior to the occurrence of a coronary thrombus. For example Kloner[39] noted that patients had better outcomes if they had angina prior to the onset of their coronary occlusion and he proposed that was because they were preconditioned by the anginal attack. A large number of coronary patients also take oral hypoglycemic drugs that are essentially K_{ATP} blockers. There has been a concern that these drugs may actually prevent any potential preconditioning effect of angina or other triggers in these patients and worsen their tolerance of a thrombosis, although that has never been proven.

6. THE TRIGGER PATHWAYS ARE DIVERGENT

It was mentioned above that at least 4 receptors, adenosine A_1/A_3, bradykinin and opioid, participate in ischemic preconditioning. Furthermore several other Gi-coupled receptors are capable of mimicking preconditioning in the presence of exogenous agonist but do not participate in the physiological response. We tested to see how many of these receptors trigger protection through a K_{ATP}/ROS-dependent pathway. Figure 2 shows that protection from a 5-min pulse of acetylcholine could be blocked if it were co-administered with either the mK_{ATP} blocker 5HD or the free radical scavenger mercaptoproprionylglycine (MPG). Bradykinin, morphine, and phenylephrine all behaved in the same manner.[40] To our surprise neither 5HD nor MPG could block protection from adenosine or the A_1-selective agonist N6-(2-phenylisopropyl) adenosine (R-PIA). Thus while bradykinin and opioids trigger protection through a pathway dependent on mK_{ATP} opening and ROS production, adenosine's pathway uses neither of these and presumably has a direct coupling to PKC, perhaps through a phospholipase C isoform. Yet all three receptor systems are dependent on PKC to mediate their protection. Figure 3 shows a diagram of these divergent trigger pathways.

The trigger pathway for the muscarinic receptor has been fairly well explored at the time of this writing and can serve as a prototype of all of the mitochondrial-dependent receptors. Figure 4 shows that the pathway between the muscarinic receptor and the mK_{ATP} is surprisingly complex. When acetylcholine binds to the receptor it causes activation of a metalloproteinase which cleaves heparin-binding epidermal growth factor (HB-EGF) from membrane-bound proHB-EGF. The HB-EGF fragment then binds to the epidermal growth factor (EGF) receptor.[41, 42] That causes formation of a signaling unit comprising the EGF receptor, Src, and phosphatidylinositol –3 kinase (PI3 kinase). The activated PI3 kinase phosphorylates membrane phosphoinositide in its 3 position which activates the phospholipid dependent kinases PDK1 and PDK2. These phosphorylate and activate Akt.

Activated Akt then phosphorylates eNOS.[43] When phosphorylated, eNOS synthesizes nitric oxide from arginine. The nitric oxide acts as a second messenger to cause guanylyl cyclase to make cGMP. The cGMP also acts as a diffusible second messenger and causes activation of protein kinase G (PKG).[44, 45] Phosphorylation of mitochondrial proteins by PKG results in mK_{ATP} opening and ROS production by the mitochondria.[46] ROS presumably act as additional second messengers to activate PKC. Evidence suggests that the pathway for the δ opioid receptor is virtually identical to that for the muscarinic receptor in the rabbit heart.[44] While bradykinin also signals through Akt[43] and eNOS,[44] we were unable to show any involvement with the EGF receptor or a

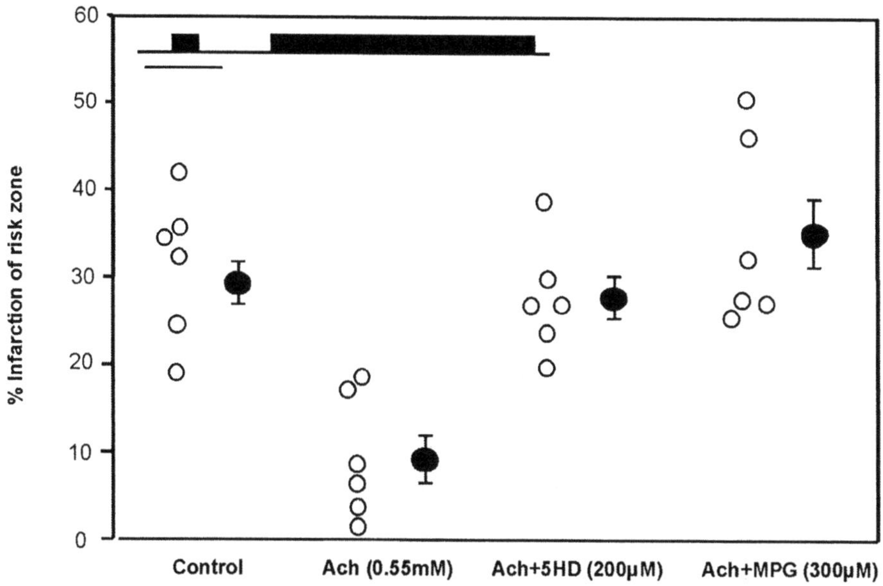

Figure 2. Infarct size is shown for rabbit hearts exposed to 30 min of regional ischemia and 2 h of reperfusion. A 5-min infusion of intracoronary acetylcholine followed by 10 min of washout puts the heart into a protected state. If the mK_{ATP} blocker 5HD or a ROS scavenger mercaptoproprionylglycine (MPG) is infused to bracket the acetylcholine pulse (see horizontal bar in the protocol diagram), protection is blocked. Adapted from[11]

metalloproteinase (unpublished observation). It is currently not known how bradykinin activates PI3 kinase.

There are alternative explanations of how the muscarinic receptor activates PI3 kinase. Tong et al.[47] propose that the coupling somehow involves receptor internalization as transgenic mutant mice in which receptor internalization was blocked could not be preconditioned. Miura's group proposes that the metalloproteinase liberates TNF rather than EGF.[48] In our rabbit cardiomyocyte model, however, the evidence for EGF coupling seems very strong.[49]

The complexity of these pathways is quite remarkable. One of the big surprises for us was the clear presence of nitric oxide in the trigger pathway. It has been known for some time that nitric oxide donors could precondition the isolated rabbit heart, although eNOS blockade with L-NAME did not block IPC in that model.[50] On the other hand, Lochner and colleagues have presented evidence for nitric oxide involvement in IPC in rat.[51] Mapping these pathways with receptor-specific agonists reveals the answer to these seemingly discrepant findings. IPC in the isolated rabbit heart is almost exclusively triggered by adenosine since there are no kininogens in the perfusate to make bradykinin and an intact innervation seems to be required for opioid release.[17] Since adenosine receptors use a nitric oxide-independent pathway, the eNOS blocker would have had no effect against IPC in the isolated rabbit heart. Elucidation of these pathways has revealed many ways in which we can pharmacologically precondition the heart. Of course, all of these agents that are involved in the trigger pathway have to be given prior to ischemia.

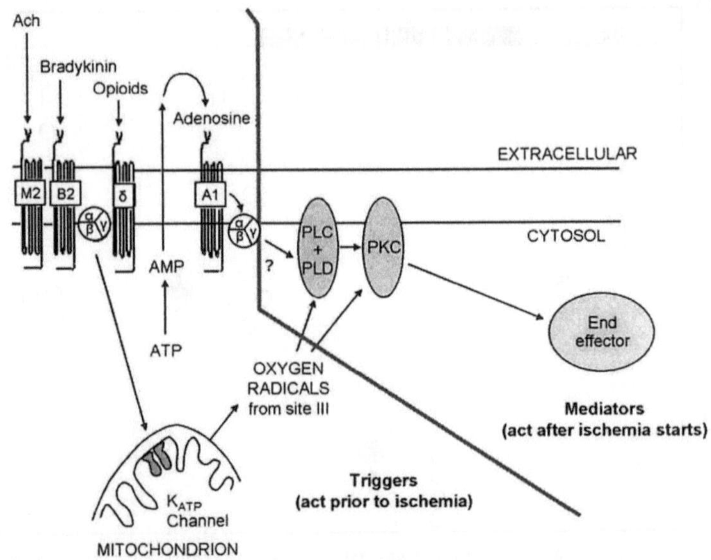

Figure 3. A diagram showing that bradykinin and opioid receptors precondition the rabbit heart through a pathway dependent on mK_{ATP} opening and oxygen radical production, while adenosine receptors do not. Yet all 3 receptors depend on PKC to mediate the protection. Note that everything prior to radical production is a trigger, while PKC acts as a mediator.

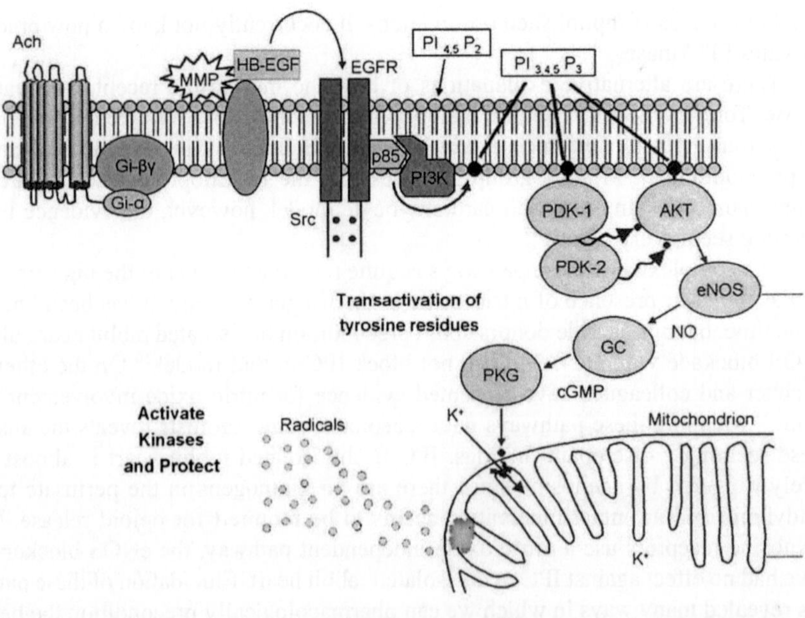

Figure 4. A flow diagram showing the signal transduction steps that couple the muscarinic receptor to the mK_{ATP} in a rabbit cardiomyocyte. Note the complexity of the pathway. See text for a detailed explanation.

7. IPC APPEARS TO EXERT ITS PROTECTION DURING REPERFUSION BY PREVENTING MPT PORE OPENING

An explanation of how IPC actually protects against infarction has been remarkably elusive. A number of hypotheses have been proposed including reduced free radical production at reperfusion, reduced osmotic swelling, reduced apoptosis, and reduced Ca^{2+} overload.[6] There is recent evidence that IPC's protection is mediated, at least in part, by preventing the formation of the mitochondrial permeability transition (MPT) pore. This high-conductance pore forms in the mitochondrial membrane during reperfusion, and when open creates a direct channel between the cytosol and the mitochondrial matrix. Channel opening acts to depolarize the matrix thus stopping energy production. The two factors known to induce MPT formation and opening are free radicals and calcium, both of which are present in reperfused myocardium. MPT opening also allows the release of cytochrome c into the cytosol which can promote apoptosis.

Recently Yellon's group has provided convincing evidence that IPC could be acting to prevent MPT pore opening during the reperfusion period. Infusion of the MPT blocker cyclosporine A at reperfusion following 35 min of ischemia mimicked the effect of IPC and protected isolated rat hearts against infarction. By contrast, infusion of atractyloside (an MPT promoter) at reperfusion in IPC-treated or pharmacologically preconditioned hearts blocked protection.[52] Along these same lines, Argaud et al.[53] found that mitochondria isolated from the ischemic zone of preconditioned hearts were much more resistant to calcium-triggered MPT formation than those from nonpreconditioned hearts. Together these results suggest that IPC protects against infarction by keeping the MPT pore closed during reperfusion.

Yellon's group also observed that activation of PI-3 kinase was critical to protecting IPC hearts at reperfusion.[54] They found that PI3 kinase or ERK 1/2 blockers given at the time of reperfusion following the index ischemia blocked IPC's anti-infarct effect but had no effect on non-preconditioned hearts. This suggests that IPC is actually exerting its protective effect during the reperfusion period rather than during ischemia. The assumption is that survival kinases, including ERK 1/2, PI3 kinase and its downstream target Akt, are steps in pathways that act to prevent MPT pore formation during reperfusion resulting in protection.

Somehow activation of PKC during ischemia causes the heart to activate ERK 1/2 and Akt during the critical first minutes of the reperfusion period. Little is known about how these kinases are arranged or how they are activated in the preconditioned heart. Juhaszova et al.[38] recently investigated isolated rat cardiomyocytes that were subjected to hypoxia/reoxygenation. MPT opening was monitored by measuring mitochondrial potential with a voltage-dependent dye, tetramethylrhodamine methyl ester (TMRM). They described a trigger pathway dependent on ROS and a mediator pathway containing PI3 kinase and ERK. They proposed that all of these converge on a kinase called GSK3β which then directly modulates MPT opening. They also found evidence that mK_{ATP} opening also inhibits MPT opening which may explain the additional mediator role of mK_{ATP}. Weiss and co-workers have also described a modulating role of mK_{ATP} on MPT opening.[55]

The molecular structure of the MPT pore is not fully understood either. Current evidence suggests that two proteins, the voltage-dependent anion channel (VDAC), located in the outer mitochondrial membrane, and the adenine nucleotide translocase (ANT-1), located in the inner mitochondrial membrane, combine to form a pore that spans both membranes.

8. DRUGS THAT PROTECT AT REPERFUSION TARGET THE SAME PATHWAYS AS IPC

The report by the Yellon group that IPC exerts its protection not during the ischemic period but rather in the first minutes of reperfusion caused a paradigm shift in our thinking about IPC. The clear implication is that the heart can still be treated at the time of reperfusion. IPC has had little clinical impact because patients with acute myocardial infarction usually present in clinic after the index ischemia has begun. Thus it is too late to precondition them. However, if the pathways that prevent MPT opening could be activated at the time of reperfusion, it should still be possible to protect those hearts. Through empirical screening a number of agents have recently been identified that are capable of protecting the ischemic heart when given at reperfusion including intracoronary insulin,[56] the A_1/A_2 adenosine agonists AMP579[57] and NECA,[58] TGF-β1,[59] urocortin,[60] bradykinin,[61, 58] CGX1051,[62] atorvastatin,[63] and very recently erythropoietin.[64] A unique feature of all of these agents is that their protection depends on activation of PI3 kinase and/or ERK. Accordingly, the latter kinases have been referred to as reperfusion injury salvage kinases (RISK).[54] Based on the available evidence it appears these agents activate the same pathways that are involved during reperfusion in IPC. Activation of PI3 kinase and ERK by these agents presumably exerts a powerful inhibition of the MPT pore.

9. DOES REPERFUSION INJURY EXIST?

The evidence that IPC exerts its protection in the reperfusion period and the fact that certain drugs that modulate the survival kinases can protect the heart when given at reperfusion has revived the concept of reperfusion injury. In 1985 Braunwald and Kloner proposed that events early in reperfusion act to kill previously ischemic heart muscle.[65] Yet reperfusion is required if survival is to occur. Reperfusion injury was originally proposed to result from reperfusion-induced free radicals and/or calcium entry. The term fell out of favor because it could not be proven that a free radical scavenger could actually limit infarct size. Now attention has turned to the MPT pore.

Is MPT opening truly the initial event of reperfusion injury or is it just an injured myocyte's response to reintroduction of oxygen? The question is largely one of semantics. The myocyte must first be injured by ischemia before it will respond to reintroduction of oxygen with MPT formation. Weiss et al.[66] refer to this as the "priming phase". Fortunately it appears that appropriate therapy can prevent MPT opening even if the myocyte has been primed. Thus as the heart emerges from ischemia we believe it contains 3 populations of cells. The first is dead and cannot be revived, the second has experienced sublethal injury during ischemia and will survive without intervention. The third is still alive but has undergone sufficient injury that MPT will open with reperfusion and it is that population which likely is targeted by IPC.

10. CLINICAL IMPLICATIONS

The future for cardioprotection currently looks very bright. Animal studies are revealing more and more interventions capable of preventing infarction when administered at the time of reperfusion. Some of these like AMP579, erythropoietin, or CGX1051 could easily be given parenterally to a patient with an ischemic heart. Others like insulin have problematic side effects that complicate their clinical use. While we, like others, found insulin to be very protective in the isolated heart, parenteral administration causes a precipitous drop in blood sugar and thus it must be co-administered with glucose. We have not been successful in finding a protective dose of insulin for the in situ rabbit heart (unpublished observation). Bradykinin causes hypotension and could only be given by the intracoronary route.

The biggest obstacle that must be overcome at present is the reluctance of the pharmaceutical industry to develop these drugs. Unfortunately a cardioprotective drug can only be used in a relatively small market since only about 500,000 candidate patients with acute myocardial infarction per year come to the hospital in the United States. Each of these patients would receive only a single dose of the drug at the time of reperfusion. Furthermore, since mortality is low in this group, a large number of patients would have to be treated to show a survival benefit and thus the phase 2 trials would be very expensive with expectation of only a modest return on the investment. Finally, industry has already invested a tremendous amount of money in this area and has little to show for it. The most recent example was the negative GUARDIAN trial in which Aventis tested whether cariporide could protect ischemic hearts.[67] Most of the animal studies with cariporide failed to demonstrate any protective effect when given at reperfusion, and it is therefore not surprising that the drug was not effective when given to patients with unstable angina. It was only found to be protective in the surgical setting where pretreatment could be provided.

In retrospect virtually all of the past clinical trials of cardioprotective agents have been based on flawed, unconvincing preclinical data. Drugs such as free radical scavengers and anti-inflammatory agents gave very discrepant results in animal studies. While some investigators reported cardioprotection, many others had negative results.[4] Enthusiasm generally caused industry to ignore those warning signs. Thus it was not surprising that those agents failed to perform in clinical trials. Fortunately the technology has greatly improved since then. AMP579, for example, has been found to be very protective in every laboratory that has tested it. Hopefully industry can be convinced that they should throw the dice one more time and begin trials with this new generation of cardioprotectants. They must select agents for which the preclinical data are both solid and thorough and they must adhere to doses and schedules that have been verified in animal studies.

REFERENCES

1. P. R. Maroko, J. K. Kjekshus, B. E. Sobel, T. Watanabe, J. W. Covell, J. Jr. Ross, and E. Braunwald, Factors influencing infarct size following experimental coronary artery occlusions, *Circulation* **43**, 67–82, (1971).
2. K. A. Reimer, J. E. Lowe, M. M. Rassmussen and R. B. Jennings, The wavefront phenomenon of ischemic cell death. I. Myocardial infarct size vs. duration of coronary occlusion in dogs, *Circulation* **56**, 786–794, (1977).
3. R. A. Kloner, K. Przyklenk and P. Whittaker, Deleterious effects of oxygen radicals in ischemia/reperfusion: resolved and unresolved issues, *Circulation* **80**, 1115–1127, (1989).
4. K. A. Reimer, C. E. Murry and C. E. Richard, The role of neutrophils and free radicals in the ischemic-reperfused heart: why the confusion and controversy? *J Mol Cell Cardiol* **21**, 1225–1239, (1989).
5. C. E. Murry, R. B. Jennings and K. A. Reimer, Preconditioning with ischemia: a delay of lethal cell injury in ischemic myocardium, *Circulation* **74**, 1124–1136, (1986).

6. D. M. Yellon and J. M. Downey, Preconditioning the myocardium: from cellular physiology to clinical cardiology, *Physiol Rev* **83**, 1113–1151, (2003).
7. G. S. Liu, J. Thornton, D. M. Van Winkle, A. W. H. Stanley, R. A. Olsson and J. M. Downey, Protection against infarction afforded by preconditioning is mediated by A1 adenosine receptors in rabbit heart, *Circulation* **84**, 350–356, (1991).
8. P. Ping, J. Zhang, Y. Qiu, X.-L. Tang, S. Manchikalapudi, X. Cao and R. Bolli, Ischemic preconditioning induces selective translocation of protein kinase C isoforms ε and η in the heart of conscious rabbits without subcellular redistribution of total protein kinase C activity, *Circ Res* **81**, 404–414, (1997).
9. K. Ytrehus, Y. Liu and J. M. Downey, Preconditioning protects ischemic rabbit heart by protein kinase C activation, *Am J Physiol* **266**, H1145–H1152, (1994).
10. X.-M. Yang, H. Sato, J. M. Downey and M. V. Cohen, Protection of ischemic preconditioning is dependent upon a critical timing sequence of protein kinase C activation, *J Mol Cell Cardiol* **29**, 991–999, (1997).
11. Liu GS, S. C. Richards, R, A. Olsson, K. Mullane, R. S. Walsh and J. M. Downey, Evidence that the adenosine A3 receptor may mediate the protection afforded by preconditioning in the isolated rabbit heart, *Cardiovasc Res* **28**, 1057–1061, (1994).
12. A. Banerjee, C. Locke-Winter, K. B. Rogers, M. B. Mitchell, E. C. Brew, C.B. Cairns, D. D. Bensard and A. H. Harken, Preconditioning against myocardial dysfunction after ischemia and reperfusion by an α1-adrenergic mechanism, *Circ Res* **73**, 656–670, (1993).
13. J. D. Thornton, J. F. Daly, M. V. Cohen, X.-M. Yang and J. M. Downey, Catecholamines can induce adenosine receptor-mediated protection of the myocardium but do not participate in ischemic preconditioning in the rabbit, *Circ Res* **73**, 649–655, (1993).
14. Y. Liu, A. Tsuchida, M. V. Cohen and J. M. Downey, Pretreatment with angiotensin II activates protein kinase C and limits myocardial infarction in isolated rabbit hearts, *J Mol Cell Cardiol* **27**, 883–892, (1995).
15. P. Wang, K. Gallagher, J. M. Downey, and M. V. Cohen, Endothelin-1 limits myocardial infarction through PKC activation, *J Mol Cell Cardiol* **27**, A44. (1995). Ref Type: Abstract
16. T. M. Wall, R. Sheehy and J. C. Hartman, Role of bradykinin in myocardial preconditioning, *J Pharmacol Exp Ther* **270**, 681–689, (1994).
17. T. Miki, M. V. Cohen and J.M. Downey, Opioid receptor contributes to ischemic preconditioning through protein kinase C activation in rabbits, *Mol Cell Biochem* **186**, 3–12, (1998).
18. J. E.J. Schultz, E. Rose, Z. Yao and G. J. Gross, Evidence for involvement of opioid receptors in ischemic preconditioning in rat hearts, *Am J Physiol* **268**, H2157–H2161, (1995).
19. M. Goto, Y. Liu, X.-M. Yang, J. L. Ardell, M. V. Cohen and J. M. Downey, Role of bradykinin in protection of ischemic preconditioning in rabbit hearts, *Circ Res* **77**, 611–621, (1995).
20. S. Kawamura, K. Yoshida, T. Miura, Y. Mizukami and M. Matsuzaki, Ischemic preconditioning translocates PKC-δ and -ε, which mediate functional protection in isolated rat heart, *Am J Physiol* **275**, H2266–H2271, (1998).
21. G. S. Liu, Cohen MV, Mochly-Rosen D and Downey JM. Protein kinase C-ε is responsible for the protection of preconditioning in rabbit cardiomyocytes, J Mol Cell Cardiol 31, 1937–1948, (1999).
22. Y. Qiu, P. Ping, X.-L. Tang, S. Manchikalapudi, A. Rizvi, J. Zhang, H. Takano, W.-J. Wu, S. Teschner and R. Bolli, Direct evidence that protein kinase C plays an essential role in the development of late preconditioning against myocardial stunning in conscious rabbits and that ε is the isoform involved, *J Clin Invest* **101**, 2182–2198, (1998).
23. J. Zhao, O. Renner, L. Wightman, P. H. Sugden, L. Stewart, A. D. Miller, D. S. Latchman and M. S. Marber, The expression of constitutively active isotypes of protein kinase C to investigate preconditioning, *J Biol Chem* **273**, 23072–23079, (1998).
24. L. Chen, H. Hahn, G. Wu, C.-H. Chen, T. Liron, D. Schechtman, G. Cavallaro, L. Banci, Y. Guo, R. Bolli, G. W. I. Dorn and D. Mochly-Rosen, Opposing cardioprotective actions and parallel hypertrophic effects of δPKC and εPKC, *Proc Natl Acad Sci* **98**, 11114–11119, (2001).
25. C. L. Murriel, E. Churchill, K. Inagaki, L. I. Szweda and D. Mochly-Rosen, Protein kinase Cdelta activation induces apoptosis in response to cardiac ischemia and reperfusion damage: a mechanism involving BAD and the mitochondria, *J Biol Chem* **279**, 47985–47991, (2004).
26. C. P. Baines, C. X. Song, Y. T. Zheng, G. W. Wang, J. Zhang, O. L. Wang, Y. Guo, R. Bolli, E. M. Cardwell and P. Ping, Protein kinase Cepsilon interacts with and inhibits the permeability transition pore in cardiac mitochondria, *Circ Res* **92**, 873–880, (2003).

27. T. Sato, B. O'Rourke and E. Marbán, Modulation of mitochondrial ATP-dependent K^+ channels by protein kinase C,. *Circ Res* **83**, 110–114, (1998).
28. Y. Wang and M. Ashraf, Role of protein kinase C in mitochondrial K_{ATP} channel-mediated protection against Ca2+ overload injury in rat myocardium, *Circ Res* **84**, 1156–1165, (1999).
29. G. J. Gross and J. A. Auchampach, Blockade of ATP-sensitive potassium channels prevents myocardial preconditioning in dogs, *Circ Res* **70**, 223–233, (1992).
30. K. D. Garlid, P. Paucek, V. Yarov-Yarovoy, H. N. Murray, R. B. Darbenzio, A. J. D'Alonzo, N. J. Lodge, M. A. Smith and G. J. Grover, Cardioprotective effect of diazoxide and its interaction with mitochondrial ATP-sensitive K^+ channels: possible mechanism of cardioprotection, *Circ Res* **81**, 1072–1082, (1997).
31. Y. Liu, T. Sato, B. O'Rourke and E. Marban, Mitochondrial ATP-dependent potassium channels: novel effectors of cardioprotection? *Circulation* **97**, 2463–2469, (1998).
32. C. P. Baines, G. S. Liu, M. Birincioglu, S. D. Critz, M. V. Cohen and J. M. Downey, Ischemic preconditioning depends on interaction between mitochondrial K_{ATP} channels and actin cytoskeleton, *Am J Physiol* **276**, H1361–H1368, (1999).
33. N. Inagaki, T. Gonoi, J. P. Clement, C. Z. Wang, L. Aguilar-Bryan, J. Bryan and S. Seino, A family of sulfonylurea receptors determines the pharmacological properties of ATP-sensitive K^+ channels, *Neuron* **16**, 1011–1017, (1996).
34. Y. Wang, K. Hirai and M. Ashraf, Activation of mitochondrial ATP-sensitive K+ channel for cardiac protection against ischemic injury is dependent on protein kinase C activity, *Circ Res* **85**, 731–741, (1999).
35. R. A. Forbes, C. Steenbergen and E. Murphy, Diazoxide-induced cardioprotection requires signaling through a redox-sensitive mechanism, *Circ Res* **88**, 802–809, (2001).
36. T. Pain, X.-M. Yang, S. D. Critz, Y. Yue, A. Nakano, G. S. Liu, G. Heusch, M. V. Cohen and J. M. Downey, Opening of mitochondrial K_{ATP} channels triggers the preconditioned state by generating free radicals, *Circ Res* **87**, 460–466, (2000).
37. S. Wang, J. Cone and Y. Liu, Dual roles of mitochondrial K_{ATP} channels in diazoxide-mediated protection in isolated rabbit hearts, *Am J Physiol* **280**, H246–H255, (2001).
38. M. Juhaszova, D. B. Zorov, S.-H. Kim, S. Pepe, Q. Fu, K. W. Fishbein, B. D. Ziman, S. Wang, K. Ytrehus, C. L. Antos, E. N. Olson and S. J. Sollott, Glycogen synthase kinase-3β mediates convergence of protection signaling to inhibit the mitochondrial permeability transition pore, *J Clin Invest* **113**, 1535–1549, (2004).
39. R. A. Kloner, T. Shook, K. Przyklenk,V. G. Davis, L. Junio, R. V. Matthews, S. Burstein, C. M. Gibson, W. K. Poole, C. P. Cannon, C. H. McCabe and E. Braunwald, Previous angina alters in-hospital outcome in TIMI 4: a clinical correlate to preconditioning? *Circulation* **91**, 37–45, (1995).
40. M. V. Cohen, X.-M. Yang, G. S. Liu, G. Heusch and J. M. Downey, Acetylcholine, bradykinin, opioids, and phenylephrine, but not adenosine, trigger preconditioning by generating free radicals and opening mitochondrial K_{ATP} channels, *Circ Res* **89**, 273–278, (2001).
41. T. Krieg, M. Landsberger, M. F. Alexeyev, S. B. Felix, M. V. Cohen and J. M. Downey, Activation of Akt is essential for acetylcholine to trigger generation of oxygen free radicals, *Cardiovasc Res* **58**, 196–202, (2003).
42. T. Krieg, Q. Qin, E. C. McIntosh, M. V. Cohen and J. M. Downey, ACh and adenosine activate PI3-kinase in rabbit hearts through transactivation of receptor tyrosine kinases, *Am J Physiol* **283**, H2322–H2330, (2002).
43. T. Krieg, Q. Qin, S. Philipp, M. F. Alexeyev, M. V. Cohen and J. M. Downey, Acetylcholine and bradykinin trigger preconditioning in the heart through a pathway that includes Akt and NOS, *Am J Physiol* **287**, H2606–H2611, (2004).
44. O. Oldenburg, Q. Qin, T. Krieg, X.-M. Yang, S. Philipp, S. D. Critz, M. V. Cohen and J. M. Downey, Bradykinin induces mitochondrial ROS generation via NO, cGMP, PKG, and mitoK_{ATP} channel opening and leads to cardioprotection, *Am J Physiol* **286**, H468–H476, (2004).
45. Q. Qin, X.-M. Yang, L. Cui, S. D. Critz, M. V. Cohen, N. C. Browner, T. M. Lincoln and J. M. Downey, Exogenous NO triggers preconditioning via a cGMP- and mitoK_{ATP}-dependent mechanism, *Am J Physiol* **287**, H712–H718, (2004).
46. K. D. Garlid, A. D. Costa, M. V. Cohen, J. M. Downey, and S. D. Critz, Cyclic GMP and PKG activate mito K_{ATP} channels in isolated mitochondrial, *Cardiovasc J S Afr* **15** (Suppl 1), S5. (2004).
47. H. Tong, H. A. Rockman, W. J. Koch, C. Steenbergen and E. Murphy, G protein-coupled receptor internalization signaling is required for cardioprotection in ischemic preconditioning, *Circ Res* **94**, 1133–1141, (2004).

48. Y. Ichikawa, T. Miura, A. Nakano, T. Miki, Y. Nakamura, K. Tsuchihashi and K. Shimamoto, The role of ADAM protease in the tyrosine kinase-mediated trigger mechanism of ischemic preconditioning, *Cardiovasc Res* **62**, 167–175, (2004).
49. Mitochondrial ROS generation following achetylcholine-induced EGF receptor transactivation requires metalloproteinase cleavage of proHB-EGF, *J Mol Cell Cardiol* **36**, 435–443, (2004).
50. A. Nakano, G. S. Liu, G. Heusch, J. M. Downey and M. V. Cohen, Exogenous nitric oxide can trigger a preconditioned state through a free radical mechanism, but endogenous nitric oxide is not a trigger of classical ischemic preconditioning, *J Mol Cell Cardiol* **32**, 1159–1167, (2000).
51. A. Lochner, E. Marais, S. Genade and J. A. Moolman, Nitric oxide: a trigger for classic preconditioning? *Am J Physiol* **279**, H2752–H2765, (2000).
52. D. J. Hausenloy, H. L. Maddock, G. F. Baxter and D. M. Yellon, Inhibiting mitochondrial permeability transition pore opening: a new paradigm for myocardial preconditioning? *Cardiovasc Res* **55**, 534–543, (2002).
53. L. Argaud, O. Gateau-Roesch, L. Chalabreysse, L. Gomez, J. Loufouat, F. Thivolet-Bejui, D. Robert and M. Ovize, Preconditioning delays Ca^{2+}-induced mitochondrial permeability transition, *Cardiovasc Res* **61**, 115–122 (2004).
54. D. J. Hausenloy and D. M. Yellow, New directions for protecting the heart against ischaemia-reperfusion injury: targeting the Reperfusion Injury Salvage Kinase (RISK)-pathway, *Cardiovasc Res* **61**, 448–460, (2004).
55. P. Korge, H. M. Honda and J. N. Weiss, Protection of cardiac mitochondria by diazoxide and protein kinase C: implications for ischemic preconditioning, *Proc Natl Acad Sci USA* **99**, 3312–3317, (2002).
56. A. K. Jonassen, M. N. Sack, O. D. Mjøs and D. M. Yellon, Myocardial protection by insulin at reperfusion requires early administration and is mediated via Akt and p70s6 kinase cell-survival signaling, *Circ Res* **89**, 1191–1198, (2001).
57. Z. Xu, X.-M. Yang, M. V. Cohen, T. Neumann, G. Heusch and J. M. Downey, Limitation of infarct size in rabbit hearts by the novel adenosine receptor agonist AMP 579 administered at reperfusion, *J Mol Cell Cardiol* **32**, 2339–2347, (2000).
58. X.-M. Yang, T. Krieg, L. Cui, J. M. Downey and M. V. Cohen, NECA and bradykinin at reperfusion reduce infarction in rabbit hearts by signaling through PI3K, ERK, and NO, *J Mol Cell Cardiol* **36**, 411–421, (2004).
59. G. F. Baxter, M. M. Mocanu, B. K. Brar, D. S. Latchman and D. M. Yellon, Cardioprotective effects of transforming growth factor-β1 during early reoxygenation or reperfusion are mediated by p42/p44 MAPK, *J Cardiovasc Pharmacol* **38**, 930–939, (2001).
60. D. Schulman, D. S. Latchman and D. M. Yellon, Urocortin protects the heart from reperfusion injury via upregulation of p42/p44 MAPK signaling pathway, *Am J Physiol* **283**, H1481–H1488, (2002).
61. R. M. Bell and D. M. Yellon, Bradykinin limits infarction when administered as an adjunct to reperfusion in mouse heart: the role of PI3K, Akt and eNOS, *J Mol Cell Cardiol* **35**, 185–193, (2003).
62. S. J. Zhang, X.-M. Yang, G. S. Liu, M. V. Cohen, K. Pemberton and J. M. Downey, CGX-1051, a peptide from Conus snail venom, attenuates infarction in rabbit hearts when administered at reperfusion, *J Cardiovasc Pharmacol* **42**, 764–771, (2003).
63. R. M. Bell and D. M. Yellon, Atorvastatin, administered at the onset of reperfusion, and independent of lipid lowering, protects the myocardium by up-regulating a pro-survival pathway, *J Am Coll Cardiol* **41**, 508–515, (2003).
64. C. J. Parsa, J. Kim, R. U. Riel, L. S. Pascal, R. B. Thompson, J. A. Petrofski, A. Matsumoto, J. S. Stamler and W. J. Koch, Cardioprotective effects of erythropoietin in the reperfused ischemic heart: a potential role for cardiac fibroblasts, *J Biol Chem* **279**, 20655–20662, (2004).
65. E. Braunwald and R. A. Kloner. Myocardial reperfusion: a double-edged sword? *J Clin Invest* **76**, 1713–1719, (1985).
66. J. N. Weiss, P. Korge, H. M. Honda and P. Ping, Role of the mitochondrial permeability transition in myocardial disease, *Circ Res* **93**, 292–301, (2003).
67. B. R. Chaitman, A review of the GUARDIAN trial results: clinical implications and the significance of elevated perioperative CK-MB on 6-month survival, *J Card Surg 18 Suppl* **1**, 13–20, (2003).

CHAPTER 4

CONNEXIN 43 AND ISCHEMIC PRECONDITIONING

Rainer Schulz, M.D., Gerd Heusch, M.D.

1. INTRODUCTION

In the heart, gap junctions play an essential role for normal contractile function, since through them major ionic fluxes between adjacent cardiomyocytes are spread, thereby allowing electrical synchronization of contraction. Each single gap junction is composed of 12 connexin 43 (Cx43) units, assembled in two hexameric connexons (hemichannels) which are contributed one each by the two participating cells[1]. Most gap junctions are located at the cells terminal intercalated disks, but they also exist at the lateral sarcolemma. A transmural gradient of Cx43 and thus gap junction expression exists across the left ventricular wall[2,3], with a higher expression in the endocardium than in the epicardium[4]. Gap junctions propagate the electrical activity in the longitudinal and transversal direction[3], and conductance in pairs of mice myocytes is similar in end-to-end (longitudinal) or side-to-side (transversal) connections[5]. Some unopposed connexons are also located at the lateral sarcolemma and connect the intracellular and extracellular space. Until recently these so-called hemichannels were thought to remain permanently closed in order to avoid cell death[6]; new data, however, have documented the existence of regulated hemichannel opening in cultured cells[7]. Hemichannels appear to be involved in cellular responses such as the release of cytosolic components, e.g. NAD+ and ATP[8], activation of cell survival pathways[9] and volume regulation[10].

Cx43 has four transmembrane, two extracellular and three cytosolic (including the amino and carboxy terminus) domains; the residues 1-242 form the plasma channel portion, while the residues 243-382 form the cytosolic tail of Cx43[11]. The length of the cytosolic tail of Cx43 slightly varies between different species and tissues[12].

Connexins interact with other proteins within the cell. Recent studies suggest an association between Cx43 and the peripheral membrane protein ZO-1 in rat cardiomyocytes.[13] ZO-1 – in turn - binds to α-spectrin, a protein which is highly expressed at

---

Institut für Pathophysiologie, Zentrum für Innere Medizin, Universitätsklinikum Essen, 45122 Essen, Germany.
Address for correspondence: Prof. Dr. med. Rainer Schulz, Institut für Pathophysiologie, Zentrum für Innere Medizin, Universitätsklinikum Essen, Hufelandstraße 55, 45122 Essen, Germany, Phone: +49 201 723 4521, FAX: +49 201 723 4481, e-mail: rainer_schulz@uni-essen.de

the intercalated disk[13,14]. Furthermore, Cx43 co-localizes with fibroblast growth factor (FGF) receptors[15] and cytoskeletal proteins[7,16].

2. REGULATION OF HEMICHANNELS AND GAP JUNCTIONS

Cx43-formed hemichannels are not ion-selective[17] and are permeable to organic ions and molecules of a molecular weight of less than 1000 Da and a maximal diameter of approximately 1.5 nm. The transport of ions and small molecules through hemichannels and gap junctions is mediated by passive diffusion and thus depends on the concentration difference between connected cells and the electrical charge of the moving ions or molecules. The transfer of ions and small molecules further depends on the number of available channels (assembly), their open-probability[18] and the individual channel conductance. The number of available channels depends on the synthesis, transport, half-life and breakdown of Cx43[7].

Cx43-formed gap junctions exhibit three conductance states: one of 20-30 pS, one of 40-60 pS and one of 70-100 pS.[1,19,20] The conductance of Cx43-formed hemichannels ranges from 31 to 352 pS.[21] More recently, the conductance of fully open hemichannels in HeLa-cells was found to be 220 pS; however, also a sub-state of approximately 75 pS exists between the fully open and the closed state,[22] suggesting that hemichannel conductance can be regulated as well.

On Western blot, Cx43 exhibits three bands with molecular weights ranging from 41 kDa to 46 kDa depending on the number and epitopes being phosphorylated.[23-26]

Single channel conductance as well as cell-cell conductance and permeability can be modulated by the intracellular pH, the intracellular calcium or ATP concentrations and the phosphorylation status of Cx43 (for details, see[27-29]). However, single channel conductance and cell-cell conductance can be affected in the opposite direction. Cell-cell conductance in the presence of decreased single channel conductance might nevertheless be increased by increased single channel open-probability or increased channel assembly. Furthermore, regulatory mechanisms can have opposite effects on cell-cell electrical coupling and dye transfer if they have divergent effects on single channel open-probability and channel pore size.[30,31] Finally, regulatory mechanisms interact and depend on the prevailing circumstances, since acidosis in normal hearts reduces dye transfer between cardiomyocytes, while the same level of acidosis during ischemia does not.[32] Protein kinases and phosphatases, which are involved in the regulation of single channel conductance and cell-cell conductance and permeability, are (figure 1):

2.1. Protein kinase A (PKA).

Cyclic adenosine monophosphate (cAMP) activates PKA, which in turn phosphorylates Cx43 in rat cardiomyocytes.[33] Increases in the cAMP concentration increase electrical conductance between paired cardiomyocytes[31,34,35] and increase cell permeability – assessed as dye transfer – in non-cardiomyocytes.[36-38] Apart from increased cell-cell conductance and permeability, cAMP also increases the extent of gap junction formation.[36-38] Increased cAMP concentration results from its enhanced production following stimulation of adenyl cyclase or from inhibition of phosphodiesterase III secondary to an increased concentration of cyclic guanosine monophosphate (cGMP).[39-41]

2.2. cGMP-dependent protein kinases (PKG).

At a higher concentration, cGMP activates PKG (for review, see[40]). cGMP decreases single channel conductance in rat cardiomyocytes[20,31] as well as cell-cell conductance[20,31,34] and permeability.[31]

2.3. Protein kinase C (PKC).

PKC isoforms (α and ε) form signaling complexes with Cx43[42,43] and phosphorylate Cx43 in cardiomyocytes,[44-46] resulting in decreased single channel conductance and cell-cell permeability.[30,31] On the other hand, electrical conductance between paired cardiomyocytes is increased following PKC activation,[30,31,47] which could be explained by differences in the single channel open-probability and pore size following channel phosphorylation.

2.4. Protein tyrosine kinase (PTK).

PTK – such as the src kinase – phosphorylates tyrosine residues 247 and 265 of Cx43. In paired rat cardiomyocytes, permeability is reduced with phosphorylation of Cx43 by PTK.[44,48] Phosphorylation of Cx43 at its tyrosine residue 265 reduces the binding of Cx43 to ZO-1 and subsequently the expression of Cx43 at the intercalated disks.[49] Reduced intercellular communication following lipopolysaccharide administration is related to Cx43 phosphorylation at tyrosine residues.[50]

2.5. Mitogen activated protein kinases (MAPKs).

More recently, MAPKs such as ERK,[51-54] BMK-1,[55] p38[43,51] and JNK[56,57] have been implicated in the regulation of Cx43 phosphorylation. BMK-1 phosphorylates the serine residue 255 of Cx43,[55] while other MAPKs contribute to Cx43 phosphorylation of the serine residues 279 and 282.[54,58,59] Increased phosphorylation of Cx43 by MAPKs increases electrical conductance of paired rat cardiomyocytes.[51]

2.6. Casein kinase (CasK).

CasK1 contributes to Cx43 phosphorylation at serine residues 325 and 330. Such increased Cx43 phosphorylation leads to increased non-junctional membrane expression of Cx43 and decreased cell-cell conductance in rat kidney cells.[60]

2.7. Protein phosphatases (PP)

PP co-localize with Cx43 in pig cardiomyocytes[61] and contribute to Cx43 dephosphorylation,[62,63] and dephosphorylation of Cx43 increases single channel conductance in rat cardiomyocytes.[20]

Apart from the fact that different protein kinases and protein phosphatases independently contribute to the regulation of single channel conductance and cell-cell conductance and permeability, there exists also a substantial cross talk between the different protein kinase/phosphatase pathways. For example, cGMP not only activates PKG but

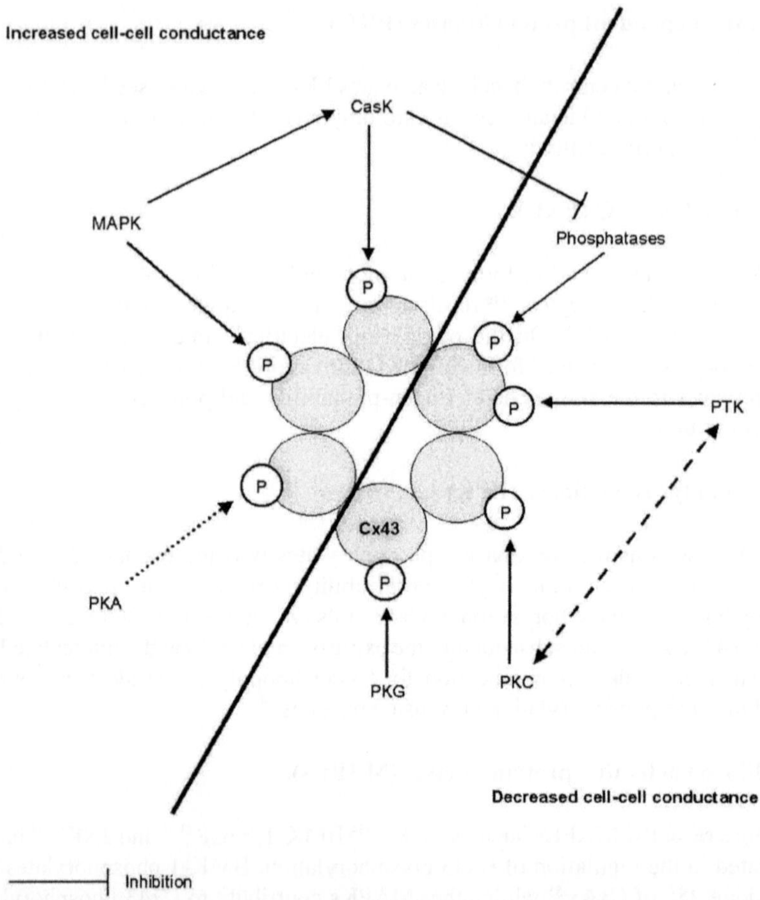

Figure 1. Schematic diagram of protein phosphatases and protein kinases (PK) on opening or closure of connexons. PTK: protein tyrosine kinase; MAPK: mitogen activated protein kinases; CasK: casein kinase; P indicates phosphorylation.

also activates p38 MAPK which, in turn, can induce PP translocation from the cytosol to the membrane.[64] Similarly, activation of PKC and/or PTK can activate MAPKs[65] which subsequently may induce activation of CasK,[66] thereby inhibiting PP.[67] Activation of PP, in turn, dephosphorylates MAPKs, thereby decreasing their activities.[68]

2.8. Proton and calcium concentration.

Apart from activation of protein kinases, increases in the intracellular proton and calcium concentrations or a decrease in the intracellular ATP concentration gradually decrease cell-cell conductance (for review, see[27]). However, while acidosis in normal hearts reduces dye transfer between cardiomyocytes, the same level of acidosis during ischemia does not,[32] pointing to an interaction of several of the above regulatory mechanisms.

3. MYOCARDIAL ISCHEMIA/REPERFUSION INJURY AND ITS MODIFICATION BY ISCHEMIC PRECONDITIONING

Cardiomyocyte death occurs during ischemia as well as during the subsequent reperfusion,[69] with both necrosis and apoptosis contributing to cell death.[70] Loss of cardiomyocyte volume regulation contributes to irreversible ischemic tissue injury,[71] and open hemichannels might contribute to the ischemia/reperfusion-induced osmotic imbalance in cardiomyocytes.[72,73]

Brief episodes of ischemia/reperfusion delay the development of irreversible tissue damage induced by a subsequent more prolonged ischemic period.[74] Apart from the delay in infarct development, ischemic preconditioning also reduces the extent of apoptosis.[75-77] The signal transduction cascade of ischemic preconditioning has been discussed in detail elsewhere.[71,78]

4. ALTERATIONS IN CX43 DURING ISCHEMIA

In normoperfused myocardium, most of the Cx43 is in a partially phosphorylated state, and it remains in a phosphorylated state within the first minutes of ischemia.[43] With prolongation of ischemia, however, Cx43 becomes dephosphorylated[43,79-81] (Figure 2), most likely due to an unaltered or increased activity of PP and a reduced energy availability for protein kinases. The time course of progressive Cx43 dephosphorylation is closely related to that of electrical uncoupling in isolated rat hearts.[79,80] However, although ischemia clearly impairs electrical cell coupling, cell-cell permeability in general – as assessed by dye transfer - can not be easily deduced from electrophysiological observations.[82] Indeed, in isolated rat hearts electrical coupling between cardiomyocytes is reduced following 10 minutes of global ischemia, while dye transfer between cardiomyocytes persists for up to 45 minutes of global ischemia.[32] In mice astrocytes, simulated ischemia reduces gap junction communication between cells, but even induces opening of non-junctional hemichannels.[6] Also in isolated cardiomyocytes, simulated ischemia causes opening of hemichannels.[72,73] Opening of hemichannels contributes to the elevation of the intracellular sodium and calcium concentrations during simulated ischemia in rabbit ventricular cardiomyocytes.[72]

With a single channel conductance of more than 100 pS,[1,20,22] only ten hemichannels need to be open to produce a millimolar cellular sodium influx,[83] and such a millimolar increase in the intracellular sodium concentration has been measured during ischemia in whole hearts.[84-86] The osmotic imbalance resulting from increased AMP, inorganic phosphate and sodium concentrations results in swelling and finally membrane rupture of the ischemic cells.

On top, an increased intracellular calcium concentration in the presence of some remaining or restored energy production can induce cardiomyocyte hypercontracture,[69] and opening of gap junctions might be involved in the transmission of factors triggering hypercontracture between adjacent cells,[32,87] such as sodium.[87,88] Indeed, cell-cell transmission of hypercontracture can be attenuated in isolated rat cardiomyocytes, in rat hearts in vitro and in pig hearts in vivo by the gap junction uncoupler heptanol (1-2 mM); in pig hearts in vivo heptanol reduces myocardial shrinkage and infarct size as well.[89] Similar results have been obtained with butanedione monoxime, another gap junction uncoupler,[90] in pig hearts in vivo.[91]

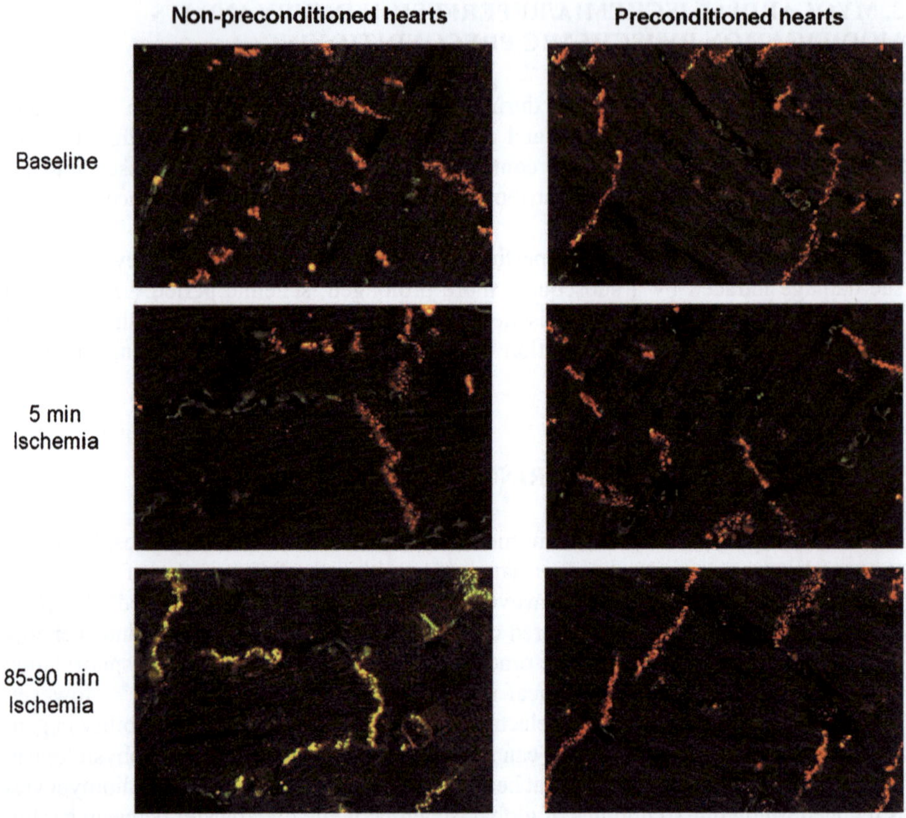

Figure 2. Representative examples of total Cx43 (red) and non-phosphorylated Cx43 (green) from a non-preconditioned heart (left side) and a preconditioned heart (right side). While in non-preconditioned hearts the density of non-phosphorylated Cx43 at the intercalated disks increased during 85-90 min ischemia (yellow color), the density remained unchanged in preconditioned hearts.

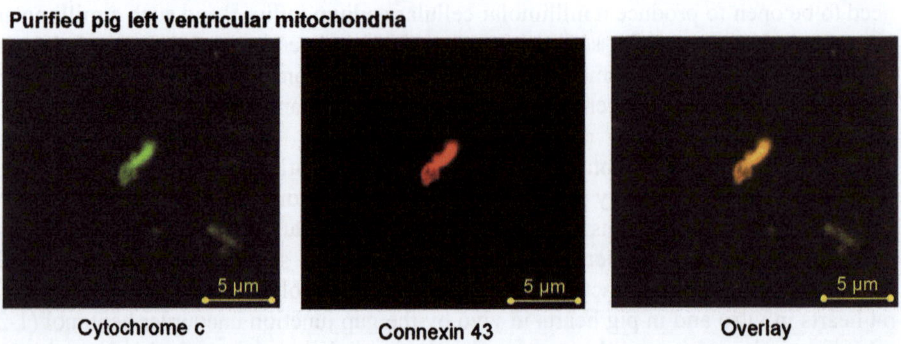

Figure 3. Purified pig left ventricular mitochondria were stained with antibodies against cytochrome c (green) and Cx43 (red) and analyzed by confocal laser scan microscopy. Merged image shows co-localization pixels in yellow.

Thus, early during ischemia gap junctions contribute to the transmission of factors triggering hypercontracture. With prolongation of ischemia, modification of gap junction conductance by dephosphorylation of Cx43 induces electrical uncoupling. While thus ion transfer through gap junctions might be impaired, the transfer of other small molecules (cell-cell permeability in general) remains unaltered. Regulation of hemichannels and gap junctions during ischemia can differ, and opening of hemichannels during simulated ischemia in isolated cells contributes to cell swelling and induction of irreversible tissue injury.

5. CX43 AND ISCHEMIC PRECONDITIONING

Both changes in the electrical coupling between cardiomyocytes and in the channel permeability have been demonstrated following ischemic preconditioning. Cx43 dephosphorylation is decreased in preconditioned compared to non-preconditioned myocardium,[43,80] and the electrical uncoupling, which is closely related to Cx43 dephosphorylation,[79] is almost completely abolished by ischemic preconditioning in rat hearts.[80] Decreased channel permeability could protect cardiomyocytes against sodium and subsequently volume overload, and indeed cardiomyocytes become more resistant towards a hypotonic challenge once they are preconditioned.[92] Also, administration of fibroblast growth factor (FGF)-2, which is known to reduce cell-cell permeability in cardiomyocytes via PTK activation and Cx43 phosphorylation,[44,48] mimics ischemic preconditioning's protection in rats[93] and pigs[94] (for review, see[95]). Finally, even the passage of a "death factor"[82,96] during the sustained ischemia between adjacent cells could be reduced in preconditioned hearts with reduced cell-cell permeability.

An alternative explanation of the protection afforded by Cx43 relates to the preconditioning ischemic period per se rather than the sustained ischemic episode. During the preconditioning ischemia, a "survival factor" [97] could pass through severely ischemic cardiomyocytes via connexons, thereby putting connected cells or cells in close proximity into a protected state. Established factors which are released from cardiomyocytes and can induce a preconditioning phenomenon in cardiomyocytes are calcium ("calcium preconditioning") and adenosine (for review, see[71]). Indeed, uncoupling of connexons with heptanol in mice[97]] or genetic Cx43-deficiency[98,99] abolishes ischemic preconditioning's protection.

It is currently unclear, whether the obvious importance of Cx43 in ischemic preconditioning's protection relates to alterations in gap junction communication or to changes in volume homeostasis. A study in pigs hearts in vivo[100] found protection but no alteration of ischemia-induced changes in cardiac impedance and therefore favored a non-gap junction mediated mechanism. More directly, we have recently seen that ischemic preconditioning's protection is also abolished in isolated cardiomyocytes from heterozygous Cx43-deficient mice, a preparation where no cell-cell communication via gap junctions exists.[101]

Although it is generally assumed that Cx43 is exclusively localized at the sarcolemma, there is some evidence that this may not be the case. It has been recently shown that the carboxy-terminus of the protein can also be localized at cardiomyocyte nuclei.[102] In cultured human endothelial cells, Cx43 was also detected in mitochondria, where its level increased in response to cellular stress.[103] Cardiomyocyte mitochondria play an important role in triggering cardioprotection and have been suggested to act as an end-effector of ischemic preconditioning's protection.[104-110] Most recently, western blot analysis on mitochondrial preparations isolated from rat, mouse, pig (Figure 3) and human left ventricular myocardium showed the presence of Cx43.[111] The preparations were not contaminated with markers for other cell compartments, and the localization of Cx43 to mitochondria was also confirmed by FACS sorting (double staining with MitoTracker Red and Cx43), immuno-electron and confocal microscopy. In mitochondria isolated from the ischemic anterior wall (AW) and the control posterior wall (PW) of pigs at the end of 90 min low-flow ischemia following a preceding preconditioning cycle of 10 min ischemia and 15 min reperfusion, the mitochondrial Cx43/adenine nucleotide transporter ratio was more than 3 fold greater in AW than in PW, whereas the ratio remained at 1 in non-preconditioned myocardium.[111] The enhancement of the mitochondrial Cx43 protein level occurred rapidly, since an increase of mitochondrial Cx43 was already detected with two cycles of 5 min ischemia/reperfusion in isolated rat hearts. These data demonstrate that Cx43 is localized at cardiomyocyte mitochondria and that ischemic preconditioning enhances such mitochondrial localization. The functional importance of mitochondrial Cx43 is unknown at present.

Thus, Cx43 is involved in ischemia/reperfusion injury and ischemic preconditioning's protection. The exact underlying mechanism(s), how in fact Cx43 mediates protection, remain to be established.

6. CLINICAL IMPLICATIONS

While IP is effective in healthy hearts of almost all animal species tested so far,[112] there is evidence that it might be no longer operative in hearts post myocardial infarction or in failing hearts,[113,114] both entities associated with a reduction in myocardial Cx43 expression.[115-118]

Concluding remarks

Cx43 appears to play an important role in ischemia and reperfusion injury and ischemic's preconditioning protection. The exact underlying mechanisms, how Cx43 mediates protection remain to be established. Cx43 deficiency abolishes ischemic preconditioning effect. Altered expression of Cx43, as it is observed in the post-infarcted or failing hearts may account for the ineffectiveness of ischemic preconditioning under certain pathological states.

REFERENCES

1. T.A.B. van Veen, H.V.M. van Rijen, T. Opthof, Cardiac gap junction channels: modulation of expression and channel properties, *Cardiovasc Res* **51**, 217–229 (2001).
2. S. Poelzing, F.G. Akar, E. Baron, D.S. Rosenbaum, Heterogenous connexin43 expression produces electrophysiological heterogeneities across ventricular wall, *Am J Physiol Heart Circ Physiol* **286**, H2001–H2009 (2004).
3. H.V.van Rijen, D. Eckardt, J. Degen, M. Theis, T. Ott, K. Willecke, H.J. Jongsma, T. Opthof, J.M. de Bakker, Slow conduction and enhanced anisotropy increase the propensity for ventricular tachyarrhythmias in adult mice with induced deletion of connexin43, *Circulation* **109**, 1048–1055 (2004).

4. K.A. Yamada, E.M. Kanter, K.G. Green, J.E. Saffitz, Transmural distribution of connexins in rodent hearts, *J Cardiovasc Electrophysiol* **15**, 710–715 (2004).
5. J.-A. Yao, Gutstein, D.E. Liu F, G.I. Fishman, A.L. Wit, Cell coupling between ventricular myocyte pairs from connexin43-deficient murine hearts, *Circ Res* **93**, 736–743 (2003).
6. J.E. Contreras, H.A. Sánchez, E.A. Eugenin, D. Speidel, M. Theis, K. Willecke, F.F. Bukauskas, M.V. Bennett, J.C. Saez, Metabolic inhibition induces opening of unopposed connexin 43 gap junction hemichannels and reduces gap junctional communication in cortical astrocytes in culture, *Proc Natl Acad Sci USA* **99**, 495–500 (2002).
7. J.C. Saez, V.M. Berthoud, M.C. Branes, A.D. Martinez, E.C. Beyer, Plasma membrane channels formed by connexins: Their regulation and functions, *Physiol Rev* **83**, 1359–1400 (2003).
8. A. De Maio, V.L. Vega, J.E. Contreras, Gap junctions, homeostasis, and injury, *J Cell Physiol* **191**, 269–282 (2002).
9. L.I. Plotkin, T. Bellido, Bisphosphonate-induced, hemichannel-mediated, anti-apoptosis through the Src/ERK pathway: a gap junction-independent action of connexin43, *Cell Commun Adhes* **8**, 377–382 (2001).
10. A.P. Quist, S.K. Rhee, H. Lin, R. Lal, Physiological role of gap-junctional hemichannels. Extracellular calcium-dependent isosmotic volume regulation, *Cell Biol* **48**, 1063–1074 (2000).
11. S.B. Yancey, S.A. John, R. Lal, B.J. Austin, J.P. Revel, The 43-kD polypeptide of heart gap junctions: immunolocalization, topology, and functional domains, *J Cell Biol* **108**, 2241–2254 (1989).
12. E.C. Beyer, J. Kistler, D.L. Paul, D.A. Goodenough, Antisera directed against connexin43 peptides react with a 43-kD protein localized to gap junctions in myocardium and other tissues, *J Cell Biol* **108**, 595–605 (1989).
13. T. Toyofuku, M. Yabuki, K. Otsu, T. Kuzuya, M. Hori, M. Tada, Direct association of the gap junction protein connexin-43 with ZO-1 in cardiac myocytes, *J Biol Chem* **273**, 12725–12731 (1998).
14. R.J. Barker, R.L. Price, R.G. Gourdie, Increased association of ZO-1 with connexin 43 during remodeling of cardiac gap junctions, *Circ Res* **90**, 317–324 (2002).
15. E. Kardami, R.M. Stoski, B.W. Doble, T. Yamamoto, E.L. Hertzberg, J.I. Nagy, Biochemical and ultrastructural evidence for the association of basic fibroblast growth factor with cardiac gap junctions, *J Biol Chem* **266**, 19551–19557 (1991).
16. B.N. Giepmans, I. Verlaan, T. Hengeveld, H. Janssen, J. Calafat, M.M. Falk, W.H. Moolenaar, Gap junction protein connexin-43 interacts directly with microtubules, *Curr Biol* **11**,1364–1368 (2001).
17. R.D. Veenstra, H.-Z. Wang, D.A. Beblo, M.G. Chilton, A.L. Harris, E.C. Beyer, P.R. Brink, Selectivity of connexin-specific gap junctions does not correlate with channel conductance, *Circ Res* **77**, 1156–1165 (1995).
18. D.C. Spray, J.M. Burt, Structure-activity relations of the cardiac gap junction channel, *Am J Physiol Cell Physiol* **258**, C195–C205 (1990).
19. L. Polontchouk, V. Valiunas, J.-A. Haefliger, H.M. Eppenberger, R. Weingart, Expression and regulation of connexins in cultured ventricular myocytes isolated from adult rat hearts, *Pflügers Arch – Eur J Physiol* **443**, 676–689 (2002).
20. B.R. Takens-Kwak, H.J. Jongsma, Cardiac gap junctions: three distinct single channel conductances and their modulation by phosphorylating treatments, *Pflügers Arch – Eur J Physiol* **422**, 198–200 (1992).
21. C.G. Nebigil, N. Etienne, N. Messaddeo, L. Maroteaux, Serotonin is a novel survival factor of cardiomyocytes : mitochondria as a target of 5-HT2B receptor signaling, *Faseb J* **17**, 1373–1375 (2003).
22. J.E. Contreras, J.C. Saez, FF. Bukauskas, M.V.L. Bennett, Gating and regulation of connexin 43 (Cx43) hemichannels, *Proc Natl Acad Sci USA* **100**, 11388–11393 (2003).
23. J.K. VanSlyke, LS. Musil, Analysis of connexin intracellular transport and assembly, *Methods* **20**, 156–164 (2000).
24. L.S. Musil, B.A. Cunningham, G.M. Edelman, D.A. Goodenough, Differential phosphorylation of the gap junction protein connexin43 in junctional communication-competent and -deficient cell-lines, *J Cell Biol* **111**, 2077–2088 (1990).
25. J.C. Saez, A.C. Nairn, A.J. Czernik, G.I. Fishman, D.C. Spray, EL. Hertzberg, Phosphorylation of connexin43 and the regulation of neonatal rat cardiac myocyte gap junctions, *J Mol Cell Cardiol* **29**, 2131–2145 (1997).
26. E.L. Hertzberg, J.C. Sáez, R.A. Corpina, C. Roy, J.A. Kessler, Use of antibodies in the analysis of connexin 43 turnover and phosphorylation, *Methods* **20**, 129–139 (2000).
27. R. Schulz, G. Heusch, Connexin 43 and ischemic preconditioning, *Cardiovasc Res* **62**, 335–344 (2004).

28. M. Delmar, W. Coombs, P. Sorgen, H. Duffy, S.M. Taffet, Structural bases for the chemical regulation of connexin43 channels, *Cardiovasc Res* **62**, 268–275 (2004).
29. A.P. Moreno, Biophysical properties of homomeric and heteromultimeric channels formed by cardiac connexins, *Cardiovasc Res* **62**, 276–286 (2004).
30. BR. Kwak, TA. van Veen, LJ. Analbers, HJ. Jongsma, TPA increases conductance but decreases permeability in neonatal rat cardiomyocyte gap junction channels, *Exp Cell Res* **220**, 56–463 (1995).
31. BR. Kwak, HJ. Jongsma, Regulation of cardiac gap junction channel permeability and conductance by several phosphorylating conditions. *Mol Cell Biochem* **157**, 93–99 (1996).
32. M. Ruiz-Meana, D. Garcia-Dorado, S. Lane, P. Pina, J. Inserte, M. Mirabet, J. Soler-Soler, Persistence of gap junction communication during myocardial ischemia, *Am J Physiol Heart Circ Physiol* **280**, H2563–H2571 (2001).
33. A.F. Lau, V. Hatch-Pigott, DS. Crow, Evidence that heart connexin43 is a phosphoprotein, *J Mol Cell Cardiol* **23**, 659–663 (1991).
34. J.M. Burt, D.C. Spray, Inotropic agents modulate gap junctional conductance between cardiac myocytes, *Am J Physiol Heart Circ Physiol* **254**, H1206–H1210 (1988).
35. W.C. De Mello, Impaired regulation of cell communication by ß-adrenergic receptor activation in the failing heart, *Hypertension* **27**, 265–268 (1996).
36. A.F. Paulson, P.D. Lampe, R.A. Meyer, E. TenBroek, M.M. Atkinson, T.F. Walseth, R.G. Johnson, Cyclic AMP and LDL trigger a rapid enhancement in gap junction assembly through a stimulation of connexin trafficking, *J Cell Science* **113**, 3037–3049 (2000).
37. P.D. Lampe, Q. Qiu, RA. Meyer, E.M. TenBroek, T.F. Walseth, T.A. Starich, H.L. Grunenwald, R.G. Johnson, Gap junction assembly: PTX-sensitive G proteins regulate the distribution of connexin43 within cells, *Am J Physiol Cell Physiol* **281**, C1211–C1222 (2001).
38. E.M. TenBroek, P.D. Lampe, J.L. Solan, J.K. Reynhout, R.G. Johnson, Ser364 of connexin43 and the upregulation of gap junction assembly by cAMP, *J Cell Biol* **155**, 1307–1318 (2003).
39. G. Kojda, K. Kottenberg, Regulation of basal myocardial function by NO, *Cardiovasc Res* **41**, 514–523 (1999).
40. M.T. Gewaltig, G. Kojda, Vasoprotection by nitric oxide: mechanisms and therapeutic potential, *Cardiovasc Res* **55**, 250–260 (2002).
41. A. Friebe, D. Koesling, Regulation of nitric oxide – sensitive guanylyl cyclase, *Circ Res* **93**, 96–105 (2003).
42. P. Ping, J. Zhang, W.M. Pierce, R. Bolli, Functional proteomic analysis of protein kinase C ε signaling complexes in the normal heart and during cardioprotection, *Circ Res* **88**, 59–62 (2001).
43. R. Schulz, P. Gres, A. Skyschally, A. Duschin, S. Belosjorow, I Konietzka, G. Heusch, Ischemic preconditioning preserves connexin 43 phosphorylation during sustained ischemia in pig hearts in vivo, *Faseb J* **17**, 1355–1357 (2003).
44. B.W. Doble, P. Ping, E. Kardami, The ε subtype of protein kinase C is required for cardiomyocyte connexin-43 phosphorylation, *Circ Res* **86**, 293–301 (2000).
45. N. Bowling, X. Huang, G.E. Sandusky, R.L. Fouts, K. Mintze, M. Esterman, P.D. Allen, R Maddi, E. McCall, C.J. Vlahos, Protein kinase C-α and -ε modulate connexin-43 phosphorylation in human heart, *J Mol Cell Cardiol* **33**, 789–798 (2001).
46. B.W. Doble, P. Ping, R.R. Fandrich, P.A. Cattani, E. Kardami, Protein kinase C-epsilon mediates phorbol ester-induced phosphorylation of connexin-43, *Cell Commun Adhes* **8**, 253–256 (2001).
47. S. Weng, M. Lauven, T. Schaefer, L. Polontchouk, R. Grover, S. Dhein, Pharmacological modification of gap junction coupling by an antiarrhythmic peptide via protein kinase C activation, *Faseb J* **16**, 1114–1116.
48. B.W. Doble, Y. Chen, D.G. Bosc, D.W. Litchfield, E. Kardami, Fibroblast growth factor-2 decreases metabolic coupling and stimulates phosphorylation as well as masking of connexin43 epitopes in cardiac myocytes, *Circ Res* **79**, 647–658 (1996).
49. T. Toyofuku, Y. Akamatsu, H. Zhang, M. Tada, M. Hori, c-Src regulates the interaction between connexin-43 and ZO-1 in cardiac myocytes, *J Biol Chem* **276**, 1780–1788 (2001).
50. D. Lidington, K. Tyml, Y. Ouellette, Lipopolysaccharide-induced reductions in cellular coupling correlate with tyrosine phosphorylation of connexin 43, *J Cell Physiol* **193**, 373–379 (2002).
51. L. Polontchouk, B. Ebelt, M. Jackels, S. Dhein, Chronic effects of endothelin 1 and angiotensin II on gap junctions and intercellular communication in cardiac cells, *Faseb J* **16**, 87–89 (2002).
52. R.P. Brandes, R. Popp, G. Ott, D. Bredenkotter, C. Wallner, R. Busse, I. Fleming, The extracellular regulated kinases (ERK) 1/2 mediate cannabinoid-induced inhibition of gap junctional communication in endothelial cells, *Br J Pharmacol* **136**, 709–716 (2002).

53. D.Y. Kim, Y. Kam, S.K. Koo, C.O. Joe, Gating connexin 43 channels reconstituted in lipid vesicles by mitogen-activated protein kinase phosphorylation, *J Biol Chem* **274**, 5581–5587 (1999).
54. B.J. Warn-Cramer, G.T. Cottrell, J.M. Burt, A.F. Lau, Regulation of connexin-43 gap junctional intercellular communication by mitogen-activated protein kinase, *J Biol Chem* **273**, 9188–9196 (1998).
55. S.J. Cameron, S. Malik, M. Akaike, N. Lerner-Marmarosh, C. Yan, JD. Lee, J Abe, J. Yang, Regulation of epidermal growth factor-induced connexin 43 gap junction communication by big mitogen-activated protein kinase 1/ERK 5 but not ERK1/2 kinase activation, *J Biol Chem* **278**, 18682–18688 (2003).
56. B.G. Petrich, X. Gong, DL. Lerner, X. Wang, JH. Brown, JE. Saffitz, Y. Wang, c-Jun N-terminal kinase activation mediates downregulation of connexin43 in cardiomyocytes, *Circ Res* **91**, 640–647 (2002).
57. RJ. Barker, RG. Gourdie, JNK bond regulation. Why do mammalian hearts invest in connexin 43? *Circ Res* **91**, 556–558 (2002).
58. B.J. Warn-Cramer, P.D. Lampe, W.E, Kurata, M.Y. Kanemitsu, L.W. Loo, W. Eckhart, A.F. Lau, Characterization of the mitogen-activated protein kinase phosphorylation sites on the connexin-43 gap junction protein, *J Biol Chem* **271**, 3779–3786 (1996).
59. A.F. Lau, W.E. Kurata, M.Y. Kanemitsu, L.W. Loo, B.J. Warn-Cramer, W. Eckhart, P.D. Lampe, Regulation of connexin43 function by activated tyrosine protein kinases, *J Bioenerg Biomembr* **28**, 359–368 (1996).
60. CD. Cooper, P.D. Lampe, Casein kinase 1 regulates connexin-43 gap junction assembly, *J Biol Chem* **277**, 4962–44968 (2003).
61. I. Konietzka, P. Gres, G. Heusch, R. Schulz, Co-localization of connexin 43 (Cx43) and protein phosphatases in preconditioned myocardium in pigs, *J Mol Cell Cardiol* 36, **757** (Abstract) (2004).
62. M. Jeyaraman, S. Tanguy, RA. Fandrich, A. Lukas, E. Kardami, Ischemia-induced dephosphorylation of cardiomyocyte connexin-43 is reduced by okadaic acid calyculin A but not fostriecin, *Mol Cell Biochem* **242**, 129–134 (2003).
63. X. Ai, S.M. Pogwizd, Connexin 43 downregulation and dephosphorylation in nonischemic heart failure is associated with enhanced colocalized protein phosphatase type 2A, *Circ Res* **96**, 54–63 (2005).
64. Q. Liu, P.A. Hofmann, Modulation of protein phosphatase 2a by adenosine A1 receptors in cardiomyocytes: role for p38 MAPK, *Am J Physiol Heart Circ Physiol* **285**, H97–H103 (2003).
65. M.C. Michel, Y. Li, G. Heusch, Mitogen-activated protein kinases in the heart. *Naunyn-Schmiedeberg's Arch Pharmacol* **363**, 245–266 (2001).
66. M. Sayed, S.O. Kim, B.S. Salh, O.-G. Issinger, S.L. Pelech, Stress-induced activation of protein kinase CK2 by direct interaction with p38 mitogen-activated protein kinase, *J Biol Chem* **275**, 16569–16573 (2000).
67. K. Cieslik, C.-M. Lee, J. Tang, K.K. Wu, Transcriptional regulation of endothelial nitric-oxide synthase by an interaction between casein kinase 2 and protein phosphatase 2A, *J Biol Chem* **274**, 34669–34675 (1999).
68. S.M. Keyse, Protein phosphatases and the regulation of mitogen-activated protein kinase signalling, *Curr Opinion Cell Biol* **12**:186–192 (2000).
69. H.M. Piper, The calcium paradox revisited: an artefact of great heuristic value. *Cardiovasc Res* **45**, 123–127 (2000).
70. G.-T. Kim, Y.-S. Chun, J.-W. Park, M.-S. Kim, Role of apoptosis-inducing factor in myocardial cell death by ischemia-reperfusion, *Biochem Biophys Res Commun* **309**, 619–624 (2003).
71. R. Schulz, M.V. Cohen, M. Behrends, J.M. Downey, G. Heusch, Signal transduction of ischemic preconditioning, *Cardiovasc Res* **52**, 181–198 (2001).
72. F. Li, K. Sugishita, Z. Su, I. Ueda, W.H. Barry, Activation of connexin-43 hemichannels can elevate $[Ca^{2+}]i$ and $[Na^{+}]i$ in rabbit ventricular myocytes during metabolic inhibition, *J Mol Cell Cardiol* **33**, 2145–2155 (2001).
73. S.A. John, R. Kondo, S.-Y. Wang, J.I. Goldhaber, J.N. Weiss, Connexin-43 hemichannels opened by metabolic inhibition. *J Biol Chem* **274**, 236–240 (1999).
74. C.E. Murry, R.B. Jennings, K.A. Reimer, Preconditioning with ischemia: a delay of lethal cell injury in ischemic myocardium, *Circulation* **74**, 1124–1136 (1986).
75. C.A. Piot, D. Padmanaban, P.C. Ursell, R.E. Sievers, C.L. Wolfe, Ischemic preconditioning decreases apoptosis in rat hearts in vivo, *Circulation* **96**, 1598–1604 (1997).
76. N. Maulik, T. Yoshida, R.M. Engelman, D. Deaton, J.E. Flack 3rd, J.A. Rousou, D.K. Das, Ischemic preconditioning attenuates apoptotic cell death associated with ischemia/reperfusion, *Mol Cell Biochem* **186**, 139–145 (1998).

77. M. Nakamura, N.-P. Wang, Z.-Q. Zhao, J.N. Wilcox, V. Thourani, R.A. Guyton, J. Vinten-Johansen, Preconditioning decreases Bax expression, PMN accumulation and apoptosis in reperfused rat heart, *Cardiovasc Res* **45**, 661–670 (2000).
78. D.M. Yellon, J.M. Downey, Preconditioning the myocardium: From cellular physiology to clinical cardiology, *Physiol Rev* **83**, 1113–1151 (2003).
79. M.A. Beardslee, D.L. Lerner, P.N. Tadros, J.G. Laing, E.C. Beyer, K.A. Yamada, A.G. Kleber, R.B. Schuessler, JE. Saffitz, Dephosphorylation and intracellular redistributoin of ventricular connexin 43 during electrical uncoupling induced by ischemia, *Circ Res* **87**, 656–662 (2000).
80. S.K. Jain, R.B. Schuessler, J.E. Saffitz, Mechanisms of delayed electrical uncoupling induced by ischemic preconditioning, *Circ Res* **92**, 1138–1144 (2003).
81. T. Miura, Y. Ohnuma, A. Kuno, M. Tanno, Y. Ichikawa, Y. Nakamura, T. Yano, T. Miki, J. Sakamoto, K. Shimamoto, Protective role of gap junctions in preconditioning against myocardial infarction, *Am J Physiol Heart Circ Physiol* **286**, H214–H221 (2004).
82. D. Garcia-Dorado, M. Ruiz-Meana, F. Padilla, A. Rodriguez-Sinovas, M. Mirabet, Gap-junction-mediated intercellular communication in ischemic preconditioning, *Cardiovasc Res* **55**, 456–465 (2002).
83. R.P. Kondo, SY. Wang, SA. John, JN. Weiss, JI. Goldhaber, Metabolic inhibition activates a non-selective current through connexin hemichannels in isolated ventricular myocytes, *J Mol Cell Cardiol* **32**, 1859–1872 (2000).
84. MM. Pike, C.S. Luo, S. Yanagida, G.R. Hageman, P.G. Anderson, ^{23}Na and ^{31}P nuclear magnetic resonance studies of ischemia- induced ventricular fibrillation. Alterations of intracellular Na^+ and cellular energy, *Circ Res* **77**, 349–406 (1995).
85. J.A. Balschi, ^{23}Na NMR demonstrates prolonged increase of intracellular sodium following transient regional ischemia in the in situ pig heart, *Basic Res Cardiol* **94**, 60–69 (1999).
86. C.J.A. van Echteld, J.H. Kirkels, M.H.J. Eijgelshoven, P. van der Meer, TJC. Ruigrok, Intracellular sodium during ischemia and calcium-free perfusion: A^{23}Na NMR Study, *J Mol Cell Cardiol* **23**, 297–307 (1991).
87. M. Ruiz-Meana, D. Garcia-Dorado, B. Hofstaetter, H.M. Piper, J. Soler-Soler, Propagation of cardiomyocyte hypercontracture by passage of Na^+ through gap junctions, *Circ Res* **85**, 280–287 (1999).
88. D. Garcia-Dorado, A. Rodriguez-Sinovas, M. Ruiz-Maena, Gap junction-mediated spread of cell injury and death during myocardial ischemia-reperfusion, *Cardiovasc Res* **61**, 386–401 (2004).
89. D. Garcia-Dorado, J. Inserte, M. Ruiz-Meana, M.A. Gonzalez, J. Solares, M. Julia, J.A. Barrabes, J. Soler-Soler, Gap junction uncoupler heptanol prevents cell-to-cell progression of hypercontracture and limits necrosis during myocardial reperfusion, *Circulation* **96**, 3579–3586 (1997).
90. F. Duthe, E. DuPont, F. Verrechia, I. Plaisance, N.J. Severs, D Sarrouilhe, J.C. Herve, Dephosphorylation agents depress gap junctional communication between rat cardiac cells without modifying the connexin 43 phosphorylation degree, *Gen Physiol Biophys* **19**, 441–449 (2000).
91. D. Garcia-Dorado, P. Théroux, J.M. Duran, J. Solares, J. Alonso, E. Sanz, R. Munoz, J. Elizaga, J. Botas, F. Fernandez-Aviles, et al. Selective inhibition of the contractile apparatus. A new approach to modification of infarct size, infarct composition, and infarct geometry during coronary artery occlusion and reperfusion, *Circulation* **85**, 1160–1174 (1992).
92. S.C. Armstrong, C. Shivell, C.E. Ganote, Sarcolemmal blebs and osmotic fragility as correlates of irreversible ischemic injury in preconditioned isolated rabbit cardiomycytes, *J Mol Cell Cardiol* **33**:149–160 (2001).
93. Z.-S. Jiang, R.R. Padua, H. Ju, B.W. Doble, Y. Jin, J. Hao, P.A. Cattini, I.M. Dixon, E. Kardami, Acute protection of ischemic heart by FGF-2: involvement of FGF-2 receptors and protein kinase C, *Am J Physiol Heart Circ Physiol* **282**, H1071–H1080 (2002).
94. P. Htun, W.D. Ito, I.E. Hoefer, J. Schaper, W. Schaper, Intramyocardial infusion of FGF-1 mimics ischemic preconditioning in pig myocardium, *J Mol Cell Cardiol* **30**, 867–877 (1998).
95. K.A. Detillieux, F. Sheikh, E. Kardami, P.A. Cattini, Biological activities of fibroblast growth factor-2 in the adult myocardium, *Cardiovasc Res* **57**, 8–19 (2003).
96. E.I. Azzam, S.M. de Toledo, J.B. Little, Direct evidence for the participation of gap junction-mediated intercellular communication in the transmission of damage signals from alpha-particle irradiated to non-irradiated cells, *Proc Natl Acad Sci USA* **98**, 473–478 (2001).
97. G. Li, P. Whittaker, M. Yao, R.A. Kloner, K. Przyklenk, The gap junction uncoupler heptanol abrogates infarct size reduction with preconditioning in mouse hearts, *Cardiovasc Pathol* **11**, 158–165 (2002).
98. U. Schwanke, I. Konietzka, A. Duschin, X. Li, R. Schulz, G. Heusch, No ischemic preconditioning in heterozygous connexin 43-deficient mice, *Am J Physiol Heart Circ Physiol* **283**, H1740–H1742 (2002).

99. U. Schwanke, X. Li, R. Schulz, G. Heusch, No ischemic preconditioning in heterozygous connexin 43-deficient mice: a further in vivo study, *Basic Res Cardiol* **98**, 181–182 (2003).
100. F. Padilla, D. Garcia-Dorado, A. Rodriguez-Sinovas, M. Ruiz-Meana, J. Inserte, J. Soler-Soler, Protection afforded by ischemic preconditioning is not mediated by effects on cell-to-cell electrical coupling during myocardial ischemia-reperfusion, *Am J Physiol Heart Circ Physiol* **285**, H1909–H1916 (2003).
101. X. Li, FR. Heinzel, K. Boengler, R. Schulz, G. Heusch, Role of connexin 43 in ischemic preconditioning does not involve intercellular communications through gap junctions, *J Mol Cell Cardiol* **36**, 161–163 (2004).
102. X. Dang, B.W. Doble, E. Kardami, The carboxy-tail of connexin-43 localizes to the nucleus and inhibits cell growth, *Mol Cell Biochem* **242**, 35–38 (2003).
103. H. Li, S. Brodsky, S. Kumari, V. Valiunas, P. Brink, J. Kaide, A. Nasjletti, M.S. Goligorsky, Paradoxical overexpression and translocation of connexin 43 in homocysteine-treated endothelial cells, *Am J Physiol Heart Circ Physiol* **282**, H2124–H2133 (2002).
104. L.H. Opie, M.N. Sack, Metabolic plasticity and the promotion of cardiac protection in ischemia and ischemic preconditioning, *J Mol Cell Cardiol* **34**, 1077–1089 (2002).
105. T. Krieg, M.V. Cohen, J.M. Downey, Mitochondria and their role in preconditioning's trigger phase, *Basic Res Cardiol* **98**, 228–234 (2003).
106. G. Taimor, Mitochondria as common endpoints in early and late preconditioning, *Cardiovasc Res* **59**, 266–267 (2003).
107. B. O'Rourke, Evidence for mitochondrial K^+ channels and their role in cardioprotection, *Circ Res* **94**, 420–432 (2004).
108. A.P. Halestrap, S.J. Clarke, S.A. Javadov, Mitochondrial permeability transition pore opening during myocardial reperfusion – a target for cardioprotection, *Cardiovasc Res* **61**, 372–385 (2004).
109. E. Murphy, Primary and secondary signaling pathways in early preconditioning that converge on the mitochondria to produce cardioprotection, *Circ Res* **94**, 7–16 (2004)
110. D. Hausenloy, A. Wynne, M. Duchen, D. Yellon, Transient mitochondrial permeability transition pore opening mediates preconditioning-induced protection, *Circulation* **109**,1714–1717 (2004).
111. K. Böngler, G. Dodoni, M. Ruiz-Maena, A. Cabestrero, A. Rodriguez-Sinovas, D. Garcia-Dorado, P. Gres, F. Di Lisa, G. Heusch, R. Schulz, Mitochondrial localization of connexin 43 in cardiomyocytes and its enhancement by ischemic preconditioning, *Circulation* **110**, III–236(Abstract) (2004)
112. G. Heusch, Nitroglycerin and delayed preconditioning in humans. Yet another new mechanism for an old drug? *Circulation* **103**, 2876–2878 (2001).
113. T. Miki, T. Miura, M. Tanno, J. Sakamoto, A. Kuno, S. Genda, T. Matsumoto, Y. Ichikawa, K. Shimamoto, Interruption of signal transduction between G protein and PKC-epsilon underlies the impaired myocardial response to ischemic preconditioning in postinfarct remodeled hearts, *Mol Cell Biochem* **247**, 185–193 (2003).
114. S. Ghosh, N.B. Standen, M. Galinanes, Failure to precondition pathological human myocardium, *J Am Coll Cardiol* **37**, 711–718 (2001).
115. E. DuPont, T. Matsushita, R.A. Kaba, C. Vozzi, S.R. Coppen, N. Khan, R. Kaprielian, M.H. NJ. Yacoub, Severs, Altered connexin expression in human congestive heart failure, *J Mol Cell Cardiol* **33**, 359–371 (2001).
116. D.D. Spragg, C. Leclercq, M. Loghmani, O.P. Faris, R.S. Tunin, D. DiSilvestre, E.R. McVeigh, G.F. Tomaselli, DA. Kass, Regional alterations in protein expression in the dyssynchronous failing heart, *Circulation* **108**, 929–932 (2003).
117. S. Kostin, M. Rieger, S. Dammer, S. Hein, M. Richter, W.P. Klovekorn, E.P. Bauer, J. Schaper, Gap junction remodeling and altered connexin43 expression in the failing human heart, *Mol Cell Biochem* **242**, 135–144 (2003).
118. H. Kitamura, Y. Ohnishi, A. Yoshida, K. Okajima, H. Azumi, A. Ishida, E.J. Galeano, S. Kubo, Y. Hayashi, H. Itoh, M. Yokoyama, Heterogeneous loss of connexin43 protein in nonischemic dilated cardiomyopathy with ventricular tachycardia, *J Cardiovasc Electrophysiol* **13**, 865–870 (2002).

CHAPTER 5

CORONARY MICROEMBOLIZATION

Andreas Skyschally, Rainer Schulz, Michael Haude*, Raimund Erbel*, Gerd Heusch

1. INTRODUCTION

Atherosclerotic plaque rupture is a key event in the pathogenesis of acute coronary syndromes and during coronary interventions. Atherosclerotic plaque rupture does not always result in complete thrombotic occlusion of the entire epicardial coronary artery with subsequent acute myocardial infarction, but may in milder forms result in the embolization of atherosclerotic and thrombotic debris into the coronary microcirculation.

This review summarizes the available morphological evidence for coronary microembolization in patients who died from coronary artery disease, most notably from sudden death. Then the experimental pathophysiology of coronary microembolization in animal models of acute coronary syndromes is detailed. Finally, the review presents the available clinical evidence for coronary microembolization in patients, highlights its key features - arrhythmias, contractile dysfunction, microinfarcts and reduced coronary reserve -, compares these features to those of the experimental model and addresses its prevention by mechanical protection devices and glycoprotein IIb/IIIa antagonism.

The rupture of an atherosclerotic plaque in an epicardial coronary artery with subsequent occlusive coronary thrombosis has been established as the decisive event in the pathogenesis of acute myocardial infarction[1,2]. Other, milder forms of plaque rupture with subsequent embolization of atherosclerotic and thrombotic debris into the coronary microcirculation have also been recognized before[2-5], but the clinical frequency and importance of microembolization have only recently been appreciated[6-8].

Post-mortem analyses revealed evidence for microemboli in the coronary circulation of patients who had died of ischemic heart disease. Platelet and fibrin microthrombi were identified in 13% of 244 patients with cardiac disease, and in 20% of the 50 patients, who died from sudden death, thromboemboli were found and associated with

Institut für Pathophysiologie und +Abteilung für Kardiologie
Zentrum für Innere Medizin, Universitätsklinikum Essen
This chapter is an updated version of an already published review: G. Heusch, R. Schulz, M. Haude, R. Erbel, Coronary microembolization, J Mol Cell Cardiol 37, 23-31 (2004).
Address for correspondence: Prof. Dr. med. Dr. h. c. Gerd Heusch Direktor des Instituts für Pathophysiologie Zentrum für Innere Medizin, Universitätsklinikum Essen, Hufelandstr. 55, 45122 Essen, Germany, Tel:+49 (201) 723 4480, Fax: +49 (201) 723 4481, gerd.heusch@uni-essen.de

focal myocardial necrosis[9]. In 54% of 25 patients who had died from acute coronary thrombosis, microemboli – containing platelet aggregates, hyalin and atherosclerotic plaque material, including cholesterol crystals - were found. Also, 38% of these patients had microinfarcts in the perfusion territories of the thrombotic coronary arteries[3]. In 30% of 90 patients who died suddenly of ischemic heart disease, platelet aggregates were found distal to an atherosclerotic epicardial coronary plaque that had developed fissuring and mural thrombosis[4]. In 24 patients who died from acute myocardial infarction, an acute coronary thrombosis was present in all hearts and in 79% of them microemboli were identified in the perfusion territory of the thrombotic artery[5]. Platelet aggregates, microemboli, and microinfarcts tended to be more frequent in patients with unstable angina prior to the fatal event[3,4] but were also found in those with stable angina[3]. Microembolization induced also a marked inflammatory reaction, characterized by cellular infiltration, particularly of eosinophils[3], and multifocal microinfarcts[4]. A relation between microemboli and arrhythmias was noted.[5] However the causal involvement of microemboli in death through malignant arrhythmias and/or cardiac failure remained unclear.

In summary, microemboli are frequently found in patients who died from ischemic heart disease. Qualitatively, the microemboli are characterized by platelet aggregates, hyalin and atherosclerotic plaque material, including cholesterol crystals. The microemboli are associated with microinfarcts and an inflammatory reaction. Unfortunately, more quantitative information is missing: the size and number of microemboli and associated microinfarcts in a given heart or perfusion territory have not been reported so far.

2. CORONARY BLOOD FLOW RESPONSE AND EXPERIMENTAL CORONARY MICROEMBOLIZATION

A frequent observation with coronary microembolization in prior animal experiments was a transient decrease in coronary blood flow immediately with the microembolization followed by a more prolonged increase in coronary blood flow[10-12].

An explanation for this biphasic pattern in coronary blood flow after microembolization was subsequently provided by Hori et al. in 1986 who induced coronary microembolization in anesthetized dogs with latex microspheres of different diameters and found increased coronary blood flow associated with a persistent release of adenosine into a coronary vein. Despite the increase in coronary blood flow, coronary microembolization reduced regional contractile function, measured using sonomicrometry, and reduced myocardial lactate extraction[13]. Apparently, a maldistribution of local myocardial blood flow developed, with ischemia in the territory of the embolized vessel and luxury hyperemia in the surrounding vessels. This luxury hyperemia did not prevent contractile dysfunction, lactate production and eventual microinfarction. Subsequently, the same laboratory prevented the release of adenosine in response to coronary microembolization by the α_1-adrenoceptor antagonist prazosin or antagonized the action of adenosine by theophylline and thus prevented hyperemia and induced a profound further decrease in regional contractile function and lactate extraction over that by microembolization per se, indicating that the adenosine-induced hyperemia in fact attenuated the regional myocardial ischemia resulting from coronary microembolization[14].

The destruction of free radicals by superoxide dismutase (SOD) enhanced the release of adenosine and the resulting coronary hyperemia and attenuated the decreases in regional contractile function and lactate extraction following coronary microembolization; these effects were again antagonized by theophylline. The authors attributed the enhanced adenosine release to protection of 5-ecto-nucleotidase from free radicals by SOD[15,16]. More recently, similar findings were reported in anesthetized pigs where coronary microembolization with 15 μm microspheres also caused a hyperemic response which was antagonized by theophylline and therefore attributed to adenosine[17]. The increase in baseline blood flow, secondary to adenosine release and hyperemia, and the decrease in maximal blood flow with pharmacological dilation or reactive hyperemia, secondary to physical obstruction of the microcirculation, act in concert to decrease coronary reserve[18]. In anesthetized dogs, non-selective systemic infusion of microspheres with a diameter of 25μm induced focal myocardial microinfarcts which were prevented by pretreatment with the α-adrenoceptor antagonist phentolamine and the calcium antagonist verapamil, possibly by preventing platelet aggregates[19]. Alternatively, an α-adrenergic coronary constrictor effect in the microcirculation might have contributed to the microinfarction[20,21].

In summary, the immediate response of coronary blood flow to coronary microembolization is a decrease secondary to mechanical obstruction followed by a delayed, more prolonged increase secondary to adenosine release. The coronary blood flow response to microembolization depends on the diameter and number of injected particles; with larger and more microspheres there is no hyperemia and the physical obstruction prevails[22].

3. PLATELETS, CYCLIC CORONARY FLOW VARIATIONS AND EXPERIMENTAL CORONARY MICROEMBOLIZATION

Folts et al.[23] first developed a model of an acute coronary syndrome/unstable angina in anesthetized dogs with a severe coronary stenosis superimposed on traumatic endothelial damage. This combination of endothelial damage and severe coronary stenosis induced typical cyclic coronary flow variations, characterized by progressively decreased coronary blood flow over several minutes followed by an abrupt increase in coronary blood flow[24]. Such cyclic flow variations were attributed to platelet aggregates[25,26] that progressively plugged the stenotic epicardial coronary artery segment and were then suddenly dislodged into the coronary microcirculation. This model of cyclic coronary blood flow variations was used subsequently by a number of investigators in anesthetized[27] and conscious dogs[28,29], and aspirin consistently prevented cyclic coronary blood flow variations[23,26,29].

Cyclic coronary blood flow variations involve thrombin as a mediator[30], and a number of substances released from aggregating platelets, such as serotonin and thromboxane A2, induce an additional coronary vasoconstriction[27]. Cyclic coronary blood flow variations cause decreased regional contractile function in the dependent myocardium[31] and arrhythmias[32]. Whereas in one study in anesthetized pigs with cyclic coronary blood flow variations there were surprisingly few platelet aggregates dislodged into the coronary microcirculation[26], another study in anesthetized dogs with cyclic coronary blood flow variations demonstrated significantly increased microcirculatory resistance[33], reflecting either platelet microembolization or/and increased microvascular tone.

Intracoronary infusion of ADP in anesthetized pigs causes microcirculatory embolization by platelet aggregates and in consequence cardiogenic shock, arrhythmias up to ventricular fibrillation, and microinfarcts with associated leukocyte infiltration[34]. Such platelet aggregates and microinfarcts are also induced by catecholamines in anesthetized dogs and prevented by aspirin[35,36].

In conclusion, the Folts model of cyclic coronary blood flow variations clearly involves platelet microembolization. However, the role of physical obstruction versus microvascular constriction in the impaired myocardial perfusion is not entirely clear. Platelet-endothelium and platelet-leukocyte interactions may also contribute to the local inflammatory response[37].

4. CORONARY MICROEMBOLIZATION AS AN EXPERIMENTAL MODEL OF UNSTABLE ANGINA: THE ROLE OF INFLAMMATORY CYTOKINES

Recognizing the importance of coronary microembolization in the pathogenesis of acute coronary syndromes and following coronary interventions,[6,7] we have studied the consequences of intracoronary infusion of microspheres with a diameter of 42 μm for the affected myocardium in anesthetized dogs. Stepwise intracoronary infusion of microspheres up to a final dose of 3.000 spheres per ml/min baseline coronary blood flow caused an immediate decrease in coronary blood flow upon infusion followed by a more prolonged reactive increase in flow. In contrast, regional systolic wall thickening (sonomicrometry) was stepwise reduced and did not recover (Figure 1).[18] Moreover, a progressive further decrease in regional systolic wall thickening was seen over several hours following the microembolization procedure which was not associated with a decrease in regional myocardial blood flow, as measured by microspheres. When comparing the consequences of an epicardial coronary artery stenosis on regional myocardial blood flow and contractile function with those of coronary microembolization at equal levels of contractile dysfunction, the stenosis was characterized by typical perfusion-contraction matching,[38] whereas the coronary microembolization induced a perfusion-contraction mismatch pattern (Figure 2).[39] Coronary microembolization caused patchy microinfarction which affected about 2% of the respective myocardium (Figure 3).[40] Less than 0.1% of cardiomyocytes were apoptotic, and apoptotic cardiomyocytes were always associated with the microinfarcts.[40] The microinfarcts were characterized by leukocyte infiltration (Figure 3), including monocytes/macrophages, but the microspheres per se proved to be inert and not chemoattractant in vitro[39]. Since there was only little infarcted myocardium and myocardial blood flow at the level which could be resolved by the microspheres technique was not reduced, we hypothesized that the observed inflammatory response might be responsible for the observed profound regional contractile dysfunction following coronary microembolization. Indeed, supporting this idea, methylprednisolone abolished the progressive contractile dysfunction, even when given as a single bolus and even when given 30 min after coronary microembolization (Figure 4).[41] More specifically, we identified a causal role for tumor necrosis factor α (TNFα) in the observed contractile dysfunction, supporting and extending prior findings by Arras et al. who reported enhanced TNFα expression and leukocyte infiltration after coronary microembolization in pigs[42]. Not only were increased myocardial TNFα concentrations associated with contractile dysfunction following coronary microembolization, but also did intracoronary infusion of exogenous TNFα induce dysfunction in the absence of microembolization, and conversely pretreatment with TNFα antibodies did prevent dysfunction following microembolization.[40] TNFα was localized to infiltrating

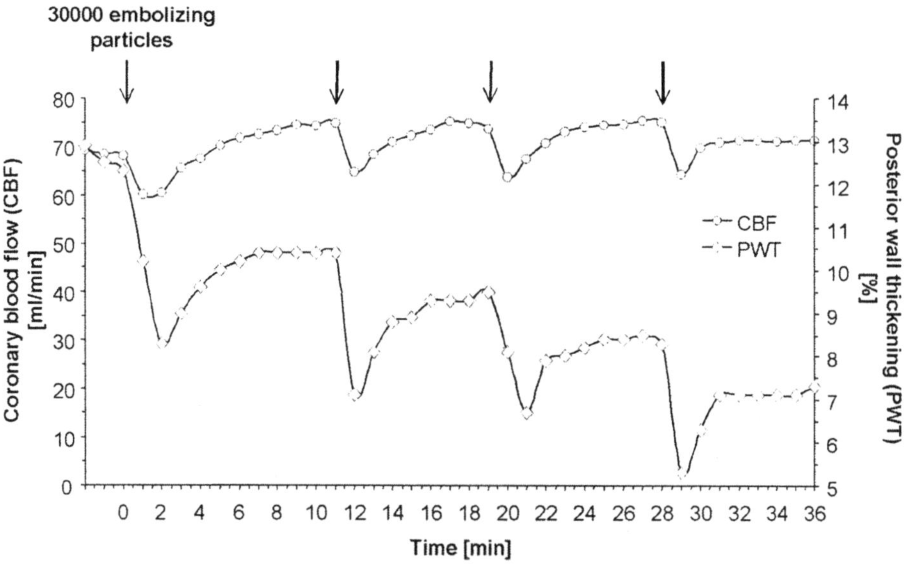

Figure 1. Coronary blood flow and regional contractile function in response to stepwise coronary microembolization. Coronary blood flow is transiently increased and then recovers, whereas regional contractile function is progressively decreased (by permission from Skyschally[18]).

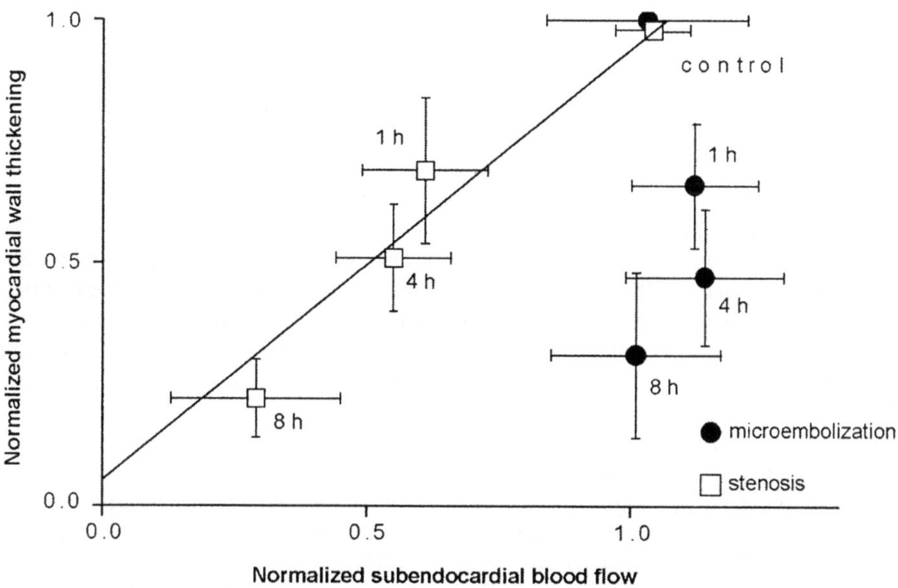

Figure 2. Coronary microembolization causes a progressive perfusion-contraction mismatch, i. e. contractile function is progressively reduced, whereas regional myocardial blood flow remains unaltered (by permission from Dorge[39]).

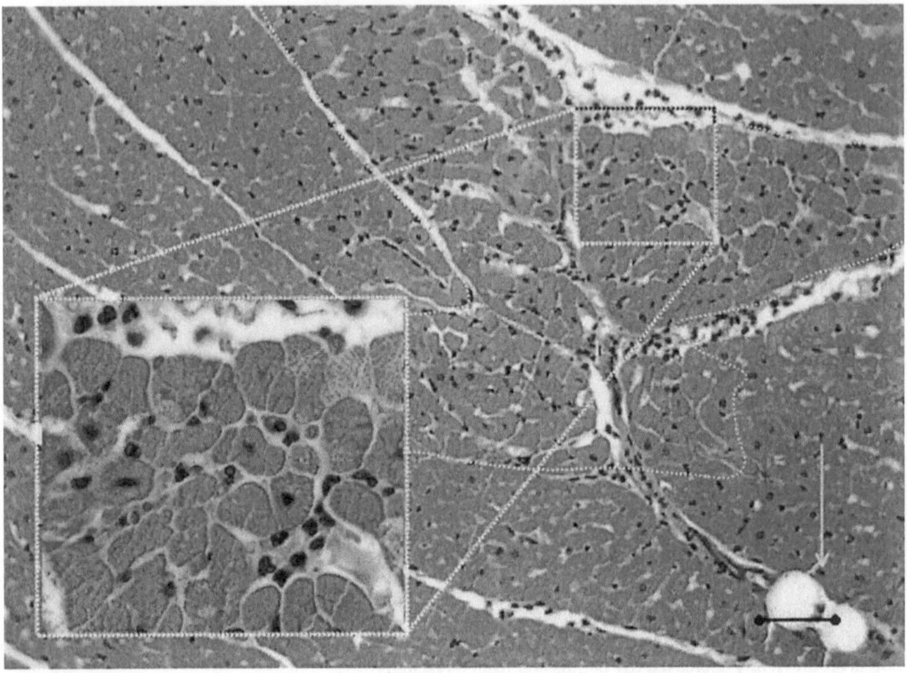

Figure 3. Microinfarct in microembolized myocardium (outlined area; 0.26±0.22 mm2; mean±SD); the arrow points to embolizing microspheres. The magnified inset displays the typical leukocyte infiltration (by permission from Dorge[39]).

leukocytes within and around microinfarcts and also to cardiomyocytes in the viable border zone around microinfarcts. In situ hybridization of TNFα-mRNA identified these viable myocytes as the major source of TNFα in microembolized myocardium.[40] To specify the signal cascade of TNFα-induced dysfunction in this model we have further studied the role of nitric oxide and sphingosine, known elements of the signal transduction of TNFα in ischemia-reperfusion injury and chronic heart failure.[43,44] Microembolization increased TNFα and sphingosine contents in the myocardium. Pretreatment with the nitric oxide-synthase inhibitor NG-nitro-L-arginine-methylester attenuated the progressive myocardial contractile dysfunction and prevented increases in TNFα and sphingosine contents.[45] N-oleoylethanolamine disrupts the sphingomyelinase pathway by blocking the enzyme ceramidase which catalyzes the conversion of ceramide to sphingosine[46,47] and it abolished the progressive contractile dysfunction following coronary microembolization; myocardial TNFα but not sphingosine content was increased.[45] These results strongly suggest that the microembolization-induced progressive contractile dysfunction is signaled through a cascade with nitric oxide located upstream of TNFα and sphingosine located downstream of TNFα.[45]

As detailed above, this experimental model of coronary microembolization is not only characterized by a perfusion-contraction mismatch pattern, but also by reduced coronary reserve. Also, the inotropic response to intracoronary infusion of dobutamine is diminished in microembolized myocardium.[18]

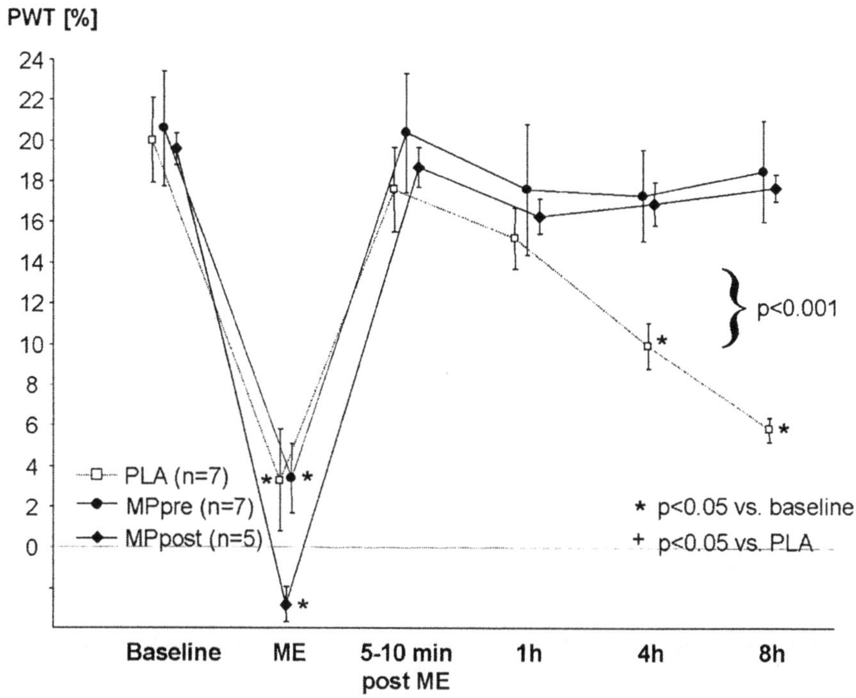

Figure 4. Posterior systolic wall thickening (PWT) at baseline, with immediate coronary microembolization (ME) and 5-10 min, 1, 4, and 8 h later. In the placebo-group (PLA), posterior systolic wall thickening after an initial recovery from microembolization was progressively decreased, whereas it remained unchanged in the groups receiving methylprednisolone before (MPpre) or after microembolization (MPpost) (by permission from Skyschally[41]).

Given the only small aggregate infarct size and the inflammatory pathogenesis of the contractile dysfunction following coronary microembolization, its eventual reversibility is not surprising. In chronically instrumented dogs, the profound contractile dysfunction which was observed several hours following coronary microembolization recovered fully over one week (Figure 5).[41]

Clearly, inflammation is important for the contractile dysfunction that develops after coronary microembolization. Whether or not the therapeutic use of cortisone can be exploited in patients who have possibly suffered coronary microembolization during a coronary intervention remains to be studied.

5. CORONARY MICROEMBOLIZATION AND ISCHEMIC PRECONDITIONING

Transient episodes of angina often precede acute myocardial infarction. Such short ischemic episodes may either protect the myocardium by ischemic preconditioning or damage it when associated with coronary microembolization. Common to

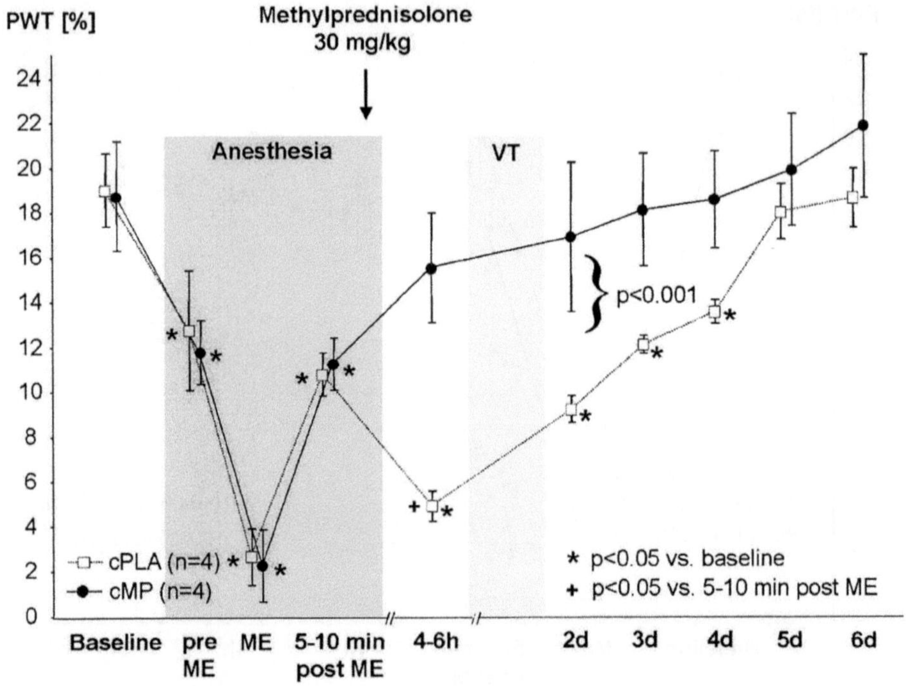

Figure 5. Posterior systolic wall thickening (PWT) at baseline, with immediate coronary microembolization (ME) and at 5-10 min, 4-6 h and at 2-6 d in chronically instrumented dogs. Between 4-6h and 2 d ventricular tachycardia (VT) did not permit functional measurements. In the placebo-group (cPLA), posterior systolic wall thickening recovered back to baseline values within 5 d, whereas it was back to baseline at 4-6 h in the group receiving methylprednisolone after microembolization (cMP) (by permission from Skyschally[41]).

both, ischemic preconditioning and coronary microembolization, is the involvement of adenosine. Adenosine is an established trigger of ischemic preconditioning[48] and the hyperemic response after coronary microembolization is caused by adenosine, released from ischemic areas in the microembolized myocardium.[13]. Thus, the surrounding non-embolized tissue may be protected against infarction from subsequent sustained ischemia/reperfusion. However, in anesthetized pigs coronary microembolization failed to protect the myocardium from infarction after 90 min sustained ischemia and 2h reperfusion.[49] This lack of protection can be attributed to the lack of increase of the interstitial adenosine concentration with coronary microembolization,[49] since a transient increase in the interstitial adenosine concentration prior to the sustained ischemia is mandatory to establish protection by ischemic preconditioning.[50] The superimposition of infarction induced by coronary microembolization per se[40] even increased the infarct size after sustained ischemia in microembolized myocardium.[49] It remains unclear whether microembolized myocardium can be classically preconditioned by a brief period of ischemia/reperfusion. Indeed, protection by ischemic preconditioning could be lost if there is a critical loss of adenosine through enhanced washout with coronary blood[13,17,49] and lymph flow[51] following coronary microembolization.

6. SOURCE AND CONSEQUENCES OF POTENTIAL THROMBOEMBOLI IN PATIENTS

Apart from coronary angiography, better resolution new imaging techniques including intravascular ultrasound[52-55] and angioscopy,[56-58] have facilitated the detection of epicardial coronary plaque rupture and ulceration and thus the potential source of coronary microembolization. Spontaneous plaque rupture is not only found in patients with unstable or stable angina at autopsy (see above). Even in a patient with a normal coronary angiogram, who developed profound, but reversible regional contractile dysfunction, plaque rupture was detected using intravascular ultrasound.[59]

Recent studies using intravascular ultrasound provided evidence that indeed the reduction in epicardial atherosclerotic plaque volume in patients undergoing a percutaneous coronary intervention in acute myocardial infarction[60] or unstable angina[61] induces microembolization and thus contributes to inadequate reperfusion, as assessed by TIMI frame count,[60] and microinfarcts, as assessed by creatine kinase (CK)-MB release.[61]

Imaging techniques reveal the potential source of coronary microemboli. Conversely, the transient elevation of CK, CK–MB isoenzyme and more sensitively troponin[62] is now regarded as a characteristic sign of micronecrosis in patients with unstable angina and may just reflect the consequences of coronary microembolization. Clearly the elevation of troponin is also a predictor of worse prognosis in patients with unstable angina.[63,64] Such considerations have found their way into the most recent consensus document on the definition of myocardial infarction by the European Society of Cardiology and the American College of Cardiology[65] which particularly acknowledges "microemboli from the atherosclerotic lesion that has been disrupted during angioplasty or from the particulate thrombus at the site of the culprit lesion". Conversely, the efficacy of glycoprotein IIb/IIIa receptor antagonists in patients with unstable angina and myocardial infarction[66,67] may not only reflect better resolution of the thrombus overlying the ruptured epicardial plaque but also that of the embolizing thromboemboli in the microcirculation.[67]

Not only in spontaneous plaque rupture and ulceration, but also and possibly more importantly during coronary interventions, microembolization is in fact induced, again leading to myocardial microinfarcts, as reflected by elevated CK and troponin[68-71] and frequently observed electrocardiographic alterations.[69] Distal coronary microembolization appears to be more common in patients undergoing rotational atherectomy[70,72,73,] as judged by CK-MB elevation,[70] persistent microvascular impairment[73] and contractile dysfunction.[72] Indeed, microinfarcts were detected by contrast-enhanced MRI technique in patients who had mild elevations of CK-MB after percutaneous coronary intervention.[74]

Supportive evidence for a causal role of thromboemboli in such complications of coronary interventions comes again from the efficacy of glycoprotein IIb/IIIa receptor antagonists[75-77] in improving microvascular function and decreasing the incidence of post-interventional troponin release, indicating less microembolization.[78]

Reminiscent of the above experimental studies, inflammatory responses are also seen in those clinical scenarios where coronary microembolization is likely to occur, i.e. nuclear factor - κB is activated in patients with unstable angina[79] and serum C-reactive protein is increased in patients who died from an acute coronary syndrome[80]. Interleukin-6 was higher up to 48 h in patients with unstable angina who experienced a major adverse cardiac event.[81] These markers of inflammation were assumed to originate from the rupturing atherosclerotic plaque, but they may be derived from microcirculatory inflammation in response to myocardial microinfarction equally well.[82]

The importance of inflammation in coronary microembolization is also supported by a recent study, in which preprocedural treatment with HMG-CoA reductase inhibitors in patients undergoing stenting of a de-novo stenosis resulted in a reduced incidence of peri-procedural myocardial injury, as assessed by analysis of CK and troponin T, and better event-free survival.[83] This beneficial effect is most likely attributable to anti-inflammatory properties of HMG-CoA reductase inhibitors,[84] such as favorably altered plaque composition and plaque stabilization.

Cyclic coronary blood flow variations, such as seen in the Folts experimental model (see above), are observed during coronary interventions[85-87] and are a sign predicting immediate complications in patients who underwent angiographically successful percutaneous transluminal coronary angioplasty.[88]

Interestingly, patients without normalization of coronary flow reserve after coronary interventions often have increased baseline coronary blood flow velocity[71,73,89-92] reminiscent of the reactive hyperemia seen with experimental microembolization (see above). In further support of a causal involvement of coronary microembolization in the observed increase in baseline blood flow velocity and reduced flow velocity reserve, such reduced coronary reserve was associated with increased coronary venous adenosine release[89] and correlated with increased serum CK and troponin.[71] Also, in patients who had increased baseline flow velocity following stent placement, the α_1 – antagonist urapidil decreased baseline flow velocity and increased coronary reserve, reminiscent of the reduction of adenosine release and hyperemia following coronary microembolization by the α_1 – antagonist prazosin in dogs.[14]

7. PROTECTION DEVICES AGAINST CORONARY MICROEMBOLIZATION

The most direct and best available clinical evidence for coronary microembolization comes probably from use of aspiration and filtration devices , i.e. “ex iuvantibus”, which can retrieve surprisingly large pieces of plaque debris and thrombotic material (Figure 6) and thus prevent it from being embolized into the microcirculation.[93-97] In the SAFER trial, an aspiration device removed embolizing debris during angioplasty of saphenous vein grafts and reduced cardiac events (a composite of death, myocardial infarction, emergency bypass surgery, target vessel revascularization).[98] Distal occlusion and aspiration permits a more complete retrieval of debris but entails myocardial ischemia and the inability of simultaneous angiographic delineation of the culprit lesion. In contrast, when using filtration devices, the extent of coronary microembolization is probably underestimated from the retrieved material since, with a filter pore size of 100 μm, particles with a size that can cause substantial microembolization in the above experimental studies are not retrieved, and side branches and tortuitous vessels may also contribute to incomplete retrieval of embolizing material.[97] In the FIRE trial, there was accordingly no difference in major adverse outcome at 30 d when using a balloon/ aspiration vs. a filter protection device in patients who underwent a coronary intervention at a diseased saphenous vein aorto-coronary bypass graft.[99] Possibly, in the future such aspiration/filtration devices should also be used to protect the coronary circulation when unclamping the aorta after cardiac surgery and other interventions, and when dissecting an atherosclerotic epicardial coronary artery segment before anastomosing a bypass vessel. Certainly, the technical feasibility of the protection devices requires further improvement. The availability of glycoprotein IIb/IIIa receptor antagonists to improve patient outcome and the efficiency of aspiration/filtration devices to reduce major adverse cardiac events during interventions on venous bypass stenosis strongly support the importance of microembolization in the clinical setting.

8. CONCLUSIONS AND REMAINING QUESTIONS

Clearly, coronary microembolization is a frequent event in ischemic heart disease, spontaneously in patients with unstable angina / acute coronary syndromes as well as artificially during coronary interventions with typical consequences, such as malignant arrhythmias and contractile dysfunction (Figure 7). The resulting microcirculatory impairment causes patchy microinfarction, and is often associated with coronary hyperemia at baseline and, conversely, transiently reduced coronary reserve. These obser-

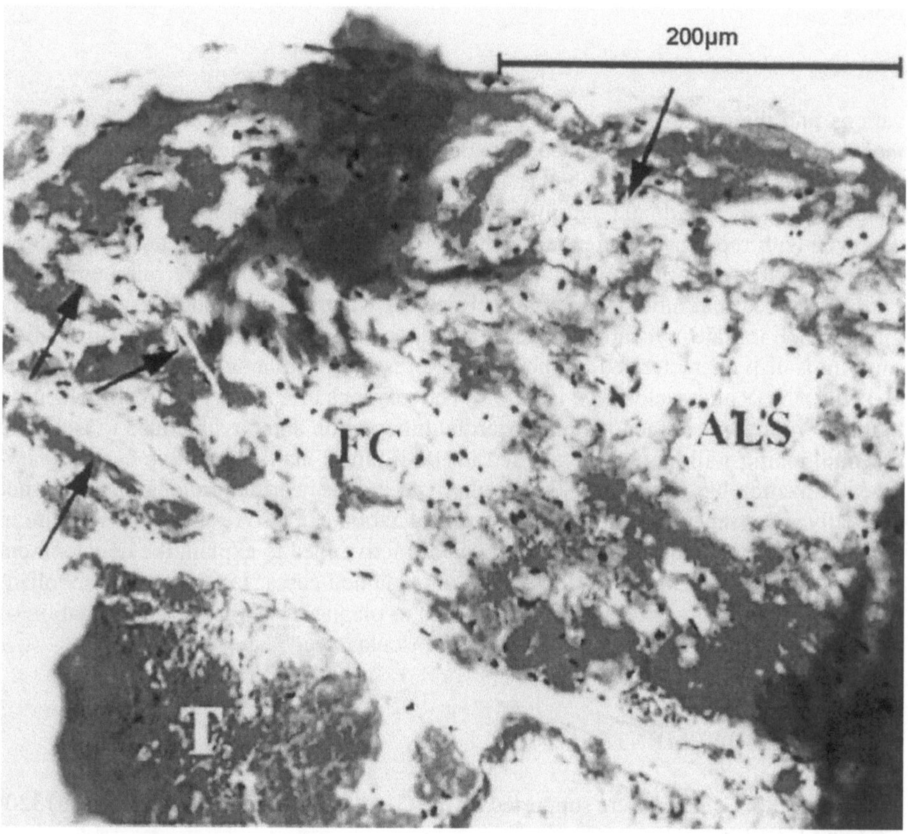

Figure 6. Characteristic plaque debris retrieved by a filtration device. ALS: amorphous lipid substance, FC: foam cell, T: thrombus. Arrows point to cholesterol crystals (by permission from Skyschally[110]).

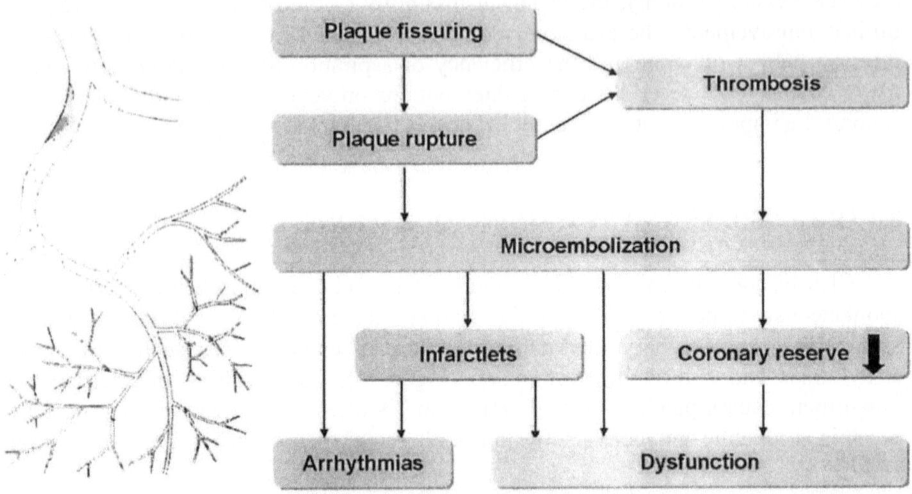

Figure 7. Schematic diagram of coronary microembolization and its consequences (by permission from Erbel[6]).

vations find their counterpart in experimental models of coronary microembolization; the contractile dysfunction induced by experimental coronary microembolization causally involves inflammation. Whether and to what extent coronary microembolization contributes to the enigmatic, but important no-reflow phenomenon[100] that is frequently observed with reperfusion of experimental[101,102] and clinical[103,104] myocardial infarction remains unclear. Another potential relation exists between coronary microembolization and myocardial hibernation.[105] Regardless of whether or not showers of coronary microemboli initiate myocardial hibernation, the phenotype of human hibernating myocardium is also characterized by increased expression of inflammatory mediators such as TNFα, iNOS and cyclooxygenase.[106,107] The relations of coronary microembolization to the no-reflow phenomenon, to myocardial hibernation and possibly also to ischemic preconditioning will have to be studied in the future. Finally, repetitive coronary microembolization has been used experimentally to induce heart failure.[108] Whether or not clinically silent repetitive coronary microembolization can also result in heart failure in humans, is currently unclear but appears an attractive idea to explain the development of heart failure in a number of otherwise unexplained cases. Finally, microembolization of coronary vasa vasorum may contribute to plaque instability and propagation of atherosclerosis into the more distal coronary vascular tree.[109]

ACKNOWLEDGEMENTS

The authors`studies were supported by the German Research Foundation (He 1320/13-1 and He 1320/14-1).

The authors are grateful to Dr. Heinz-Horst Deichmann for his generous sponsorship.

REFERENCES

1. E. Falk, Plaque rupture with severe pre–existing stenosis precipitating coronary thrombosis. Characteristics of coronary atherosclerotic plaques underlying fatal occlusive thrombi, *Br Heart J* **50**, 127–134 (1983).
2. M. J. Davies and A. C. Thomas, Plaque fissuring – the cause of acute myocardial infarction, sudden ischaemic death, and crescendo angina, *Br Heart J* **53**, 363–373 (1985).
3. E. Falk, Unstable angina with fatal outcome: dynamic coronary thrombosis leading to infarction and/or sudden death. Autopsy evidence of recurrent mural thrombosis with peripheral embolization culminating in total vascular occlusion, *Circulation* **71**, 699–708 (1985).
4. M. J. Davies, A. C. Thomas, P. A. Knapman and J. R. Hangartner, Intramyocardial platelet aggregation in patients with unstable angina suffering sudden ischemic cardiac death, *Circulation* **73**, 418–427 (1986).
5. R. J. Frink, P. A. Rooney, J. O. Trowbridge and J. P. Rose, Coronary thrombosis and platelet/fibrin microemboli in death associated with acute myocardial infarction, *Br Heart J* **59**, 196–200 (1988).
6. R. Erbel and G. Heusch, Brief review: coronary microembolization, *J Am Coll Cardiol* **36**, 22–24 (2000).
7. E. J. Topol, J. S. Yadav, Recognition of the importance of embolization in atherosclerotic vascular disease, *Circulation* **101**, 570–580 (2000).
8. G. Heusch, R. Schulz, M. Haude and R. Erbel, Coronary microembolization, *J Mol Cell Cardiol* **37**, 23–31 (2004).
9. N. El-Maraghi, E. Genton, The relevance of platelet and fibrin thrombembolism of the coronary microcirculation, with special reference to sudden cardiac death, *Circulation* **62**, 936–944 (1980).
10. R. J. Bing, A. Castellanos, E. Gradel, C. Lupton and A. Siegel, Experimental myocardial infarction: Circulatory biochemical and pathologic changes, *Am J Med Sci* **232**, 533–554 (1956).
11. J. W. West, T. Kobayashi and F. S. Anderson, Effects of selective coronary embolization on coronary blood flow and coronary sinus venous blood oxygen saturation in dogs, *Circ Res* **10**, 722–738 (1962).
12. R. M. Herzberg, R. Rubio and R. M. Berne, Coronary occlusion and embolization: effect on blood flow in adjacent arteries, *Am J Physiol* **210**, 169–175 (1966).
13. M. Hori, M. Inoue, M. Kitakaze, Y. Koretsune, K. Iwai, J. Tamai, H. Ito, A. Kitabatake, T. Sato and T. Kamada, Role of adenosine in hyperemic response of coronary blood flow in microcirculation., *Am J Physiol Heart Circ Physiol* **250**, H509–H518 (1986).
14. M. Hori, J. Tamai, M. Kitakaze, K. Iwakura, K. Gotoh, K. Iwai, Y. Koretsune, T. Kagiya, A. Kitabatake and T. Kamada, Adenosine-induced hyperemia attenuates myocardial ischemia in coronary microembolization in dogs, *Am J Physiol Heart Circ Physiol* **257**, H244–H251 (1989).
15. M. Hori, K. Gotoh, M. Kitakaze, K. Iwai, K. Iwakura, H. Sato, Y. Koretsune, M. Inoue, A. Kitabatake and T. Kamada, Role of oxygen–derived free radicals in myocardial edema and ischemia in coronary microvascular embolization, *Circulation* **84**, 828–840 (1991).
16. S. Takashima, M. Hori, M. Kitakaze, H. Sato, M. Inoue and T. Kamada, Superoxide dismutase restores contractile and metabolic dysfunction through augmentation of adenosine release in coronary microembolization, *Circulation* **87**, 982–995 (1993).
17. F. Grund, H. T. Sommerschild, T. Lyberg, K. Kirkeboen and A. Ilebekk, Microembolization in pigs: effects on coronary blood flow and myocardial ischemic tolerance, *Am J Physiol Heart Circ Physiol* **277**, H533–H542 (1999).
18. A. Skyschally, R. Schulz, R. Erbel and G. Heusch, Reduced coronary and inotropic reserves with coronary microembolization, *Am J Physiol Heart Circ Physiol* **282**, H611–H614 (2002).
19. C. Eng, S. Cho, S. M. Factor, E. H. Sonnenblick and E. S. Kirk, Myocardial micronecrosis produced by microsphere embolization. Role of an alpha-adrenergic tonic influence on the coronary microcirculation, *Circ Res* **54**, 74–82 (1984).
20. G. Heusch, α-Adrenergic mechanisms in myocardial ischemia, *Circulation* **81**, 1–13 (1990).
21. G. Heusch, Emerging importance of alpha-adrenergic coronary vasoconstriction in acute coronary syndromes and its genetic background, *J Am Coll Cardiol* **41**, 195–196 (2003).
22. S. Mohlenkamp, P. E. Beighley, E. A. Pfeifer, T. R. Behrenbeck, P. F. Sheedy II and E. L. Ritman, Intramyocardial blood volume, perfusion and transit time in response to embolization of different sized microvessels, *Cardiovasc Res* **57**, 843–852 (2003).

23. J. D. Folts, E. B. Crowell and G. G. Rowe, Platelet aggregation in partially obstructed vessels and its elimination with aspirin, *Circulation* **54**, 365–370 (1976).
24. J. T. Willerson, P. Golino, J. Eidt, W. B. Campbell and L. M. Buja, Specific platelet mediators and unstable coronary artery lesions. Experimental evidence and potential clinical implications, *Circulation* **80**, 198–205 (1989).
25. J. D. Folts, Deleterious hemodynamic effects of thrombotic/embolic materials on the distal myocardial vasculature, *Cardiovasc Res* **42**, 6–7 (1999).
26. J. A. Barrabus, D. Garcia-Dorado, B. Soriano, J. Solares, Y. Puigfel, L. Trobo, A. Garcia-Lafuente and J. Soler–Soler, Dynamic intracoronary thrombosis does not cause significant downstream platelet embolization, *Cardiovasc Res* **47**, 265–273 (2000).
27. P. Golino, M. Buja, Y. Sheng-Kun, J. McNatt and J. T. Willerson, Failure of nitroglycerin and diltiazem to reduce platelet-mediated vasoconstriction in dogs with coronary artery stenosis and endothelial injury: further evidence for thromboxane A_2 and serotonin as mediators of coronary artery vasoconstriction in vivo, *J Am Coll Cardiol* **15**, 718–726 (1990).
28. J. D. Folts, K. Gallagher and G. G. Rowe, Blood flow reductions in stenosed canine coronary arteries: vasospasm or platelet aggregation?, *Circulation* **65**, 248–255 (1985).
29. K. P. Gallagher, G. Osakada, W. S. Kemper and J. Ross Jr., Cyclical coronary flow reductions in conscious dogs equipped with ameroid constrictors to produce severe coronary narrowing, *Basic Res Cardiol* **80**, 100–106 (1985).
30. J. F. Eidt, P. Allison, J. Ashton, P. Golino, J. McNatt, L. M. Buja and J. T. Willerson, Thrombin is an important mediator of platelet aggregation in stenosed canine coronary arteries with endothelial injury, *J Clin Invest* **84**, 18–27 (1989).
31. B. G. Bertha and J. D. Folts, Subendocardial and subepicardial segmental function changes in the dog heart due to gradual coronary flow reduction by an acutely developing thrombus, *Cardiovasc Res* **19**, 495–506 (1985).
32. P. R. Kowey, R. L. Verrier, B. Lown and R. I. Handin, Influence of intracoronary platelet aggregation on ventricular electrical properties during partial coronary artery stenosis, *Am J Cardiol* **51**, 596–602 (1983).
33. M. Mansaray, P. R. Belcher, I. Vergroesen, Z. M. Wright, J. W. Hynd, A. J. Drake–Holland and M. I. M. Noble, Downstream resistance effects of intracoronary thrombosis in the stenosed canine coronary artery, *Cardiovasc Res* **42**, 193–200 (1999).
34. L. Jorgensen, H. C. Rowsell, T. Hovig, M. F. Glynn and J. F. Mustard, Adenosine diphosphate–induced platelet aggregation and myocardial infarction in swine, *Lab Invest* **17**, 616–644 (1967).
35. J. I. Haft, P. D. Kranz, F. J. Albert and K. Fani, Intravascular platelet aggregation in the heart induced by norepinephrine, *Circulation* **46**, 698–708 (1972).
36. J. I. Haft, K. Gershengorn, P. D. Kranz and R. Oestreicher, Protection against epinephrine-induced myocardial necrosis by drugs that inhibit platelet aggregation, *Am J Cardiol* **30**, 838–843 (1972).
37. M. Gawaz, Role of platelets in coronary thrombosis and reperfusion of ischemic myocardium, *Cardiovasc Res* **61**, 498–511 (2004).
38. J. Ross Jr., Myocardial perfusion-contraction matching, *Circulation* **83**, 1076–1083 (1991).
39. H. Dφrge, T. Neumann, M. Behrends, A. Skyschally, R. Schulz, C. Kasper, R. Erbel and G. Heusch, Perfusion-contraction mismatch with coronary microvascular obstruction: role of inflammation, *Am J Physiol Heart Circ Physiol* **279**, H2587–H2592 (2000).
40. H. Dorge, R. Schulz, S. Belosjorow, H. Post, A. van de Sand, I. Konietzka, S. Frede, T. Hartung, J. Vinten-Johansen, K. A. Youker, M. L. Entman, R. Erbel and G. Heusch, Coronary microembolization: the role of TNFα in contractile dysfunction, *J Mol Cell Cardiol* **34**, 51–62 (2002).
41. A. Skyschally, M. Haude, H. Dorge, M. Thielmann, A. Duschin, A. van de Sand, I. Konietzka, A. Bóchert, S. Aker, P. Massoudy, R. Schulz, R. Erbel and G. Heusch, Glucocorticoid treatment prevents progressive myocardial dysfunction resulting from experimental coronary microembolization, *Circulation* **109**, 2337–2342 (2004).
42. M. Arras, R. Strasser, M. Mohri, R. Doll, P. Eckert, W. Schaper and J. Schaper, Tumor necrosis factor-alpha is expressed by monocytes/macrophages following cardiac microembolization and is antagonized by cyclosporine, *Basic Res Cardiol* **93**, 97–107 (1998).
43. T. Yokoyama, L. Vaca, W. Durante, P. Hazarika and D. L. Mann, Cellular basis for the negative inotropic effects of tumor necrosis factor-α in the adult mammalian heart, *J Clin Invest* **92**, 2303–2312 (1993).

44. D. R. Meldrum, Tumor necrosis factor in the heart, *Am J Physiol Regul Integ Comp Physiol* **274**, R577–R595 (1998).
45. M. Thielmann, H. Dorge, C. Martin, S. Belosjorow, U. Schwanke, A. van de Sand, I. Konietzka, A. Bóchert, A. Króger, R. Schulz and G. Heusch, Myocardial dysfunction with coronary microembolization: signal transduction through a sequence of nitric oxide, tumor necrosis factor-α and sphingosine, *Circ Res* **90**, 807–813 (2002).
46. Y. A. Hannun and R. M. Bell, Functions of sphingolipids and sphingolipid breakdown products in cellular regulation, *Science,* **S 243**, 500–507 (1989).
47. E. Coroneos, M. Martinez, S. McKenna and M. Kester, Differential regulation of sphingomyelinase and ceramidase activities by growth factors and cytokines, *J Biol Chem* **270**, 23305–23309 (1995).
48. R. Schulz, M. V. Cohen, M. Behrends, J. M. Downey and G. Heusch, Signal transduction of ischemic preconditioning, *Cardiovasc Res* **52**, 181–198 (2001).
49. A. Skyschally, R. Schulz, P. Gres, I. Konietzka, C. Martin, M. Haude, R. Erbel and G. Heusch, Coronary microembolization does not induce acute preconditioning against infarction in pigs – the role of adenosine, *Cardiovasc Res* **63**, 313–322 (2004).
50. R. Schulz, J. Rose, H. Post and G. Heusch, Involvement of endogenous adenosine in ischaemic preconditioning in swine, *Pflógers Arch* **430**, 273–282 (1995).
51. D. Saito, M. Hasui, T. Shiraki and H. Kono, Effects of coronary blood flow, myocardial contractility, and heart rate on cardiac lymph circulation in open-chest dogs. Use of a direct cannulation method for subepicardial lymph vessel, *Arzneimittelforschung* **47**, 119–124 (1997).
52. J. Zamorano, R. Erbel, J. Ge, G. Gorge, P. Kearney, L. Koch, A. Scholte and J. Meyer, Spontaneous plaque rupture visualized by intravascular ultrasound, *Eur Heart J* **15**, 131–133 (1994).
53. J. Ge, F. Liu, P. Kearney, G. Gorge, M. Haude, D. Baumgart, M. Ashry and R. Erbel, Intravascular ultrasound approach to the diagnosis of coronary artery aneurysm, *Am Heart J* **130**, 765–771 (1995).
54. J. Ge, F. Chirillo, J. Schwedtmann, G. Gorge, M. Haude, D. Baumgart, V. Shah, C. von Birgelen, S. Sack, H. Boudoulas and R. Erbel, Screening of ruptured plaques in patients with coronary artery disease by intravascular ultrasound, *Heart* **81**, 621–627 (1999).
55. M. Gossl, C. von Birgelen, G. S. Mintz, D. Bose, H. Eggebrecht, D. Baumgart, M. Haude and R. Erbel, Volumetric assessment of ulcerated ruptured coronary plaques with three–dimensional intravascular ultrasound in vivo, *Am J Cardiol* **91**, 992–996 (2003).
56. Y. Ueda, M. Asakura, A. Hirayama, K. Komamura, M. Hori and K. Kodama, Intracoronary morphology of culprit lesions after reperfusion in acute myocardial infarction: Serial angioscopic observations, *J Am Coll Cardiol* **27**, 606–610 (1996).
57. E. van Belle, J.-M. Lablanche, C. Bauters, N. Renaud, E. P. McFadden and M. E. Bertrand, Coronary angioscopic findings in the infarct–releated vessel within 1 month of acute myocardial infarction. Natural history and the effect of thrombolysis, *Circulation* **97**, 26–33 (1998).
58. K. Okamatsu, M. Takano, S. Sakai, F. Ishibashi, R. Uemura, T. Takano and K. Mizuno, Elevated troponin T levels and lesion characteristics in non-ST-elevation acute coronary syndromes, *Circulation* **109**, 465–470 (2004).
59. D. Baumgart, F. Liu, M. Haude, G. Gorge, J. Ge and R. Erbel, Acute plaque rupture and myocardial stunning in patient with normal coronary arteriography, *Lancet* **346**, 193–194 (1995).
60. J. Kotani, G. S. Mintz, J. Pregowski, L. Kalinczuk, A. D. Pichard, L. F. Satler, W. O. Suddath, R. Waksman and N. J. Weissman, Volumetric intravascular ultrasound evidence that distal embolization during acute infarct intervention contributes to inadequate myocardial perfusion grade, *Am J Cardiol* **92**, 728–732 (2003).
61. F. Prati, T. Pawlowski, R. Gil, A. Labellarte, A. Gziut, E. Caradonna, A. Manzoli, A. Pappalardo, F. Burzotta, A. Boccanelli, Stenting of culprit lesions in unstable angina leads to a marked reduction in plaque burden: A major role of plaque embolization?, *Circulation* **107**, 2320–2325 (2003).
62. C. W. Hamm, J. Ravkilde, W. Gerhardt, P. Jorgensen, E. Peheim, L. Ljungdahl, B. Goldmann and H. A. Katus, The prognostic value of serum troponin T in unstable angina, *N Engl J Med* **327**, 146–150 (1992).
63. S. J. Brener and E. J. Topol, Troponin, embolization and restoration of microvascular integrity, *Eur Heart J* **21**, 1117–1119 (2000).
64. J. Herrmann, L. Volbracht, M. Haude, H. Eggebrecht, N. Malyar, K. Mann and R. Erbel, Biochemische Marker bei ischðmischen und nicht ischðmischen Myokardschðdigungen, *Med Klin* **96**, 144–156 (2001).

65. J. S. Alpert and K. Thygesen, Myocardial infarction redefined – a consensus document of the Joint European Society of Cardiology/American College of Cardiology committee for the redefinition of myocardial infarction, *Eur Heart J* **21**, 1502–1513 (2000).
66. PRISM-PLUS Study Investigators, Inhibition of the platelet glycoprotein IIb/IIIa receptor with tirofiban in unstable angina and Non-Q-Wave myocardial infarction, *N Engl J Med* **338**, 1488–1497 (1998).
67. C. W. Hamm, C. Heeschen, B. Goldmann, A. Vahanian, J. Adgey, C. Macaya Miguel, W. Rutsch, J. Berger, J. Koostra and M. L. Simoons, Benefit of abciximab in patients with refractory unstable angina in relation to serum troponin T levels., *N Engl J Med* **340**, 1623–1629 (1999).
68. A. E. Abdelmeguid, E. J. Topol, P. L. Whitlow, S. K. Sapp and S. G. Ellis, Significance of mild transient release of creatine kinase-MB fraction after percutaneous coronary interventions, *Circulation* **94**, 1528–1536 (1996).
69. R. M. Califf, A. E. Abdelmeguid, R. E. Kuntz, J. J. Popma, C. J. Davidson, E. A. Cohen, N. S. Kleiman, K. W. Mahaffey, E. J. Topol, C. J. Pepine, R. J. Lipicky, C. B. Granger, R. A. Harrington, B. E. Tardiff, B. S. Crenshaw, R. P. Bauman, B. D. Zuckerman, B. R. Chaitman, J. A. Bittl and E. M. Ohman, Myonecrosis after revascularization procedures, *J Am Coll Cardiol* **31**, 241–251 (1998).
70. R. Mehran, G. Dangas, G. S. Mintz, A. J. Lansky, A. D. Pichard, L. F. Satler, K. M. Kent, G. W. Stone and M. B. Leon, Atherosclerotic plaque burden and CK-MB enzyme elevation after coronary interventions, *Circulation* **101**, 604–610 (2000).
71. J. Herrmann, M. Haude, A. Lerman, R. Schulz, L. Volbracht, J. Ge, A. Schmermund, H. Wieneke, C. von Birgelen, H. Eggebrecht, D. Baumgart, G. Heusch and R. Erbel, Abnormal coronary flow velocity reserve following coronary intervention is associated with cardiac marker elevation, *Circulation* **103**, 2339–2345 (2001).
72. M. J. A. Williams, C. J. Dow, J. B. Newell, I. F. Palacios and M. H. Picard, Prevalence and timing of regional myocardial dysfunction after rotational coronary atherectomy, *J Am Coll Cardiol* **28**, 861–869 (1996).
73. T. R. Bowers, R. E. Stewart, W. W. O'Neill, V. M. Reddy and R. D. Safian, Effect of Rotablator atherectomy and adjunctive balloon angioplasty on coronary blood flow, *Circulation* **95**, 1157–1164 (1997).
74. M. J. Ricciardi, E. Wu, C. J. Davidson, K. M. Choi, F. J. Klocke, R. O. Bonow, R. M. Judd, R. J. Kim, Visualization of discrete microinfarction after percutaneous coronary intervention associated with mild creatine kinase–MB elevation, *Circulation* **103**, 2780–2783 (2001).
75. K.-H. Mak, R. Challapalli, M. J. Eisenberg, K. M. Anderson, R. M. Califf and E. J. Topol, Effect of platelet glycoprotein IIb/IIIa receptor inhibition on distal embolization during percutaneous revascularization of aortocoronary saphenous vein grafts, *Am J Cardiol* **80**, 985–988 (1997).
76. F.-J. Neumann, R. Blasini, C. Schmitt, E. Alt, J. Dirschinger, M. Gawaz, A. Kastrati and A. Schomig, Effect of glycoprotein IIb/IIIa receptor blockade on recovery of coronary flow and left ventricular function after placement of coronary-artery stents in acute myocardial infarction, *Circulation* **98**, 2695–2701 (1998).
77. A. Schomig, A. Kastrati, J. Dirschinger, J. Mehilli, U. Schricke, J. Pache, S. Martinoff, F.-J. Neumann and M. Schwaiger, Coronary stenting plus platelet glycoprotein IIb/IIIa blockade compared with tissue plasminogen activator in acute myocardial infarction, *N Engl J Med* **343**, 385–391 (2000).
78. A. Bonz, B. Lengfelder, J. Strotmann, S. Held, O. Turschner, K. Harre, C. Wacker, C. Waller, N. Kochsiek, M. Meesmann, L. Neyses, P. Schanzenbacher, G. Ertl and W. Voelker, Effect of additional temporary glycoprotein IIb/IIIa receptor inhibition on troponin release in elective percutaneous coronary interventions after pretreatment with aspirin and clopidogrel (TOPSTAR trial), *J Am Coll Cardiol* **40**, 662–628 (2002).
79. M. E. Ritchie, Nuclear factor-ϰB is selectively and markedly activated in humans with unstable angina pectoris, *Circulation* **98**, 1707–1713 (1998).
80. A. R. Burke, R. Tracy and R. Virmani, C-reactive protein as a risk factor for atherothrombosis: a postmortem study. *Laboratory Investigation* **81**, 43A (2001).
81. M. R. Cusack, M. S. Marber, P. D. Lambiase, C. A. Bucknall and S. R. Redwood, Systemic inflammation in unstable angina is the result of myocardial necrosis, *J Am Coll Cardiol* **39**, 1917–1923 (2002).
82. G. Heusch, R. Schulz and R. Erbel, Inflammatory markers in coronary heart disease: Coronary vascular versus myocardial origin? *Circulation* **108**, e4 (2003).
83. J. Herrmann, A. Lerman, D. Baumgart, L. Volbracht, R. Schulz, C. von Birgelen, M. Haude, G. Heusch and R. Erbel, Pre-procedural statin medication reduces the extent of peri-procedural non-Q-wave myocardial infarction, *Circulation* **106**, 2180–2183 (2002).

84. N. Werner, G. Nickenig and U. Laufs, Pleiotropic effects of HMG-CoA reductase inhibitors, *Basic Res Cardiol* **97**, 105–116 (2002).
85. E. Eichhorn, P. A. Grayburn, J. E. Willard, V. Anderson, J. B. Bedotto, Carry M., J. K. Kahn and J. T. Willerson, Spontaneous alterations in coronary blood flow velocity before and after coronary angioplasty in patients with severe angina, *J Am Coll Cardiol* **17**, 43–52 (1991).
86. H. V. Anderson, R. L. Kirkeeide, A. Krishnaswami, L. A. Weigelt, M. Revana, H. F. Weisman and J. T. Willerson, Cyclic flow variations after coronary angioplasty in humans: clinical and angiographic characteristics and elimination with 7E3 monoclonal platelet antibody, *J Am Coll Cardiol* **23**, 1031–1037 (1994).
87. M. S. Flynn, M. J. Kern, F. V. Aguirre, R. G. Bach, E. A. Caracciolo and T. J. Donohue, Alterations in coronary blood flow velocity during intracoronary thrombolysis and rescue coronary angioplasty for acute myocardial infarction, *Cath Cardiovasc Diag* **31**, 219–224 (1994).
88. M. Sunamura, C. Di Mario, J. J. Piek, E. Schroeder, C. Vrints, P. Probst, G. R. Heyndrickx, E. Fleck and P. W. Serruys, Cyclic flow variations after angioplasy: A rare phenomenon predictive of immediate complications, *Am Heart J* **131**, 843–848 (1996).
89. S. Nanto, K. Kodama, M. Hori, M. Mishima, A. Hirayama, M. Inoue and T. Kamada, Temporal increase in resting coronary blood flow causes an impairment of coronary flow reserve after coronary angioplasty, *Am Heart J* **123**, 28–36 (1992).
90. R. A. M. Van Liebergen, J. J. Piek, K. T. Koch, R. J. de Winter and K. I. Lie, Immediate and long-term effect of balloon angioplasty or stent implantation on the absolute and relative coronary blood flow velocity reserve, *Circulation* **98**, 2133–2140 (1998).
91. M. J. Kern, S. Puri, R. G. Bach, T. J. Donohue, P. Dupouy, E. A. Caracciolo, R. Craig, F. Aguirre, E. Aptecar, T. L. Wolford, C. J. Mechem and J.–L. Dubois–Rande, Abnormal coronary flow velocity reserve after coronary artery stenting in patients. Role of relative coronary reserve to assess potential mechanisms, *Circulation* **100**, 2491–2498 (1999).
92. L. Gregorini, J. Marco, B. Farah, M. Bernies, C. Palombo, M. Kozakova, I. M. Bossi, B. Cassagneau, J. Fajadet, C. Di Mario, R. Albiero, M. Cugno, A. Grossi and G. Heusch, Effects of selective α1- and α2-adrenergic blockade on coronary flow reserve after coronary stenting, *Circulation* **106**, 2901–2907 (2002).
93. M. Carlino, J. De Gregorio, C. Di Mario, A. Anzuini, F. Airoldi, R. Albiero, C. Briguori, A. Dharmadhikari, I. Sheiban and A. Colombo, Prevention of distal embolization during saphenous vein graft lesion angioplasty, *Circulation* **99**, 3221–3223 (1999).
94. E. Grube, U. Gerckens, A. C. Yeung, S. Rowold, N. Kirchhof, J. Sedgewick, J. S. Yadav and S. Stertzer, Prevention of distal embolization during coronary angioplasty in saphenous vein grafts and native vessels using porous filter protection, *Circulation* **104**, 2436–2441 (2001).
95. E. Grube, J. Schofer, J. Webb, G. Schuler, A. Colombo, H. Sievert, U. Gerckens and G. W. Stone, The Saphenous Vein Graft Angioplasty Free of Emboli (SAFE) Trial Study Group, Evaluation of a balloon occlusion and aspiration system for protection from distal embolization during stenting in saphenous vein grafts, *Am J Cardiol* **89**, 941–945 (2002).
96. U. Limbruno, A. Micheli, M. De Carlo, G. Amoroso, R. Rossini, C. Palagi, V. Di Bello, A. S. Petronia, G. Fontanini and M. Mariani, Mechanical prevention of distal embolization during primary angioplasty. Safety, feasibility, and impact on myocardial reperfusion, *Circulation* **108**, 171–176 (2003).
97. G. Sangiorgi and A. Colombo, Embolic protection devices, *Heart* **89**, 990–992 (2003).
98. D. S. Baim, D. Wahr, B. George, M. B. Leon, J. Greenberg, D. E. Cutlip, U. Kaya, J. J. Popma, K. K. L. Ho and R. E. Kuntz, Randomized trial of a distal embolic protection device during percutaneous intervention of saphenous vein aorto-coronary bypass grafts, *Circulation* **105**, 1285–1290 (2002).
99. G. W. Stone, C. Rogers, J. Hermiller, R. Feldman, P. Hall, R. Haber, A. Masud, P. Cambier, R. P. Caputo, M. Turco, R. Kovach, B. Brodie, H. C. Herrmann, R. E. Kuntz, J. J. Popma, S. Ramee and D. A. Cox, Randomized comparison of distal protection with a filter-based catheter and a balloon occlusion and aspiration system during percutaneous intervention of diseased saphenous vein aorto–coronary bypass grafts, *Circulation* **108**, 548–553 (2003).
100. L. Thuesen and E. Falk, Pathology of coronary microembolisation and no reflow, *Heart* **89**, 983–985 (2003).
101. R. A. Kloner, C. E. Ganote and R. B. Jennings, The "no-reflow" phenomenon after temporary coronary occlusion in the dog, *J Clin Invest* **54**, 1496–1508 (1974).

102. G. Ambrosio, H. F. Weisman, J. A. Mannisi and L. C. Becker, Progressive impairment of regional myocardial perfusion after initial restoration of postischemic blood flow, *Circulation* **80**, 1846–1861 (1989).
103. M. Marzilli, E. Orsini, P. Marraccini and R. Testa, Beneficial effects of intracoronary adenosine as an adjunct to primary angioplasty in acute myocardial infarction, *Circulation* **101**, 2154–2159 (2000).
104. E. Eeckhout and M. J. Kern, The coronary no-reflow phenomenon: a review of mechanisms and therapies, *Eur Heart J* **22**, 729–739 (2001).
105. G. Heusch and R. Schulz, Hibernating myocardium. New answers, still more questions!, *Circ Res* **91**, 863–865 (2002).
106. C. S. B. Baker, D. P. Dutka, D. Pagano, O. Rimoldi, M. Pitt, R. J. C. Hall, J. M. Polak, R. S. Bonser and P. G. Camici, Immunocytochemical evidence for inducible nitric oxide synthase and cylooxygenase-2 expression with nitrotyrosine formation in human hibernating myocardium, *Basic Res Cardiol* **97**, 409–415 (2002).
107. D. K. Kalra, X. Zhu, M. K. Ramchandani, G. Lawrie, M. J. Reardon, D. Lee-Jackson, W. L. Winters, N. Sivasubramanian, D. L. Mann and W. A. Zoghbi, Increased myocardial gene expresssion of tumor necrosis factor-α and nitric oxide synthase-2. A potential mechanism for depressed myocardial function in hibernating myocardium in humans, *Circulation* **105**, 1537–1540 (2002).
108. H. N. Sabbah, P. D. Stein, T. Kono, M. Gheorghiade, T. B. Levine, S. Jafri, E. T. Hawkins and S. Goldstein, A canine model of chronic heart failure produced by multiple sequential coronary microembolizations, *Am J Physiol Heart Circ Physiol* **29**, H1379–H1384 (1991).
109. M. Gossl, N. M. Malyar, M. Rosol, P. E. Beighley and E. L. Ritman, Impact of coronary vasa vasorum functional structure on coronary vessel wall perfusion distribution, *Am J Physiol Heart Circ Physiol* **285**, H2019–H2026 (2003).
110. A. Skyschally, R. Erbel and G. Heusch, Coronary microembolization, *Circ J* **67**, 279–286 (2003).

CHAPTER 6

FIBROBLAST GROWTH FACTOR-2

As a therapeutic agent against heart disease

Elissavet Kardami[1, 2, 3], Karen A. Detillieux[3], Sarah K. Jimenez[3], Peter A. Cattini[3]

1. INTRODUCTION

The treatment of ischemic heart disease remains a major challenge facing the medical community. Preventative medicine aiming for vascular health through lifestyle changes and appropriate medications can be viewed as a first and fundamental line of defense. It is nevertheless an incontestable fact that building a 'second line of defense', i.e., the management/treatment of ischemic heart disease and its short- and long-term consequences, will remain an essential and urgent need for the foreseeable future. Since blockage of a coronary artery can result in myocardial tissue loss due to lack of oxygen and other critical metabolites, an obvious approach is to increase or restore blood flow to the affected area as quickly as possible. While there is some evidence that the development of collateral vessels occurs naturally to some degree as a response to coronary artery occlusion[1, 2] the nature of the occlusion usually demands that flow be restored more immediately and completely than natural processes would allow. Current therapies to restore flow include physical and invasive procedures, such as balloon angioplasty, arterial stents, coronary bypass surgery, as well as use of thrombolytic agents. Recently, the prospect of enhancing collateral development or increasing blood flow to an ischemic region through therapeutic angiogenesis has been gaining momentum. While these approaches serve the valuable purpose of restoring blood flow and improving prognosis and quality of life of cardiac patients to a considerable degree, they do require some time to take effect and during that delay myocardial tissue continues to be subjected to the ischemic insult and thus the extent of injury progresses. Furthermore, the act of restoring flow itself has been associated with exacerbated injury – known as

[1] Institute of Cardiovascular Sciences, St. Boniface Hospital Research Centre,
[2] Department of Human Anatomy and Cell Sciences
[3] Department of Physiology, University of Manitoba, Winnipeg, Manitoba, Canada
Correspondence to: Dr. Elissavet Kardami, Professor, Institute of Cardiovascular Sciences, St. Boniface Hospital Reseach Centre, 351 Tache Avenue, Winnipeg, MB R2H 2A6 Canada, Phone: (204) 235-3411 Fax: (204), Email: ekardami@sbrc.ca

the reperfusion injury (or secondary injury) phenomenon, which occurs as myocytes are forced to resume contraction under conditions of decreased pH, increased intracellular calcium, and increased osmotic pressure[3]. Consequently, therapies using so-called "cardioprotective agents", preserving the viability of the myocardium and limiting the extent of infarction during an ischemic episode, and even reducing the extent of injury upon reperfusion, would be of significant benefit. The term cardioprotection, although used in the past in a more general sense, more recently has been applied specifically to the effect of increasing myocyte viability under conditions of ischemia[4]. This chapter will examine how fibroblast growth factor-2 (FGF-2) can play a significant role in ameliorating the consequences of ischemia-reperfusion injury, through both acute (cardioprotective) and chronic (regenerative and/or angiogenic) effects . The ongoing transition from experimental evidence to clinical application will be discussed.

2. FGF-2 IN THE HEART

FGF-2 is one of 23 structurally related polypeptide growth factors (FGF-1 to FGF-23)[5], but because of its high affinity for heparin is also considered a member of the larger heparin binding growth factor family, which includes vascular endothelial growth factor (VEGF) and heparin-binding epidermal growth factor-like growth factor[6-8]. It is a highly conserved, basic protein that exists in AUG-initiated 18 kDa (lo-FGF-2), and CUG-initiated 20-34 kDa isoforms (four in the human; three in the rat or mouse), termed by us as hi-FGF-2, deriving from alternate translation initiation sites[9]. The N-terminal extension of hi-FGF-2 contains a nuclear localization signal (NLS), mediating its predominantly nuclear distribution. Lo-FGF-2 has been localized to cytosolic, nuclear and extracellular sites[5, 9]. The vast majority of studies to-date have described or implicated the extracellular (autocrine/paracrine) action of lo-FGF-2. Nevertheless, there is increasing evidence that hi-FGF-2 has significant, distinct and sometimes opposing effects to the lo-FGF-2 isoform[10]. All clinical studies to-date have used the lo-FGF-2 isoform.

FGF-2 expression is upregulated during stress and injury, at both the transcriptional and translational level, and this factor is implicated in most aspects (and cell types) associated with the injury-repair-regeneration response, including chemotaxis, cell motility, mitogenicity, survival, plus effects on differentiation and gene expression[11]. Translational regulation of FGF-2 is still incompletely understood, but has several relatively unique characteristics[12]. The presence of IRES (internal ribosome entry sites) elements in its mRNA sequence contributes to regulation of translation initiation: in the human FGF-2 mRNA, the regular cap-dependent mechanism initiates translation at the first cap-proximal CUG site (34 kDa FGF-2)[13], while a single IRES element initiates translation from the three CUG (21-25 kDa) and one AUG (18 kDa) sites[14]. IRES-mediated translation leads to FGF-2 accumulation in stressed cells[15]. In addition, FGF-2 isoform expression is highly tissue specific in vivo[16, 17] resulting, in part, from tissue specific FGF-2 IRES activity[18]. Multiple agents including angiotensin II (AngII), endothelin, and FGF-2 itself[19, 20] stimulate FGF-2 expression at the transcriptional level in different cell types, including cardiomyocytes[21]. All cardiac cells, including cardiomyocytes, express FGF-2 and both isoform types are present in the heart[16]. A transient upregulation in hi-FGF-2 accumulation is detected after isoproterenol-induced cardiac injury[22].

FGF-2 protein, lacking any "classical" hydrophobic export signal peptide, is secreted to the extracellular environment by a non-conventional, Golgi-independent pathway[11, 23]. In the postnatal heart, there is also evidence to support a passive mechanism of FGF-2 release from adult cardiac myocytes on a beat-to-beat basis through contraction-induced transient remodeling or "wounding" of the plasma membrane under normal physiological conditions[24, 25]. Cardiac fibroblasts are also considered an important source of FGF-2, playing a major role in the development of hypertrophy[26]. Endothelial and vascular smooth muscle cells also release FGF-2 through a mechanism involving non-lethal plasma membrane disruptions[27-29]. Increased contractility, or increased expression of FGF-2[30], result in increased FGF-2 release. While most studies implicate or assume lo-FGF-2 as the secreted species, increasing evidence indicates that hi-FGF-2 can also be released from cell[31, 32], including cardiac myocytes[33]. It follows that, once released, both types of isoforms are likely to interact with plasma membrane receptors.

FGF-2 signal transduction is mediated via two major pathways: (1) through membrane-bound cell surface receptors and (2) by transport of FGF-2 (and its receptor) to the nucleus. At the cell surface, the biological functions of FGF-2 (as well as many other members of the FGF family) are mediated primarily by high-affinity FGF receptors of the tyrosine kinase family, of which there are four members (FGFR1-4), each existing in multiple variants due to alternative splicing[8]. FGFR-1 is the predominant FGFR in embryonic, neonatal and adult cardiomyocytes[34, 35]. Heparan sulphate proteoglycans (HSPGs), which function partly to sequester FGF-2 in the extracellular matrix until signaling is triggered, also act as lower affinity 'receptors' to facilitate interaction of the ligand with FGFR[8, 36]. Activated FGFRs recruit and phosphorylate other signaling molecules culminating in the activation of major signal transduction pathways such as all three branches of the MAPK pathway (via Ras activation), the phosphoinositide/PKC pathway and Src-associated pathways[11]. There are no systematic studies at present as to whether extracellular hi or lo FGF-2 can stimulate similar early and/or late signal transduction pathways. Both isoforms can stimulate cell proliferation and survival, but they can have different effects on cell migration[31]. In addition, there is increasing evidence that hi-FGF-2, but not lo-FGF-2, preferentially promotes cardiac hypertrophy when acting at the cell surface[37].

The second major pathway for FGF-2-FGFR-1 signaling also begins with extracellular FGF-2 binding and activating FGFR-1 at the plasma membrane. This is then followed by FGF-2-FGFR1 internalization and nuclear translocation. Activated nuclear FGFR-1 can then activate a number of genes directly[38, 39]. A variation of this mode of signaling, exclusively intracrine FGF-2-FGFR1, has also been documented[37]. Internalization followed by nuclear translocation appears to be essential for the mitogenic response by lo-FGF-2. It occurs during the G1 stage of the cell cycle and is mediated by lo-FGF-2 binding to translokin, a ubiquitous cytosolic protein[40]. Activation of casein kinase 2 (CK2) through the interaction of its beta-subunit with lo-FGF-2 in the nucleus is essential for the induction of the mitogenic response[40-42]. Hi FGF-2 does not bind translokin but is directed to the nucleus by its own NLS[43]. Nuclear localization of ectopically expressed hi FGF-2 causes (in contrast to lo FGF-2) nuclear disruption[33, 44, 45] and cell death[46].

The vast majority of work done to examine FGF-2 as a cardioprotective or angiogenic agent has focused on lo-FGF-2 acting at the cell surface. As more information is collected with respect to the specific actions of hi-FGF-2, as well as the mitogenic consequences of nuclear signaling, the relative importance of hi vs. lo-FGF-2 and cell surface vs. nuclear signaling in the context of cardioprotection will come to light. For now, we will focus on what is known about the acute and chronic effects of lo-FGF-2 in ischemia-reperfusion injury; to simplify matters, the term FGF-2 will refer to lo-FGF-2 for the remaining of this chapter. We will examine the evidence that FGF-2, when administered appropriately, can exert a beneficial effect on the ischemic heart at not less than four points of intervention: (1) prior to an ischemic insult (preconditioning-like cardioprotection), (2) at the time of reflow (reperfusion or "secondary" injury prevention), (3) as an agent of myocardial regeneration through recruitment and/or amplification of cardiac stem cells, and (4) as a potent enhancer of angiogenesis to increase blood flow to a chronically ischemic region of the myocardium.

3. PRECONDITIONING-LIKE CARDIOPROTECTION BY FGF-2

Ischemic preconditioning is a naturally occurring cardioprotective mechanism in which a series of short bursts of ischemia prior to an extended episode results in significant preservation of myocardial viability and function. A hallmark of ischemic preconditioning is that it consists of two distinct phases: an early phase of protection developing within minutes of the onset of the brief ischemic episode and lasting 2 to 3 hours, and a delayed or late phase ("second window") that appears 12 to 24 hours later and lasts several days[47]. The connection between these two phases seems to be that molecular "triggers", which are directly responsible for the early phase, also launch signaling cascades which eventually result in the appearance or up-regulation of "mediators" of delayed preconditioning. The time required for this upregulation results in the biphasic nature of the phenomenon. Considerable research has focused on triggers, molecular pathways and endpoints of preconditioning, with a view to exploiting their therapeutic potential by "mimicking" the preconditioning response.

FGF-2 and its relative FGF-1 can elicit a preconditioning-type response. This is a well-documented effect that has been reviewed elsewhere[11, 48]. FGF-2 infused into the coronary circulation prior to global ischemia resulted in significantly improved recovery of left ventricular (LV) function upon reperfusion of the ex vivo perfused rat heart[49]. This result was subsequently confirmed in isolated mouse hearts, infused with FGF-2 in a similar manner[30]. In both cases, improved recovery of LV function was accompanied by decreased myocardial loss. Chronic overexpression of FGF-2 in transgenic mouse myocardium also resulted in decreased myocardial injury[30]. In a separate study using isolated work-performing hearts and low-flow ischemia, cardiac-specific overexpression of human FGF-2 in mice resulted in improved post-ischemic contractile function compared to wild-type hearts[50], while hearts devoid of FGF-2 showed impaired functional recovery. In an in vivo pig model, the infusion of FGF-1 or FGF-2 directly to the myocardium prior to coronary occlusion and reperfusion resulted in decreased infarct size and increased survival[51].

Among the intracellular signals involved in preconditioning (early and late phases), the best characterized are protein kinase C (especially the ε isoform), map kinases, the transcription factors AP-1 and NFκB, and nitric oxide and its synthases (Figure 1, reviewed by Bolli[47]). Interestingly, FGF-2 activates and/or is upregulated by each of these mediators[52-57]. While the data do not prove that FGF-2 is involved in the endogenous preconditioning response, there is sufficient evidence that FGF-2 could at least mimic the preconditioning response in both the early and late phases; therefore, we can envision a therapeutic strategy employing FGF-2 to induce such an effect.

4. REPERFUSION (SECONDARY) INJURY PREVENTION

The potential of the preconditioning approach for clinical use would by necessity be limited to those patients who present at high risk of infarction without having had such an episode. One application may be in cases of planned ischemic episodes, such as in preparation for cardiac surgery or transplantation. However, the clinical limitations of a preconditioning agent are such that it would still be desirable to identify molecules that would exert their cardioprotective effect even when administered after the onset of ischemia. Thus, cytoprotective agents administered during an evolving myocardial infarction and/or during re-establishment of blood flow, along with thrombolytic agents, would decrease the extent of cardiac injury and improve prognosis. A variety of protein factors that include FGF-2, acting by binding and activating plasma membrane receptors, have been identified as candidate molecules for cardioprotective therapy[58].

FGF-2 is capable of conferring protections of ischemic myocardium irrespectively of whether it is administered prior to or during reperfusion[52, 53, 59]. In a rat model of myocardial infarction (MI), FGF-2 administered directly to the ischemic left ventricle in rats after irreversible coronary ligation, exerted significant protection from tissue loss and contractile dysfunction, assessed 4-24 hours and 6-8 weeks post-MI[59]. While long-term protection might be attributed to an angiogenic effect[60-63], acute protection reflects direct beneficial effects to the myocardium. This was shown conclusively in a recent study demonstrating that a mutant non-angiogenic FGF-2 retains acute cardioprotective properties[53]. Protection by FGF-2 (including its non-angiogenic mutant) administered during the reperfusion phase was linked to PKC activation, including the ε subtype, and the PKC inhibitor chelerythrine blocked protection from secondary injury[59]. Thus, as in the preconditioning response, it is likely that the ability of FGF-2 to stimulate PKC (in particular PKCε) during reperfusion mediates its protective activity. Indeed, delivery of a peptide PKCε agonist into intact hearts reduced ischemic damage when delivered during the reperfusion phase[64]. The protective effects of FGF-2 and its non-angiogenic mutant during reperfusion are likely to include prevention of apoptotic cell death, since they were shown to prevent the release of cytochrome c to the cytosol[53].

The concept of lethal reperfusion injury (or secondary injury) as a separate phenomenon from ischemic injury is controversial[58] but its existence is strongly supported by reduction of myocardial loss through interventions administered at the time of reperfusion, thus excluding preconditioning-like response[65]. Two forms of cell death are implicated in ischemia-reperfusion injury. Necrosis is characterized by cell swelling and membrane disruption and an associated inflammatory response, while apoptosis is distinguished by chromatin condensation and apoptotic body formation with preserved membrane integrity. Apoptosis is distinct from necrosis in that it appears to be a tightly regulated, energy dependent process. There is significant evidence to suggest that the apoptotic process is accelerated during the reperfusion phase, possibly due to forced reflow under conditions of low pH and accumulated reactive oxygen species[3, 65]. Additionally, considerable evidence indicates that interventions in apoptotic signaling can enhance myocyte survival during reperfusion. These pathways have been collectively termed the Reperfusion Injury Salvage Kinase pathways, or RISK[58]. They include the phosphatidylinositol-3-OH kinase (PI3K) – Akt axis and the extracellular signal related kinases Erk1/2. Both PI3K-Akt and Erk1/2 pathways have been implicated in cellular survival through the recruitment of anti-apoptotic pathways[66]. The RISK pathway is linked to the cardioprotective action of several growth factors or bioactive molecules

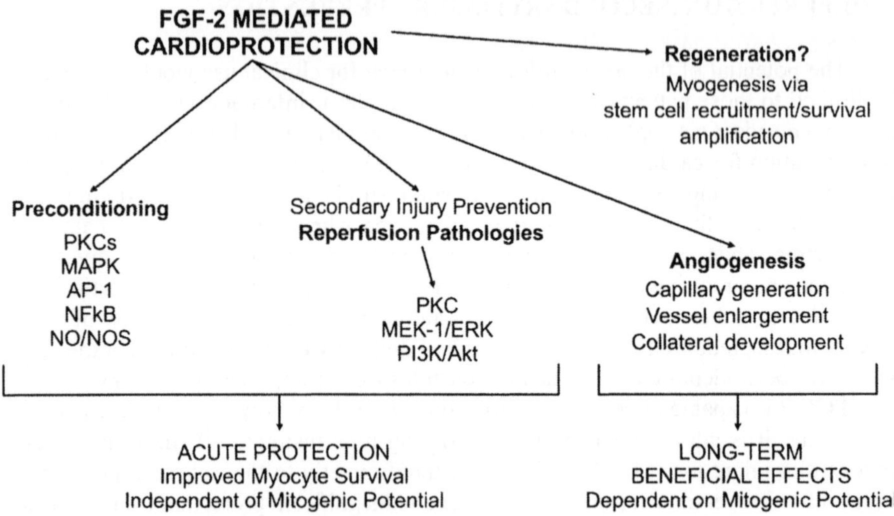

Figure 1. Schematic indicating the various ways in which FGF-2 can exert a protective influence on the myocardium, and possible mediators of these effects. Acute cardioprotection by FGF-2 occurs independently of its mitogenic activity and results in direct effects on myocyte survival. In contrast, chronic 'protection' requires mitogenic potential and manifests as smaller scars, preservation of contractile function and is characterized by increased vascularization and blood flow to the heart. Long-term beneficial effects may also include recruitment and expansion of myogenic stem cell populations, and thus true regeneration. Figure adapted from [Detillieux et al., 2004]. Abbreviations: PKC, protein kinase C; MAPK, mitogen-activating protein kinase, AP-1; activating protein-1, NFkB, nuclear factor kappa B; NO, nitric oxide; nitric oxide synthase, MEK-1, map-erk kinase-1; ERK, externally regulated kinase (analogous to MAPK), PI3K, phosphatidyl inositol-3-OH kinase; Akt, Akt8 viral oncogene, synonymous with protein kinase B.

including insulin, insulin-like growth factor-1 (IGF-1), transforming growth factor β1 (TGFβ1), and cardiotrophin-1 (CT-1) in addition to FGF-2 and its close relative FGF-1[58]. The evidence for the cardioprotective effects of insulin, IGF-1, TGFβ1, CT-1, FGF-2 and FGF-1 when administered at the time of reperfusion are summarized in Table 1. All of these factors have an anti-apoptotic effect via the salvage kinase pathway (PI3K-Akt or Erk1/2 or both). The protective effect of FGF-2 against iNOS induced cardiomyocyte apoptosis was mediated by ERK1/2[67], and FGF-2 protection during reperfusion of the isolated heart was associated with Akt activation [unpublished observations]. Furthermore, a proteomics approach has identified a signaling module consisting of a three-way link between Akt, PKC and eNOS[68], suggesting that the salvage kinase pathway is also dependent on PKC, which is consistent with the role of PKC in FGF-2-mediated reperfusion injury protection[59]; Figure 1.

It would appear that numerous ligands can activate similar pathways that are protective in the context of reperfusion injury. It would be tempting to consider all of these agents, and possible others that activate the RISK pathway, and the PKC pathway, as interchangeable if aiming to increase cardiac resistance to reperfusion or ischemia-reperfusion injury and dysfunction. Extreme caution needs to be exercised when considering a particular ligand for therapy, however, since these factors are associated with a diverse

Table 1. Growth Factors and Reperfusion Injury Protection

Growth Factor	Receptor	RISK Pathway	Experimental Model	Clinical Studies
Insulin	Ins. Receptor (TK)	PI3K-Akt Erk1/2	Neonatal rat cardiac myocytes[137] In vivo rat heart[138, 139] Isolated perfused rat heart[140]	Reviewed in[135]
IGF-1	IGFR (TK)	PI3K-Akt Erk1/2	Neonatal rat cardiac myocytes[141, 142] In vivo rat hear[143] Transgenic mouse heart[144] Isolated perfused rat heart[145] Isolated perfused mouse heart[146]	
TGFβ	TGFβR (S/TK)	Erk1/2	Neonatal rat cardiac myocytes[147] Isolated perfused rat heart[147, 148] In vivo rat heart (coronary ligation)[148]	
CT-1	gp130	PI3K-Akt Erk1/2	Neonatal rat cardiac myocytes[149, 150] Adult rat cardiac myocytes[151] Isolated perfused rat heart[151] In vivo rat heart (coronary ligation)[152]	
FGF-2	FGFR1	Erk1/2 PKC	Isolated perfused rat hearts[53, 59] Transgenic mouse heart[30]	
FGF-1	FGFR1	not determined	In vivo rat heart (coronary ligation)[153-155] Transgenic mouse heart[156]	

CT, cardiotrophin; FGF, fibroblast growth factor; IGF, insulin-like growth factor; RISK, reperfusion injury salvage kinase; S/TK, serine-threonine kinase; TK, tyrosine kinase

range of cellular responses, including effects on glucose metabolism, immune responses and hypertrophy. Before bringing a given factor or compound to the next level (clinical trials) issues of dosage, and corresponding short- as well as long-term effects should be very carefully evaluated.

5. THERAPEUTIC ANGIOGENESIS AND FGF-2

In addition to its action directly on myocytes, FGF-2 plays a key role in the vascular response to myocardial ischemia and reperfusion[11]. During development, the formation of the vasculature involves two separate but overlapping processes: (1) vasculogenesis, or the formation of major vessels through the proliferation and migration of smooth muscle cells, fibroblasts and endothelial cells, and (2) angiogenesis, a process specific to endothelial cells and resulting in the formation of small vessels and capillaries[69]. Through the use of antisense strategies, FGF-2 was demonstrated to be essential for embryonic mouse vascular development[70]. FGF-2 can stimulate proliferation of all three principal vascular cell types (endothelial cells, vascular smooth muscle cells and fibroblasts), and its role in both developmental vasculogenesis and angiogenesis is well established[69, 71, 72].

Extensive studies in canine[73-76] as well as porcine[63, 77, 78] models of chronic ischemia point to the ability of FGF-2 to promote vessel formation, in the context of collateral development, as well as capillarization. FGF-2 induces VEGF expression in vascular endothelial cells via both paracrine and autocrine pathways to mediate angiogenesis[79]. In fact, the roles of FGF-2 and VEGF in angiogenesis are inextricably linked and dependent one upon the other[80, 81], a relationship which is believed to relate to the observed synergistic response when both growth factors are used in combination[82, 83]; Figure 1. A series of phase I clinical trials (summarized in Table 2), using FGF-2 to promote therapeutic angiogenesis in patients with chronic myocardial ischemia, have shown promise with respect to safety and efficacy[84-89], although a recent double-blind, placebo-controlled phase II study (FIRST), while indicating no safety concerns, failed to corroborate the beneficial therapeutic effect shown previously[90]. While disappointing in its functional outcome, much consideration has been given to the lessons learned form this trial[91, 92]. The main difficulty in the clinical application of therapeutic angiogenesis lies in the choice and measurement of appropriate endpoints. Indeed, in the case of FIRST, the major endpoints were exercise tolerance tests (ETT) and quality of life questionnaire surveys[90]. While these may represent the best available functional endpoints at this time, the results rely on much more than myocardial blood flow alone, and this was confounded even further by the fact that the patient population in FIRST was largely asymptomatic even at the outset of the study[91, 92]. All this draws particular attention to the complexity and importance of clinical trial design (see section 7).

6. REPAIR AND REGENERATION: REBUILDING, IN ADDITION TO PRESERVING, THE DAMAGED MYOCARDIUM

Following an acute myocardial infarction and irreversible tissue damage lost tissue is replaced mostly by scar; viable myocytes become hypertrophic as part of a compensa-

Table 2. FGF-2 Therapeutic Angiogenesis Clinical Trials

Reference	Design	Delivery	Dose (μg/kg)	Size (n)	Primary Endpoints	Results
Sellke et al.[84]	Ph I, open label (pilot study)	HA beads	0, 1, 10 μg	8	Mortality, toxicity, angina, stress perfusion scans	Safety and technical feasibility demonstrated
Laham et al.[85] Ruel et al.[85, 89]	Ph I/II, R, DB, PC	HA beads	0, 10, 100 μg	24	CCS, SPECT	Safety and technical feasibility demonstrated in short and long term
Unger et al.[88]	Ph I, open label, (dose escalation)	ic bolus	0 – 100	25	ETT, angiography	Acute hypotension, some sustained hypotension, bradycardia, transient mild thrombocytopenia and proteinuria in upper dose
Udelson et al.[87]	Ph I, open label, (dose escalation)	ic, iv	0.33 – 48	59	ETT	stress-induced ischemia, resting myocardial perfusion
Laham et al.[86]	Ph I, open label, (dose escalation)	ic bolus	0.33 – 48	52	SAQ, ETT, MRI	Dose-limiting hypotension (max. 36 μg/kg)
Simons et al. "FIRST"[90]	Ph II, R, DB, PC	ic bolus	0.3, 3, 30	337	SAQ, ETT, SPECT	Placebo effect significant, no lasting increased improvement with FGF-2 treatment
Lederman et al. "TRAFFIC"[119]	Ph II, R, DB, PC	ia, bolus or double	30	190	ABI	Serious adverse effects similar in all groups, including control. Single dose as effective as double dose.

ABI, ankle-brachial index; CCS, Canadian Cardiovascular Society; DB, double-blind; ETT, exercise tolerance test; ia, intra-arterial; ic, intracoronary; iv, intravenous; MRI, magnetic resonance imaging; SAQ, Seattle Angina Questionnaire; SPECT, single photon

tory response. Depending on the degree of initial damage and the ensuing hypertrophy this series of events leads to maladaptive hypertrophy, remodeling and heart failure[93]. The adult heart does contain, at any time, small populations of myocytes, derived from a local 'renewal' pool, or homing in from the bone marrow, that are capable of proliferating and replacing lost tissue[94]. Indeed, probing normal adult heart tissue sections with an antibody marker of mitotic chromatin condensation reveals a small number of positive cardiomyocytes that may represent actively dividing cells (Figure 2). The adult heart also contains small numbers of cells with stem-cell-like characteristics that can be mobilized to repair and replace injured tissue (Figure 3). Endogenous heart repair remains however inadequate to replace substantial myocardial loss due to myocardial infarction. Engraftment of various types of stem cells to the ischemic myocardium is one strategy that has shown (in most if not all studies) exceptional promise in replacing lost tissue[94-103]. Another, and perhaps parallel, strategy is to boost the endogenous repair process by identifying and using factors that can stimulate repair/regeneration, while, conversely, limiting the action of inhibitory factors. In this scenario it is highly probable that FGF-2 can boost stem-cell based heart repair/regeneration, because of its potent chemotactic, cytoprotective and mitogenic properties[5, 11]. FGF-2 is a mitogen for: immature cardiomyocytes[33, 35, 104]; stem cell-like populations,[105-107] including skeletal muscle satellite cells[108] and cardiac resident stem cells[96]; bone marrow derived stem cells of various lineages[105, 109-112]. In addition, FGF-2 can stimulate DNA synthesis in neonatal cardiac myocytes, an effect that is antagonized by TGFβ signaling[113], and points to regenerative potential. FGF-2 gene and protein expression is stimulated during myocardial ischemia[11], and although there is no information as to the prevailing FGF-2 isoforms or mode of action, it is clear that local increases in extracellular lo FGF-2 levels would be highly beneficial[11, 52, 53, 59].

We thus propose that FGF-2 is capable of stimulating a 'global' repair response that includes attracting endogenous stem-cell-like populations to the infarct (circulating bone marrow derived cells; resident cells with stem-cell properties), promoting their proliferation as well as survival, but also allowing them to differentiate into different lineages, to produce new muscle and new vessels. Such global effects may be responsible for the smaller infarcts as well as the sustained and significant functional improvement that have been detected in hearts subjected to a single FGF-2 treatment[53, 59]. The homing of stem cells to sites of injury is not fully understood but stem cell factor, the ligand for the stem cell surface receptor, c-kit, plays an important role[114]. FGF-2, itself a potent chemoattractant, has also been shown to stimulate stem cell factor expression[111] and may thus promote homing in of endogenous stem cell like populations. In view of its cytoprotective properties, FGF-2 may also contribute to improved survival of native or implanted mesenchymal stem cells (MSC) in the myocardium. Implanted cells have limited survival capabilities, unless they are engineered to resist apoptotic demise: Akt-overexpressing MSC were used to prevent cell death and achieve an effective regenerative response in the rat myocardium[99]. It is therefore important to determine whether FGF-2 –based therapy increases MSC-like cells at the injury site. Preliminary experiments in our laboratory have suggested that this is indeed the case.

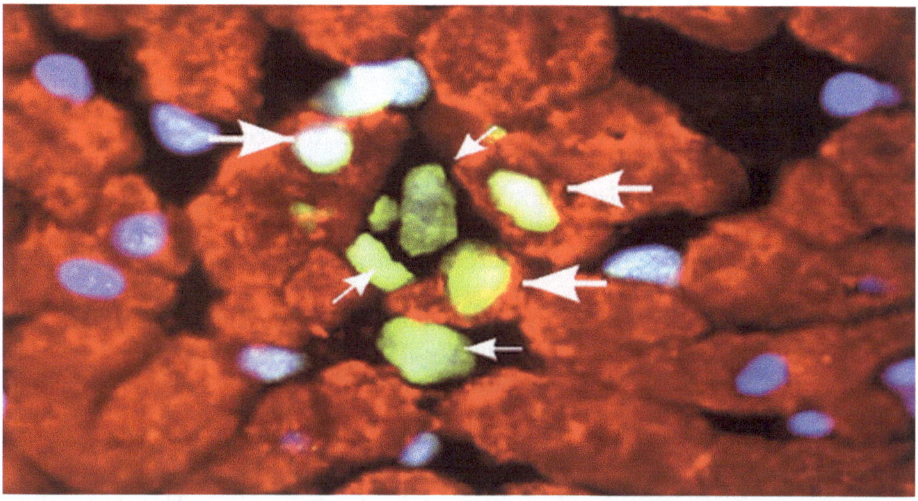

Figure 2: Identification of adult cardiomyocytes with mitotic features. Immunofluorescence staining of transverse tissue sections from normal adult rat heart ventricles for phosphorylated histone 3 (bright green), striated muscle myosin (red), and counterstained for DNA (Hoechsst 33342, blue). Presence of bright 'green' nuclei, surrounded by 'red' cytoplasmic staining, identifies cardiomyocytes with mitotic features (thick arrows), while lack of red staining identifies non-myocytes (thin arrows).

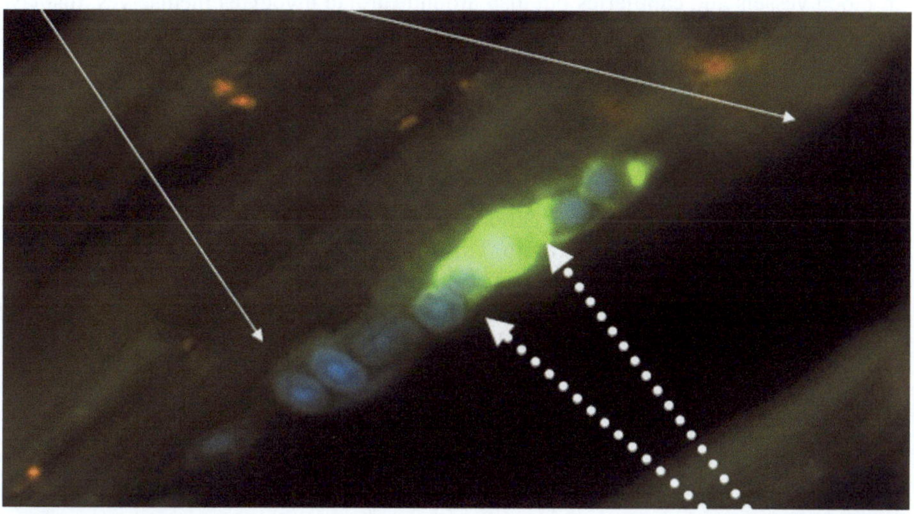

Figure 3: Identification of potential mesenchymal stem cells in the heart. Immunofluorescence staining of longitudinal tissue sections from normal adult rat heart ventricles for the cell-surface marker c-kit (or CD117), associated with mesenchymal stem cells, reveals the presence of clusters of immunopositive cells with bright membrane-associated green staining (dotted arrows) attached to the surface of cardiomyocytes. Blue staining identifies nuclei. Thin arrows point to cardiomyocyte fibers, presenting faint green (background) staining. Red lines/dots represent staining with an antibody to beta-catenin, that recognizes intercalated disks between myocytes, as well as fibroblastic cells.

7. CLINICAL APPLICATIONS

7.1. Delivery Methods

Several modalities of FGF-2-based therapy need to be considered; these include issues of dosage, sustained versus bolus treatments, and local or systemic (intracoronary or intravenous) administration[48]. All of these issues are dependent on the desired outcome of the treatment. Even before these pragmatic factors are dealt with, however, we must first take into account certain characteristics of FGF-2 that would dictate its behaviour once it enters the body. The first of these is the ability of FGF-2 to regulate its own synthesis. FGF-2 can regulate its own expression in cardiac myocytes in a positive feedback loop[21]. Such a trait could potentially affect the persistence of FGF-2 once it is administered. The second pertinent characteristic of FGF-2 in this context is its affinity for heparin and heparan sulfate proteoglycans (HSPGs). Binding of FGF-2 to HSPGs is required to form a three way complex between FGF-2, FGFR1 and HSPG to thus activate subsequent signaling[8, 36, 48]. As components of the basement membrane, HSPGs act as storage sites for FGF-2 and serve to protect it from proteolysis. This characteristic could be seen as a considerable advantage in clinical use, for several reasons. Even in situations where retention of total FGF-2 administered is low, the amount that is retained would theoretically be stored in the matrix and be protected from rapid degradation, increasing the time frame in which it is available to act. The proportion of FGF-2 administered via intracoronary routes that is reported to be retained in the myocardium varies from 1.5% in pigs[115] to 3-5% in dogs[116]. Nevertheless, in rodent models where FGF-2 is introduced by retrograde perfusion in isolated hearts, it was found to distribute not only in blood vessels and capillaries but also around cardiac myocytes themselves, displaying a basal-lamina-like pattern of localization[30, 52]. Similar distribution, demonstrating retention by matrix components, was seen in an in vivo rat model of coronary ligation where FGF-2 was injected directly into the ischemic myocardium during surgery[59], and included both viable and irreversibly injured myocytes. Retention of FGF-2 by the extracellular matrix would affect its availability for signaling, perhaps even mimicking a slow-release mechanism even after a bolus injection or infusion. Finally, HSPG binding to FGF-2 would promote spatial retention around the site of injection, allowing targeting to a specific region of the myocardium. This is of most advantage where direct myocardial injection allows spatial targeting of the dose; however, if for example FGF-2 was administered via intracoronary routes used for angioplasty or other procedures targeting an occlusion, this same precision could be attained perhaps by less invasive means.

In the treatment of chronic myocardial ischemia by the promotion of therapeutic angiogenesis, it has generally been assumed that sustained treatment with FGF-2 would be beneficial, since a permanent, long-term effect is desired. Interestingly, this assumption has virtually no basis in experimental evidence[117, 118]. However, the results of clinical trials in both myocardial and peripheral angiogenesis (the FIRST and TRAFFIC trials) would indicate otherwise, at least for long-term, angiogenic benefits[90, 92, 119, 120]. This discrepancy may be explained by the relative youth and general good health of animal subjects used in experimental studies versus the aged and ailing patient populations selected for clinical trials[92]. However, for short-term cardioprotective benefits, the retention of FGF-2 by the extracellular matrix, combined with its positive feedback autoregulation, could well prove to be sufficient for a single FGF-2 bolus to be therapeutic in acute cases of myocardial ischemia and reperfusion.

In the context of cardioprotection, whether as a preconditioning mimetic or in secondary injury prevention, the major factor to consider is the urgency of treatment and immediate effect desired for acute clinical situations, as opposed to chronic myocardial ischemia. The exception to this may be in cases where ischemia is planned for surgical purposes, when a preconditioning mimetic can be administered under more controlled conditions. However, in patients with unstable angina or an evolving myocardial infarction, speedy delivery and action of FGF-2 is most desirable. Based on what we know from angiogenesis studies, several effective delivery methods are possible. In the context of balloon angioplasty, FGF-2 could be delivered via catheter directly to the area of concern. Alternatively, percutaneous intramyocardial injection is being explored for clinical use[121, 122]. However, this method would need to be accompanied by some form of angiography in order to determine the target region. Thus, although most effective for retention of FGF-2[123, 124], the technical and pragmatic limitations may make catheter delivery more appealing, at least initially.

7.2. Safety considerations.

The safety concerns that have been raised in the clinical use of FGF-2 have been focused on its so-called "bystander" effects, which are to be expected given the multipotent nature of this growth factor (reviewed by Detillieux et al.[48]). These include renal insufficiency (proteinuria), hypotension, atherosclerotic effects, inflammation, fibrosis and oncogenic effects[117, 125]. Patients that were excluded from the angiogenesis trials include those with history of malignancy, retinopathy, renal dysfunction, recent myocardial infarction, or new onset of unstable angina[84, 86-88, 90, 115, 117]. Concerns about oncogenicity have been thus far unfounded in angiogenesis trials, presumably because of the short-term dosing with appropriate patient selection and local drug delivery[2, 117]. Likewise, no adverse effects on atherosclerotic plaque formation or stability, or immune cell effects, have been reported in clinical trials, even though these effects are well documented in experimental systems[125-127]. Nevertheless, it is noteworthy that certain types of genetically engineered non-mitogenic FGF-2[53] retain acute cardioprotective activity; thus modified FGFs may allow a wider selection of patients for treatment in the context of reperfusion-associated pathologies.

The major clinical side effects to manifest themselves in FGF-2 clinical trials have been hypotension (acute or sustained) and renal dysfunction demonstrated by significant proteinuria (see Table 2). Other minor effects have included bradycardia, transient mild thrombocytopenia and some transient retinal effects. In myocardial angiogenesis trials, these effects were dose-related and could be controlled by limiting the dose administered[86, 88, 90]. Notably, a limb ischemia trial where FGF-2 was administered by repeated intravenous infusion was abandoned prematurely because of a high rate of severe proteinuria[128], pointing to the importance of controlled, targeted dosing. Regardless of the final clinical outcome with respect to angiogenesis[91, 92], these trials have given significant insight into the safety and tolerability of FGF-2, showing that effective doses can be administered while keeping side effects within the acceptable range.

7.3. Clinical Trial Design.

The need for properly and rationally designed clinical trials for cardioprotection cannot be overstated and has been discussed elsewhere[4, 48, 129]. One criticism that has been made of past clinical trials using cardioprotective agents (specifically, preconditioning mimetics) is that the clinical application of a particular molecule (for example, the administration of adenosine along with thrombolytic agents, as in the AMISTAD trial[130]) does not reflect the experimental circumstances under which it was determined to be effective (for adenosine, as a preconditioning mimetic)[4]. However, the recent success with the expanded ATTACC trial using adenosine[131] may be explained by the connection that is being made between preconditioning and the salvage kinase pathway in experimental systems[68, 132]. Indeed, recent experimental evidence would suggest that adenosine can indeed directly protect the myocyardium against reperfusion injury in a clinical setting[133]. Despite these advances, the need for improved cardioprotective therapy continues[134].

Concluding Remarks

To date, the only growth factor to be tested in the clinical setting for its acutely cardioprotective effect is insulin (reviewed by Sack and Yellon[135]). In fact, insulin therapy in the treatment of myocardial infarction was first proposed in 1962 because of its metabolic effects[136]. It has been only since then that the direct cytoprotective properties of insulin have been discovered. Indeed, we now have a growing list of factors, including FGF-2, that show significant promise as therapeutic agents if delivered in combination with thrombolytic therapy or some other form of reperfusion (see Table 2). The particular appeal of FGF-2 is its relative clinical safety, its tissue retention, the fact that its cardioprotective effectiveness has been evidenced in numerous experimental models when administered prior to ischemia, to ischemic non-reperfused hearts, and during reperfusion, and this in addition to its strong potential for a true regenerative response, of which angiogenesis may be an aspect. This translates to a wide window of clinical opportunity for FGF-2-derived beneficial effects, whether given early (as a preconditioning mimetic), after the onset of ischemia (for secondary injury prevention;stimulation of a stem-cell based regenerative response), or late (for angiogenesis and collateral development).

As additional information is collected (for example, with respect to the relative importance of the different FGF-2 isoforms in the management of hypertrophy, or the role of mitogenicity in long-term protection), particular isoforms or engineered species of FGF-2 may become the best candidates for a particular desired endpoint. Likewise, other growth factors will fit into the picture of cardioprotective approaches according to what is known about them from experimental studies. Finally, moving from the experimental to clinical setting will require comprehensive data from animal models, astute trial design and patient selection, both of which need to reflect what is known from experimental studies with respect to such things as age, gender, and symptoms upon presentation.

REFERENCES

1. T. Pohl, C. Seiler, M. Billinger, E. Herren, K. Wustmann, H. Mehta, S. Windecker, F.R. Eberli, and B. Meier, Frequency distribution of collateral flow and factors influencing collateral channel development. Functional collateral channel measurement in 450 patients with coronary artery disease, *J Am Coll Cardiol* **38**, 1872–1878 (2001).

2. S.E. Epstein, S. Fuchs, Y.F. Zhou, R. Baffour, and R. Kornowski, Therapeutic interventions for enhancing collateral development by administration of growth factors: basic principles, early results and potential hazards, *Cardiovasc Res* **49**, 532–542 (2001).
3. H.M. Piper, and D. Garcia–Dorado, Prime causes of rapid cardiomyocyte death during reperfusion, *Ann Thorac Surg* **68**, 1913–1919 (1999).
4. D.M. Yellon, and G.F. Baxter, Protecting the ischaemic and reperfused myocardium in acute myocardial infarction: distant dream or near reality? *Heart* **83**, 381–387 (2000).
5. D.M. Ornitz, and N. Itoh, Fibroblast growth factors, *Genome Biol* **2**, REVIEWS3005 (2001).
6. N. Ferrara, K.A. Houck, L.B. Jakeman, J. Winer, and D.W. Leung, The vascular endothelial growth factor family of polypeptides, *J Cell Biochem* **47**, 211–218 (1991).
7. M. Piepkorn, M.R. Pittelkow, and P.W. Cook, Autocrine regulation of keratinocytes: the emerging role of heparin–binding, epidermal growth factor–related growth factors, *J Invest Dermatol* **111**, 715–721 (1998).
8. G. Szebenyi, and J.F. Fallon, Fibroblast growth factors as multifunctional signaling factors, *Int Rev Cytol* **185**, 45–106 (1999).
9. I. Delrieu, The high molecular weight isoforms of basic fibroblast growth factor (FGF–2): an insight into an intracrine mechanism, *FEBS Lett* **468**, 6–10 (2000).
10. B.W. Doble, X. Dang, P. Ping, R.R. Fandrich, B.E. Nickel, Y. Jin, P.A. Cattini, and E. Kardami, Phosphorylation of serine 262 in the gap junction protein connexin–43 regulates DNA synthesis in cell–cell contact forming cardiomyocytes, *J Cell Sci* **117**, 507–514 (2004).
11. K.A. Detillieux, F. Sheikh, E. Kardami, and P.A. Cattini, Biological activities of fibroblast growth factor–2 in the adult myocardium, *Cardiovasc Res* **57**, 8–19 (2003).
12. C. Touriol, S. Bornes, S. Bonnal, S. Audigier, H. Prats, A.C. Prats, and S. Vagner, Generation of protein isoform diversity by alternative initiation of translation at non–AUG codons, *Biol Cell* **95**, 169–178 (2003).
13. E. Arnaud, C. Touriol, C. Boutonnet, M.C. Gensac, S. Vagner, H. Prats, and A.C. Prats, A new 34–kilodalton isoform of human fibroblast growth factor 2 is cap dependently synthesized by using a non–AUG start codon and behaves as a survival factor, *Mol Cell Biol* **19**, 505–514 (1999).
14. S. Bonnal, C. Schaeffer, L. Creancier, S. Clamens, H. Moine, A.C. Prats, and S. Vagner, A single internal ribosome entry site containing a G quartet RNA structure drives fibroblast growth factor 2 gene expression at four alternative translation initiation codons, *J Biol Chem* **278**, 39330–39336 (2003).
15. A.C. Prats, and H. Prats, Translational control of gene expression: role of IRESs and consequences for cell transformation and angiogenesis, *Prog Nucleic Acid Res Mol Biol* **72**, 367–413 (2002).
16. J.D. Coffin, R.Z. Florkiewicz, J. Neumann, T. Mort–Hopkins, G.W. Dorn, 2nd, P. Lightfoot, R. German, P.N. Howles, A. Kier, B.A. O'Toole, et al. Abnormal bone growth and selective translational regulation in basic fibroblast growth factor (FGF–2) transgenic mice, *Mol Biol Cell* **6**, 1861–1873 (1995).
17. L. Liu, B.W. Doble, and E. Kardami, Perinatal phenotype and hypothyroidism are associated with elevated levels of 21.5– to 22–kDa basic fibroblast growth factor in cardiac ventricles, *Dev Biol* **157**, 507–516 (1993).
18. L. Creancier, D. Morello, P. Mercier, and A.C. Prats, Fibroblast growth factor 2 internal ribosome entry site (IRES) activity ex vivo and in transgenic mice reveals a stringent tissue–specific regulation, *J Cell Biol* **150**, 275–281 (2000).
19. M.K. Stachowiak, X. Fang, J.M. Myers, S.M. Dunham, R. Berezney, P.A. Maher, and E.K. Stachowiak, Integrative nuclear FGFR1 signaling (INFS) as a part of a universal "feed–forward–and–gate" signaling module that controls cell growth and differentiation, *J Cell Biochem* **90**, 662–691 (2003).
20. H. Peng, J. Myers, X. Fang, E.K. Stachowiak, P.A. Maher, G.G. Martins, G. Popescu, R. Berezney, and M.K. Stachowiak, Integrative nuclear FGFR1 signaling (INFS) pathway mediates activation of the tyrosine hydroxylase gene by angiotensin II, depolarization and protein kinase C, *J Neurochem* **81**, 506–524 (2002).
21. S.K. Jimenez, F. Sheikh, Y. Jin, K.A. Detillieux, J. Dhaliwal, E. Kardami, and P.A. Cattini, Transcriptional regulation of FGF–2 gene expression in cardiac myocytes, *Cardiovasc Res* **62**, 548–557 (2004).
22. R.R. Padua, and E. Kardami, Increased basic fibroblast growth factor (bFGF) accumulation and distinct patterns of localization in isoproterenol–induced cardiomyocyte injury, *Growth Factors* **8**, 291–306 (1993).
23. R. Friesel, and T. Maciag, Fibroblast growth factor prototype release and fibroblast growth factor receptor signaling, *Thromb Haemost* **82**, 748–754 (1999).

24. D. Kaye, D. Pimental, S. Prasad, T. Maki, H.J. Berger, P.L. McNeil, T.W. Smith, and R.A. Kelly, Role of transiently altered sarcolemmal membrane permeability and basic fibroblast growth factor release in the hypertrophic response of adult rat ventricular myocytes to increased mechanical activity in vitro, *J Clin Invest* **97**, 281–291 (1996).
25. M.S. Clarke, R.W. Caldwell, H. Chiao, K. Miyake, and P.L. McNeil, Contraction–induced cell wounding and release of fibroblast growth factor in heart, *Circ Res* **76**, 927–934 (1995).
26. C. Pellieux, A. Foletti, G. Peduto, J.F. Aubert, J. Nussberger, F. Beermann, H.R. Brunner, and T. Pedrazzini, Dilated cardiomyopathy and impaired cardiac hypertrophic response to angiotensin II in mice lacking FGF–2, *J Clin Invest* **108**, 1843–1851 (2001).
27. P.L. McNeil, L. Muthukrishnan, E. Warder, and P.A. D'Amore, Growth factors are released by mechanically wounded endothelial cells, *J Cell Biol* **109**, 811–822 (1989).
28. P.T. Ku, and P.A. D'Amore, Regulation of basic fibroblast growth factor (bFGF) gene and protein expression following its release from sublethally injured endothelial cells, *J Cell Biochem* **58**, 328–343 (1995).
29. G.C. Cheng, W.H. Briggs, D.S. Gerson , P. Libby, A.J. Grodzinsky, M.L. Gray, and R.T. Lee, Mechanical strain tightly controls fibroblast growth factor–2 release from cultured human vascular smooth muscle cells, *Circ Res* **80**, 28–36 (1997).
30. F. Sheikh, D.P. Sontag, R.R. Fandrich, E. Kardami, and P.A. Cattini, Overexpression of FGF–2 increases cardiac myocyte viability after injury in isolated mouse hearts, *Am J Physiol Heart Circ Physiol* **280**, H1039–1050 (2001).
31. R.S. Piotrowicz, P.A. Maher, and E.G. Levin, Dual activities of 22–24 kDA basic fibroblast growth factor: inhibition of migration and stimulation of proliferation, *J Cell Physiol* **178**, 144–153 (1999).
32. S. Taverna, G. Ghersi, A. Ginestra, S. Rigogliuso, S. Pecorella, G. Alaimo, F. Saladino, V. Dolo, P. Dell'Era, A. Pavan, et al. Shedding of membrane vesicles mediates fibroblast growth factor–2 release from cells, *J Biol Chem* **278**, 51911–51919 (2003).
33. K.B. Pasumarthi, B.W. Doble, E. Kardami, and P.A. Cattini, Over–expression of CUG– or AUG–initiated forms of basic fibroblast growth factor in cardiac myocytes results in similar effects on mitosis and protein synthesis but distinct nuclear morphologies, *J Mol Cell Cardiol* **26**, 1045–1060 (1994).
34. L. Liu, K.B. Pasumarthi, R.R. Padua, H. Massaeli, R.R. Fandrich, G.N. Pierce, P.A. Cattini, and E. Kardami, Adult cardiomyocytes express functional high–affinity receptors for basic fibroblast growth factor, *Am J Physiol* **268**, H1927–1938 (1995).
35. Y. Jin, K.B. Pasumarthi, M.E. Bock, A. Lytras, E. Kardami, and P.A. Cattini, Cloning and expression of fibroblast growth factor receptor–1 isoforms in the mouse heart: evidence for isoform switching during heart development, *J Mol Cell Cardiol* **26**, 1449–1459 (1994).
36. A.C. Rapraeger, A. Krufka, and B.B. Olwin, Requirement of heparan sulfate for bFGF–mediated fibroblast growth and myoblast differentiation, *Science* **252**, 1705–1708 (1991).
37. E. Kardami, Z.S. Jiang, S.K. Jimenez, C.J. Hirst, F. Sheikh, P. Zahradka, and P.A. Cattini, Fibroblast growth factor 2 isoforms and cardiac hypertrophy, *Cardiovasc Res* **63**, 458–466 (2004).
38. P.A. Maher, Nuclear Translocation of fibroblast growth factor (FGF) receptors in response to FGF–2, *J Cell Biol* **134**, 529–536 (1996).
39. J.F. Reilly, and P.A. Maher, Importin beta–mediated nuclear import of fibroblast growth factor receptor: role in cell proliferation, *J Cell Biol* **152**, 1307–1312 (2001).
40. C. Bossard, H. Laurell, L. Van den Berghe, S. Meunier, C. Zanibellato, and H. Prats, Translokin is an intracellular mediator of FGF–2 trafficking, *Nat Cell Biol* **5**, 433–439 (2003).
41. H. Bonnet, O. Filhol, I. Truchet, P. Brethenou, C. Cochet, F. Amalric, and G. Bouche, Fibroblast growth factor–2 binds to the regulatory beta subunit of CK2 and directly stimulates CK2 activity toward nucleolin, *J Biol Chem* **271**, 24781–24787 (1996).
42. G. Bouche, V. Baldin, P. Belenguer, H. Prats, and F. Amalric, Activation of rDNA transcription by FGF–2: key role of protein kinase CKII, *Cell Mol Biol Res* **40**, 547–554 (1994).
43. V. Patry, E. Arnaud, F. Amalric, and H. Prats, Involvement of basic fibroblast growth factor NH2 terminus in nuclear accumulation, *Growth Factors* **11**, 163–174 (1994).
44. K.B. Pasumarthi, E. Kardami, and P.A. Cattini, High and low molecular weight fibroblast growth factor–2 increase proliferation of neonatal rat cardiac myocytes but have differential effects on binucleation and nuclear morphology. Evidence for both paracrine and intracrine actions of fibroblast growth factor–2, *Circ Res* **78**, 126–136 (1996).

45. G. Sun, B.W. Doble, J.M. Sun, R.R. Fandrich, R. Florkiewicz, L. Kirshenbaum, J.R. Davie, P.A.Cattini, and E. Kardami, CUG–initiated FGF–2 induces chromatin compaction in cultured cardiac myocytes and in vitro, *J Cell Physiol* **186**, 457–467 (2001).
46. C.J. Hirst, M. Herlyn, P.A. Cattini, and E. Kardami, High levels of CUG–initiated FGF–2 expression cause chromatin compaction, decreased cardiomyocyte mitosis, and cell death, *Mol Cell Biochem* **246**, 111–116 (2003).
47. R. Bolli, The late phase of preconditioning, *Circ Res* **87**, 972–983 (2000).
48. K.A. Detillieux, P.A. Cattini, and E. Kardami, Beyond angiogenesis: the cardioprotective potential of fibroblast growth factor–2, *Can J Physiol Pharmacol* **82**, 1044–1052 (2004).
49. R.R. Padua, R. Sethi, N.S. Dhalla, and E. Kardami, Basic fibroblast growth factor is cardioprotective in ischemia–reperfusion injury, *Mol Cell Biochem* **143**, 129–135 (1995).
50. S.L. House, C. Bolte, M. Zhou, T. Doetschman, R. Klevitsky, G. Newman, and J. Schultz Jel, Cardiac–specific overexpression of fibroblast growth factor–2 protects against myocardial dysfunction and infarction in a murine model of low–flow ischemia, *Circulation* **108**, 3140–3148 (2003).
51. P. Htun, W.D. Ito, I.E. Hoefer, J. Schaper, and W. Schaper, Intramyocardial infusion of FGF–1 mimics ischemic preconditioning in pig myocardium, *J Mol Cell Cardiol* **30**, 867–877 (1998).
52. R.R. Padua, P.L. Merle, B.W. Doble, C.H. Yu, P. Zahradka, G.N. Pierce, V. Panagia, and E. Kardami, FGF–2–induced negative inotropism and cardioprotection are inhibited by chelerythrine: involvement of sarcolemmal calcium–independent protein kinase C, *J Mol Cell Cardiol* **30**, 2695–2709 (1998).
53. Z.S. Jiang, W. Srisakuldee, F. Soulet, G. Bouche, and E. Kardami, Non–angiogenic FGF–2 protects the ischemic heart from injury, in the presence or absence of reperfusion, *Cardiovasc Res* **62** 154–166 (2004).
54. S. Hoshi, M. Goto, N. Koyama, K. Nomoto, and H. Tanaka, Regulation of vascular smooth muscle cell proliferation by nuclear factor–kappaB and its inhibitor, I–kappaB, *J Biol Chem* **275**, 883–889 (2000).
55. N. Wakisaka, S. Murono, T. Yoshizaki, M. Furukawa, and J.S. Pagano, Epstein–barr virus latent membrane protein 1 induces and causes release of fibroblast growth factor–2, *Cancer Res* **62**, 6337–6344 (2002).
56. M. Bond, A.H. Baker, and A.C. Newby, Nuclear factor kappaB activity is essential for matrix metalloproteinase–1 and –3 upregulation in rabbit dermal fibroblasts, *Biochem Biophys Res Commun* **264**, 561–567 (1999).
57. H. Li, T. Wallerath, and U. Forstermann, Physiological mechanisms regulating the expression of endothelial–type NO synthase, *Nitric Oxide* **7**, 132–147 (2002).
58. D.J. Hausenloy, and D.M. Yellon, New directions for protecting the heart against ischaemia–reperfusion injury: targeting the Reperfusion Injury Salvage Kinase (RISK)–pathway, *Cardiovasc Res* **61**, 448–460 (2004).
59. Z.S. Jiang, R.R. Padua, H. Ju, B.W. Doble, Y. Jin, J. Hao, P.A. Cattini, I.M. Dixon, and E. Kardami, Acute protection of ischemic heart by FGF–2: involvement of FGF–2 receptors and protein kinase C, *Am J Physiol Heart Circ Physiol* **282**, H1071–1080 (2002).
60. M. Miyataka, K. Ishikawa, and R. Katori, Basic fibroblast growth factor increased regional myocardial blood flow and limited infarct size of acutely infarcted myocardium in dogs, *Angiology* **49**, 381–390 (1998).
61. Y. Uchida, A. Yanagisawa–Miwa, F. Nakamura, K. Yamada, T. Tomaru, K. Kimura, and T. Morita, Angiogenic therapy of acute myocardial infarction by intrapericardial injection of basic fibroblast growth factor and heparin sulfate: an experimental study, *Am Heart J* **130**, 1182–1188 (1995).
62. M. Kawasuji, H. Nagamine, M. Ikeda, N. Sakakibara, H. Takemura, S. Fujii, and Y. Watanabe, Therapeutic angiogenesis with intramyocardial administration of basic fibroblast growth factor, *Ann Thorac Surg* **69**, 1155–1161 (2000).
63. E. Watanabe, D.M. Smith, J. Sun, F.W. Smart, J.B. Delcarpio, T.B. Roberts, C.H. Van Meter, Jr., and W.C. Claycomb, Effect of basic fibroblast growth factor on angiogenesis in the infarcted porcine heart, *Basic Res Cardiol* **93**, 30–37 (1998).
64. L. Chen, L.R. Wright, C.H. Chen, S.F. Oliver, P.A. Wender, and D. Mochly–Rosen, Molecular transporters for peptides: delivery of a cardioprotective epsilonPKC agonist peptide into cells and intact ischemic heart using a transport system, R(7), *Chem Biol* **8**, 1123–1129 (2001).
65. F. Eefting, B. Rensing, J. Wigman, W.J. Pannekoek, W.M. Liu, M.J. Cramer, D.J. Lips, and P.A. Doevendans, Role of apoptosis in reperfusion injury, *Cardiovasc Res* **61** 414–426 (2004).

66. T.G. Cross, D. Scheel–Toellner, N.V. Henriquez, E. Deacon, M. Salmon, and J.M. Lord, Serine/threonine protein kinases and apoptosis, *Exp Cell Res* **256**, 34–41 (2000).
67. E. Iwai–Kanai, K. Hasegawa, M. Fujita, M. Araki, T. Yanazume, S. Adachi, and S. Sasayama, Basic fibroblast growth factor protects cardiac myocytes from iNOS–mediated apoptosis, *J Cell Physiol* **190**, 54–62 (2002).
68. J. Zhang, C.P. Baines, N.C. Zong, E.M. Cardwell, G. Wang, T.M. Vondriska, and P. Ping, Functional proteomic analysis of a three tier PKC{epsilon}–Akt—eNOS signaling module in cardiac protection, *Am J Physiol Heart Circ Physiol.* **288(2)**, 954–961 (2005).
69. T.J. Poole, E.B. Finkelstein, and C.M. Cox? The role of FGF and VEGF in angioblast induction and migration during vascular development, *Dev Dyn* **220**, 1–17 (2001).
70. I. Leconte, J.C. Fox, H.S. Baldwin, C.A. Buck, and J.L. Swain, Adenoviral–mediated expression of antisense RNA to fibroblast growth factors disrupts murine vascular development, *Dev Dyn* **213**, 421–430 (1998).
71. C.M. Cox, and T.J. Poole, Angioblast differentiation is influenced by the local environment: FGF–2 induces angioblasts and patterns vessel formation in the quail embryo, *Dev Dyn* **218**, 371–382 (2000).
72. P. Parsons–Wingerter, K.E. Elliott, J.I. Clark, and A.G. Farr, Fibroblast growth factor–2 selectively stimulates angiogenesis of small vessels in arterial tree, *Arterioscler Thromb Vasc Biol* **20**, 1250–1256 (2000).
73. E.F. Unger, S. Banai, M. Shou, D.F. Lazarous, M.T. Jaklitsch, M. Scheinowitz, R. Correa, C. Klingbeil, and S.E. Epstein, Basic fibroblast growth factor enhances myocardial collateral flow in a canine model, *Am J Physiol* **266**, H1588–1595 (1994).
74. A. Yanagisawa–Miwa, Y. Uchida, F. Nakamura, T. Tomaru, H. Kido, T. Kamijo, T. Sugimoto, K. Kaji, M. Utsuyama, C. Kurashima, et al, Salvage of infarcted myocardium by angiogenic action of basic fibroblast growth factor, *Science* **257**, 1401–1403 (1992).
75. D.F. Lazarous, M. Scheinowitz, M. Shou, E. Hodge, S. Rajanayagam, S. Hunsberger, W.G. Robison, Jr., J.A. Stiber, R. Correa, S.E. Epstein, et al, Effects of chronic systemic administration of basic fibroblast growth factor on collateral development in the canine heart, *Circulation* **91**, 145–153 (1995).
76. M. Shou, V. Thirumurti, S. Rajanayagam, D.F. Lazarous, E. Hodge, J.A. Stiber, M. Pettiford, E. Elliott, S.M. Shah, and E.F. Unger, Effect of basic fibroblast growth factor on myocardial angiogenesis in dogs with mature collateral vessels,, *J Am Coll Cardiol* **29**, 1102–1106 (1997).
77. K. Harada, W. Grossman, M. Friedman, E.R. Edelman, P.V. Prasad, C.S. Keighley, W.J. Manning, F.W. Sellke, and M. Simons, Basic fibroblast growth factor improves myocardial function in chronically ischemic porcine hearts, *J Clin Invest* **94**, 623–630 (1994).
78. A. Battler, M. Scheinowitz, A. Bor., D. Hasdai, Z. Vered, E. Di Segni, N. Varda–Bloom, D. Nass, S. Engelberg, M. Eldar, et al, Intracoronary injection of basic fibroblast growth factor enhances angiogenesis in infarcted swine myocardium, *J Am Coll Cardiol* **22** 2001–2006 (1993).
79. G. Seghezzi, S. Patel, C.J. Ren, A. Gualandris, G. Pintucci, E.S. Robbins, R.L. Shapiro, A.C. Galloway, D.B. Rifkin, and P. Mignatti, Fibroblast growth factor–2 (FGF–2) induces vascular endothelial growth factor (VEGF) expression in the endothelial cells of forming capillaries: an autocrine mechanism contributing to angiogenesis, *J Cell Biol* **141**, 1659–1673 (1998).
80. S.J. Mandriota, and M.S. Pepper, Vascular endothelial growth factor–induced in vitro angiogenesis and plasminogen activator expression are dependent on endogenous basic fibroblast growth factor, *J Cell Sci* **110** (Pt 18), 2293–2302 (1997).
81. M.S. Pepper, S.J. Mandriota, M. Jeltsch, V. Kumar, and K. Alitalò, Vascular endothelial growth factor (VEGF)–C synergizes with basic fibroblast growth factor and VEGF in the induction of angiogenesis in vitro and alters endothelial cell extracellular proteolytic activity, *J Cell Physiol* **177**, 439–452 (1998).
82. M.S. Pepper, N. Ferrara, L. Orci, and R. Montesano, Potent synergism between vascular endothelial growth factor and basic fibroblast growth factor in the induction of angiogenesis in vitro, *Biochem Biophys Res Commun* **189**, 824–831 (1992).
83. T. Asahara, C. Bauters, L.P. Zheng, S. Takeshita, S. Bunting, N. Ferrara, J.F. Symes, and J.M. Isner, Synergistic effect of vascular endothelial growth factor and basic fibroblast growth factor on angiogenesis in vivo, *Circulation* **92**, II365–371 (1995).
84. F.W. Sellke, R.J. Laham, E.R. Edelman, J.D. Pearlman, and M. Simons, Therapeutic angiogenesis with basic fibroblast growth factor: technique and early results, *Ann Thorac Surg* **65**, 1540–1544 (1998).
85. R.J. Laham, F.W. Sellke, E.R. Edelman, J.D. Pearlman, J.A. Ware, D.L. Brown, J.P. Gold, and M. Simons, Local perivascular delivery of basic fibroblast growth factor in patients undergoing coronary

bypass surgery: results of a phase I randomized, double–blind, placebo–controlled trial, *Circulation* **100**, 1865–1871 (1999).

86. R.J. Laham, N.A. Chronos, M. Pike, M.E. Leimbach, J.E. Udelson, J.D. Pearlman, R.I. Pettigrew, M.J. Whitehouse, C. Yoshizawa, and M. Simons, Intracoronary basic fibroblast growth factor (FGF–2) in patients with severe ischemic heart disease: results of a phase I open–label dose escalation study, *J Am Coll Cardiol* **36**, 2132–2139 (2000).
87. J.E. Udelson, V. Dilsizian, R.J. Laham, N. Chronos, J. Vansant, M. Blais, J.R. Galt, M. Pike, C. Yoshizawa, and M. Simons, Therapeutic angiogenesis with recombinant fibroblast growth factor–2 improves stress and rest myocardial perfusion abnormalities in patients with severe symptomatic chronic coronary artery disease, *Circulation* **102**, 1605–1610 (2000).
88. E.F. Unger, L. Goncalves, S.E. Epstein, E.Y. Chew, C.B. Trapnell, R.O. Cannon, 3rd, and A.A. Quyyumi, Effects of a single intracoronary injection of basic fibroblast growth factor in stable angina pectoris, *Am J Cardiol* **85**, 1414–1419 (2000).
89. M. Ruel, R.J. Laham, J.A. Parker, M.J. Post, J.A. Ware, M. Simons, and F.W. Sellke, Long–term effects of surgical angiogenic therapy with fibroblast growth factor 2 protein, *J Thorac Cardiovasc Surg* **124**, 28–34 (2002).
90. M. Simons, B.H. Annex, R.J. Laham, N. Kleiman, T. Henry, H. Dauerman, J.E. Udelson, E.V. Gervino, M. Pike, M.J. Whitehouse, et al, Pharmacological treatment of coronary artery disease with recombinant fibroblast growth factor–2: double–blind, randomized, controlled clinical trial, *Circulation* **105**, 788–793 (2002).
91. R.J. Aviles, B.H. Annex, and R.J. Lederman, Testing clinical therapeutic angiogenesis using basic fibroblast growth factor (FGF–2), *Br J Pharmacol* **140**, 637–646 (2003).
92. R. Khurana, and M. Simons, Insights from angiogenesis trials using fibroblast growth factor for advanced arteriosclerotic disease, *Trends Cardiovasc Med* **13**, 116–122 (2003).
93. M.A. Pfeffer, Left ventricular remodeling after acute myocardial infarction, *Annu Rev Med* **46**, 455–466 (1995).
94. P. Anversa, and B. Nadal–Ginard, Myocyte renewal and ventricular remodelling, *Nature* **415**, 240–243 (2002).
95. C.E. Murry, M.H. Soonpaa, H. Reinecke, H. Nakajima, H.O. Nakajima, M. Rubart, K.B. Pasumarthi, J.I. Virag, S.H. Bartelmez, V. Poppa, et al, Haematopoietic stem cells do not transdifferentiate into cardiac myocytes in myocardial infarcts, *Nature* **428**, 664–668 (2004).
96. A.P. Beltrami, L. Barlucchi, D. Torella, M. Baker, F. Limana, S. Chimenti, H .Kasahara, M. Rota, E. Musso, K. Urbanek, et al, Adult cardiac stem cells are multipotent and support myocardial regeneration, *Cell* **114**, 763–776 (2003).
97. R.C. Chiu, Bone–marrow stem cells as a source for cell therapy, *Heart Fail Rev* **8**, 247–251 (2003).
98. J.S. Forrester, M.J.Price, and R.R. Makkar, Stem cell repair of infarcted myocardium: an overview for clinicians, *Circulation* **108**, 1139–1145 (2003).
99. A.A. Mangi, N. Noiseux, D. Kong, H. He, M. Rezvani, J.S. Ingwall, and V.J. Dzau, Mesenchymal stem cells modified with Akt prevent remodeling and restore performance of infarcted hearts, *Nat Med* **9**, 1195–1201 (2003).
100. D. Orlic, J.M. Hill, and A.E. Arai, Stem cells for myocardial regeneration, *Circ Res* **91**, 1092–1102 (2002).
101. D. Orlic, J. Kajstura, S. Chimenti, D.M. Bodine, A. Leri, and P. Anversa, Transplanted adult bone marrow cells repair myocardial infarcts in mice, *Ann N Y Acad Sci* **938**, 221–229; discussion 229–230 (2001).
102. D. Orlic, J. Kajstura, S. Chimenti, D.M. Bodine, A. Leri, and P. Anversa, Bone marrow stem cells regenerate infarcted myocardium, *Pediatr Transplant 7 Suppl* **3**, 86–88 (2003).
103. Y. Schwartz, and R. Kornowski, Autologous stem cells for functional myocardial repair, *Heart Fail Rev* **8**, 237–245 (2003).
104. E. Kardami, Stimulation and inhibition of cardiac myocyte proliferation in vitro, *Mol Cell Biochem* **92**, 129–135 (1990).
105. K. Wada, H. Sugimori, P.G. Bhide, M.A. Moskowitz, and S.P. Finklestein, Effect of basic fibroblast growth factor treatment on brain progenitor cells after permanent focal ischemia in rats, *Stroke* **34**, 2722–2728 (2003).
106. I. Kashiwakura, and T.A. Takahashi, Basic fibroblast growth factor–stimulated ex vivo expansion of haematopoietic progenitor cells from human placental and umbilical cord blood, *Br J Haematol* **122**, 479–488 (2003).

107. K. Cairns, and S.P. Finklestein, Growth factors and stem cells as treatments for stroke recovery, *Phys Med Rehabil Clin N Am* **14**, S135–142 (2003).
108. M.E. Doumit, D.R. Cook, and R.A. Merkel, Fibroblast growth factor, epidermal growth factor, insulin-like growth factors, and platelet–derived growth factor–BB stimulate proliferation of clonally derived porcine myogenic satellite cells, *J Cell Physiol* **157**, 326–332 (1993).
109. E. Moroni, P. Dell'Era, M. Rusnati, and M. Presta, Fibroblast growth factors and their receptors in hematopoiesis and hematological tumors, *J Hematother Stem Cell Res* **11**, 19–32 (2002).
110. C. van den Bos, J.D. Mosca, J. Winkles, L. Kerrigan, W.H. Burgess, and D.R. Marshak, Human mesenchymal stem cells respond to fibroblast growth factors, *Hum Cell* **10**, 45–50 (1997).
111. Y. Sugimoto, T. Koji, and S. Miyoshi, Modification of expression of stem cell factor by various cytokines, *J Cell Physiol* **181**, 285–294 (1999).
112. P.E. Burger, S. Coetzee, W.L. McKeehan, M. Kan, P. Cook, Y. Fan, T. Suda, R.P. Hebbel, N. Novitzky, W.A. Muller, et al, Fibroblast growth factor receptor–1 is expressed by endothelial progenitor cells, *Blood* **100**, 3527–3535 (2002).
113. F. Sheikh, C.J. Hirst, Y. Jin, M.E. Bock, R.R. Fandrich, B.E. Nickel, B.W. Dobl, E. Kardami, and P.A. Cattini, Inhibition of TGFbeta signaling potentiates the FGF–2–induced stimulation of cardiomyocyte DNA synthesis, *Cardiovasc Res* **64**, 516–525 (2004).
114. B. Heissig, Z. Werb, S. Rafii, and K. Hattori, Role of c–kit/Kit ligand signaling in regulating vasculogenesis, *Thromb Haemost* **90**, 570–576 (2003).
115. R.J. Laham, M. Rezaee, M. Post, F.W. Sellke, R.A. Braeckman, D. Hung, and M. Simons, Intracoronary and intravenous administration of basic fibroblast growth factor: myocardial and tissue distribution, *Drug Metab Dispos* **27**, 821–826 (1999).
116. D.F. Lazarous, M. Shou, J.A. Stiber, D.M. Dadhania, V. Thirumurti, E. Hodge, and E.F. Unger, Pharmacodynamics of basic fibroblast growth factor: route of administration determines myocardial and systemic distribution, *Cardiovasc Res* **36**, 78–85 (1997).
117. M. Simons, R.O. Bonow, N.A. Chronos, D.J. Cohen, F.J. Giordano, H.K. Hammond, R.J. Laham, W. Li, M. Pike, F.W. Sellke, et al, Clinical trials in coronary angiogenesis: issues, problems, consensus: An expert panel summary, *Circulation* **102**, E73–86 (2000).
118. K. Sato, R.J. Laham, J.D. Pearlman, D. Novicki, F.W. Sellke, M. Simons, and M.J. Post, Efficacy of intracoronary versus intravenous FGF–2 in a pig model of chronic myocardial ischemia, *Ann Thorac Surg* **70**, 2113–2118 (2000).
119. R.J. Lederman, F.O. Mendelsohn, R.D. Anderson, J.F. Saucedo, A.N. Tenaglia, J.B. Hermiller, W.B. Hillegass, K. Rocha–Singh, T.E. Moon, M.J. Whitehouse, et al, Therapeutic angiogenesis with recombinant fibroblast growth factor–2 for intermittent claudication (the TRAFFIC study): a randomised trial, *Lancet* **359**, 2053–2058 (2002).
120. M.A. Bush, E. Samara, M.J. Whitehouse, C. Yoshizawa, D.L. Novicki, M. Pike, R.J. Laham, M. Simons, and N.A. Chronos, Pharmacokinetics and pharmacodynamics of recombinant FGF–2 in a phase I trial in coronary artery disease, *J Clin Pharmacol* **41**, 378–385 (2001).
121. H.C. Gwon, J.O. Jeong, H.J. Kim, S.W. Park, S.H. Lee, S.J. Park, J.E. Huh, Y. Lee, S. Kim, and D.K. Kim, The feasibility and safety of fluoroscopy–guided percutaneous intramyocardial gene injection in porcine heart, *Int J Cardiol* **79**, 77–88 (2001).
122. M. Rezaee, A.C. Yeung, P. Altman, D. Lubbe, S. Takeshi, R.S. Schwartz, S. Stertzer, and J.D. Altman, Evaluation of the percutaneous intramyocardial injection for local myocardial treatment, *Catheter Cardiovasc Interv* **53**, 271–276 (2001).
123. M.J. Post, R. Laham, F.W. Sellke, and M. Simons, Therapeutic angiogenesis in cardiology using protein formulations, *Cardiovasc Res* **49**, 522–531 (2001).
124. R.J. Laham, M. Rezaee, M. Post, X. Xu, and F.W. Sellke, Intrapericardial administration of basic fibroblast growth factor: myocardial and tissue distribution and comparison with intracoronary and intravenous administration, *Catheter Cardiovasc Interv* **58**, 375–381 (2003).
125. S.E. Epstein, R. Kornowski, S. Fuchs, and H.F. Dvorak, Angiogenesis therapy: amidst the hype, the neglected potential for serious side effects, *Circulation* **104**, 115–119 (2001).
126. S.L. Woodley, M. McMillan, J. Shelby, D.H. Lynch, L.K. Roberts, R.D. Ensley and W.H. Barry, Myocyte injury and contraction abnormalities produced by cytotoxic T lymphocytes, *Circulation* **83**, 1410–1418 (1991).

127. J.T. Meij, F. Sheikh, S.K. Jimenez, P.W. Nickerson, E. Kardami, and P.A. Cattini, Exacerbation of myocardial injury in transgenic mice overexpressing FGF–2 is T cell dependent, *Am J Physiol Heart Circ Physiol* **282**, H547–555 (2002).
128. L.T. Cooper, Jr., W.R. Hiatt, M.A. Creager, X. Regensteiner, W. Casscells, J.M. Isner, J.P. Cooke, and A.T. Hirsch, Proteinuria in a placebo–controlled study of basic fibroblast growth factor for intermittent claudication, *Vasc Med* **6**, 235–239 (2001).
129. R.A. Kloner, M.T. Speakman, and K. Przyklenk, Ischemic preconditioning: a plea for rationally targeted clinical trials, *Cardiovasc Res* **55**, 526–533 (2002).
130. K.W. Mahaffey, J.A. Puma, N.A. Barbagelata, M.F. DiCarli, M.A. Leesar, K.F. Browne, P.R. Eisenberg, R. Bolli, A.C. Casas, V. Molina–Viamonte, et al, Adenosine as an adjunct to thrombolytic therapy for acute myocardial infarction: results of a multicenter, randomized, placebo–controlled trial: the Acute Myocardial Infarction STudy of ADenosine (AMISTAD) trial, *J Am Coll Cardiol* **34**, 1711–1720 (1999).
131. M. Quintana, P. Hjemdahl, A. Sollevi, T. Kahan, M. Edner, N. Rehnqvist, E. Swahn, A.C. Kjerr, and P. Nasman, Left ventricular function and cardiovascular events following adjuvant therapy with adenosine in acute myocardial infarction treated with thrombolysis, results of the ATTenuation by Adenosine of Cardiac Complications (ATTACC) study, *Eur J Clin Pharmacol* **59**, 1–9 (2003).
132. D.J. Hausenloy, M.M. Mocanu, and D.M. Yellon, Ischemic Preconditioning Protects by Activating Pro–Survival Kinases at Reperfusion, *Am J Physiol Heart Circ Physiol* **288(2)**, 971–976 (2005).
133. M. Quintana, T. Kahan, and P. Hjemdahl, Pharmacological prevention of reperfusion injury in acute myocardial infarction. A potential role for adenosine as a therapeutic agent, *Am J Cardiovasc Drugs* **4**, 159–167 (2004).
134. R.A. Kloner, and S.H. Rezkalla, Cardiac protection during acute myocardial infarction: where do we stand in 2004? *J Am Coll Cardiol* **44**, 276–286 (2004).
135. M.N. Sack, and D.M. Yellon, Insulin therapy as an adjunct to reperfusion after acute coronary ischemia: a proposed direct myocardial cell survival effect independent of metabolic modulation, *J Am Coll Cardiol* **41**, 1404–1407 (2003).
136. D. Sodi–Pallares, M.R. Testelli, B.L. Fishleder, A. Bisteni, G.A. Medrano, C. Friedland, and A. De Micheli, Effects of an intravenous infusion of a potassium–glucose–insulin solution on the electrocardiographic signs of myocardial infarction. A preliminary clinical report, *Am J Cardiol* **9**, 166–181 (1962).
137. A.K. Jonassen, B.K. Brar, O.D. Mjos, M.N. Sack, D.S. Latchman, and D.M. Yellon, Insulin administered at reoxygenation exerts a cardioprotective effect in myocytes by a possible anti–apoptotic mechanism, *J Mol Cell Cardiol* **32**, 757–764 (2000).
138. A.K. Jonassen, E. Aasum, R.A. Riemersma, O.D. Mjos, and T.S. Larsen, Glucose–insulin–potassium reduces infarct size when administered during reperfusion, *Cardiovasc Drugs Ther* **14**, 615–623 (2000).
139. F. Gao, E. Gao, T.L. Yue, E.H. Ohlstein, B.L. Lopez, T.A. Christopher, and X.L. Ma, Nitric oxide mediates the antiapoptotic effect of insulin in myocardial ischemia–reperfusion: the roles of PI3–kinase, Akt, and endothelial nitric oxide synthase phosphorylation, *Circulation* **105**, 1497–1502 (2002).
140. A.K. Jonassen, M.N. Sack, O.D. Mjos and D.M. Yellon, Myocardial protection by insulin at reperfusion requires early administration and is mediated via Akt and p70s6 kinase cell–survival signaling, *Circ Res* **89**, 1191–1198 (2001).
141. L. Wang, W. Ma, R. Markovich, J.W. Chen, and P.H. Wang, Regulation of cardiomyocyte apoptotic signaling by insulin–like growth factor I, *Circ Res* **83**, 516–522 (1998).
142. Y. Fujio, T. Nguyen, D. Wencker, R.N. Kitsis, and K. Walsh, Akt promotes survival of cardiomyocytes in vitro and protects against ischemia–reperfusion injury in mouse heart, *Circulation* **101**, 660–667 (2000).
143. M. Buerke, T. Murohara, C. Skurk, C. Nuss, K. Tomaselli, and A.M. Lefer, Cardioprotective effect of insulin–like growth factor I in myocardial ischemia followed by reperfusion, *Proc Natl Acad Sci USA* **92**, 8031–8035 (1995).
144. K. Yamashita, J. Kajstura, D.J. Discher, B.J. Wasserlauf, N.H. Bishopric, P. Anversa, and K.A. Webster, Reperfusion–activated Akt kinase prevents apoptosis in transgenic mouse hearts overexpressing insulin–like growth factor–1, *Circ Res* **88**, 609–614 (2001).
145. H. Otani, T. Yamamura, Y. Nakao, R. Hattori, H. Kawaguchi, M. Osako, and H. Imamura, Insulin–like growth factor–I improves recovery of cardiac performance during reperfusion in isolated rat heart by a wortmannin–sensitive mechanism, *J Cardiovasc Pharmacol* **35**, 275–281 (2000).

146. E.Y. Davani, Z. Brumme, G.K. Singhera, H.C. Cote, P.R. Harrigan, and D.R. Dorscheid, Insulin–like growth factor–1 protects ischemic murine myocardium from ischemia/reperfusion associated injury, *Crit Care* 7, R176–183 (2003).
147. G.F. Baxter, M.M. Mocanu, B.K. Brar, D.S. Latchman and D.M. Yellon, Cardioprotective effects of transforming growth factor–beta1 during early reoxygenation or reperfusion are mediated by p42/p44 MAPK, *J Cardiovasc Pharmacol* **38**, 930–939 (2001).
148. A.M. Lefer, P. Tsao, N. Aoki, and M.A. Palladino, Jr. Mediation of cardioprotection by transforming growth factor–beta, *Science* **249**, 61–64 (1990).
149. Z. Sheng, K. Knowlton, J. Chen, M. Hoshijima, J.H. Brown and K.R. Chien, Cardiotrophin 1 (CT–1) inhibition of cardiac myocyte apoptosis via a mitogen–activated protein kinase–dependent pathway. Divergence from downstream CT–1 signals for myocardial cell hypertrophy, *J Biol Chem* **272**, 5783–5791 (1997).
150. B.K. Brar, A. Stephanou, D. Pennica, and D.S. Latchman, CT–1 mediated cardioprotection against ischaemic re–oxygenation injury is mediated by PI3 kinase, Akt and MEK1/2 pathways, *Cytokine* **16**, 93–96 (2001).
151. Z. Liao, B.K. Brar, Q. Cai, A. Stephanou, R.M. O'Leary, D. Pennica, D.M. Yellon, and D.S. Latchman, Cardiotrophin–1 (CT–1) can protect the adult heart from injury when added both prior to ischaemia and at reperfusion, *Cardiovasc Res* **53**, 902–910 (2002).
152. Y. Ruixing, Y. Dezhai, and L. Jiaquan, Effects of cardiotrophin–1 on hemodynamics and cardiomyocyte apoptosis in rats with acute myocardial infarction, *J Med Invest* **51**, 29–37 (2004).
153. P. Cuevas, F. Carceller, R.M. Lozano, A. Crespo, M. Zazo, and G. Gimenez–Gallego, Protection of rat myocardium by mitogenic and non–mitogenic fibroblast growth factor during post–ischemic reperfusion, *Growth Factors* **15**, 29–40 (1997).
154. P. Cuevas, D. Reimers, F. Carceller, V. Martinez–Coso, M. Redondo–Horcajo, I. Saenz de Tejada, and G. Gimenez–Gallego, Fibroblast growth factor–1 prevents myocardial apoptosis triggered by ischemia reperfusion injury, *Eur J Med Res* **2**, 465–468 (1997).
155. P. Cuevas, F. Carceller, V. Martinez–Coso, B. Cuevas, A. Fernandez–Ayerdi, D. Reimers, E. Asin–Cardiel, and G. Gimenez–Gallego, Cardioprotection from ischemia by fibroblast growth factor: role of inducible nitric oxide synthase, *Eur J Med Res* **4**, 517–524 (1999).
156. A. Buehler, A. Martire, C. Strohm, S. Wolfram, B. Fernandez, M. Palmen, X.H. Wehrens, P.A. Doevendans, W.M. Franz, W. Schaper, et al, Angiogenesis–independent cardioprotection in FGF–1 transgenic mice, *Cardiovasc Res* **55**, 768–777 (2002).

CHAPTER 7

MYOCARDIAL PROTECTION – FROM CONCEPTS TO CLINICAL PRACTICE

Dennis V. Cokkinos

1. BACKGROUND

The protection of the myocardium is of self-evident importance: Loss of myocardial function is the main factor responsible for cardiovascular morbidity and mortality, whether it concerns primary myocardial or coronary artery disease.

What is not adequately appreciated is that both the influence of noxious factors but also the protection against them can be cross – influencing. Thus protection against ischemia may encompass arrhythmias, but also myocardial damage through chemical agents; myocardial ischemic preconditioning can protect against H_2O_2 damage.[1] Conversely, heat shock can protect against ischemia.[2] Finally, although in the "bench" an impressive array of observations has provided abundant data as "concepts", their translation to the bedside of "clinical practice" remains meager.

In this review I shall try to touch upon this discrepancy between research findings and the need for their wider and more effective clinical application.

2. MYOCARDIAL PROTECTION

The discovery of the phenomenon of ischemic preconditioning by Murry and his coworkers[3] has led to an unbelievable waterfall of further explorations. However, the application of this very potent protective mechanism remains limited in the clinical setting for the following obvious reasons:

The main reason is that the need for preconditioning cannot be foreseen. Acute myocardial infarction most frequently strikes unannounced. Thus, the application of preconditioning usually cannot be pre-ordered at will. Indeed, a body of evidence has accumulated that pre-infarction angina, which comes as close to preconditioning as possible, can be protective as regards limiting myocardial necrosis and protective against ventricular arrhythmias.[4-10]

Professor of Cardiology, Medical School, University of Athens, Greece
Address for correspondence: Chairman, department of Cardiology, Onassis Cardiac Surgery Center, 356 Sygrou Ave. 176 74 Kallithea, Athens, Greece. E-mail: cokkinol@otenet.gr

An interesting discrepancy has not been adequately addressed: While most studies showing a benefit of pre-infarction angina have been prospective,[4-9] retrospective studies have not shown such a clear-cut benefit.[11,12] In my view this discrepancy stems from the difficulty inherent in retrospective studies in correctly identifying the duration and severity of pre-infarction angina. Thus, it can be reasonably postulated that if preceding angina is too long and severe, it can lead not to preconditioning but to stunning and necrosis. We have previously shown that the effect of two preconditioning cycles can, as expected, be quite effective when it precedes two long cycles – twenty minutes each – of ischemia, but they are ineffective if "sandwiched" between these two cycles.[13]

Another factor, which is not usually addressed in the discussion of clinical paradigms of preconditioning, is the state of the patient, that of the myocardium, and the previous or current use of drugs.

2.1. Patient status

Abete et al[14] very elegantly showed that in elderly patients, Holter-documented ischemia does not offer protection against a subsequent myocardial infarction. The abrogating effect of ageing on myocardial protection through ischemic preconditioning has also been stressed in many experimental studies.[15] However, it must be admitted that the full elucidation of how this mechanism operates is still lacking. Equally incomplete is the delineation of techniques to re-instate the protection in aged myocardium; some of these will be subsequently discussed in a more general way. Exercise has been found to be effective.[16]

A diametrically different picture exists in the immature heart: The chronic hypoxia to which it is subjected, renders it more resistant against ischemia.[17,18] Another intriguing aspect in this state is that ischemic preconditioning is not as effective.[19,20] However, it has not been adequately clarified if preconditioning does not really exist or if it is difficult to demonstrate additional protection in an intrinsically resistant heart.

2.1.1. Diabetes mellitus

This quite common condition has been intensely studied but concrete conclusions have not been forthcoming. Thus, many authors have reported that not very long-term pre-existing diabetes protects the myocardium, yielding a "preconditioned-like" state,[21,22] but that long-existing diabetes finally abrogates preconditioning.[23] The exact mechanism of this discrepancy remains unknown. Probably further insight into the behavior of free radicals – a subject which will be subsequently addressed – will yield more information.[24]

2.1.2. Hypercholesterolemia-atherosclerosis

Again the mechanisms through which this state operates has not been adequately elucidated. Some authors have stated that it abrogated preconditioning,[25] however others have shown that it is still present in the hypercholesterolemic rabbit.[26]

2.1.3. Hyperthyroidism

Hyperthyroidism is shown to increase tolerance of the myocardium to ischemia and reperfusion injury. The mechanisms of this phenomenon are diverse. Hyperthyroidism produces an increase of PKCδ, Hsp70 and Hsp27 and a decrease of p38 MAPK and JNK in response to ischemia and reperfusion[28-30] which is cardioprotective, according to many authors.[31] Here it must be admitted that although the use of thyroid analogues has been tried under many modalities over many years, it has never been proven clinically successful or practicable. Thus, initially encouraging results in cardiomyopathy,[32-35] after acute myocardial infarction and in the post-infarction remodeling state[36] have not had further clinical application.

It is interesting that after an acute myocardial infarction T3 administration has been found to cause a normalization of the abnormal gene expression and cardiac function.[37] Friberg et al38 reported a very interesting finding; studying patients after an acute myocardial infarction, they noted that antecedent pre-infarction angina was associated with lower levels of T3 and a smaller myocardial infarction and lower levels of interleukin-6. However, mortality was increased. They consider this a maladaptive phenomenon. This finding after an acute myocardial infarction refer to the finding found in chronic heart failure. In this state, a low fT3 is associated with a worse prognosis,39 and a low fT3/fT4 ratio as well as a high TSH are correlated with a low ejection fraction and higher levels of right atrial and capillary wedge pressures.40 Interestingly, these unfavorable findings can be reversed with exercise.41 However, no established therapy exists for this syndrome.32,33

The findings of Suzuki et al[42] are interesting in this context. They found that increased free fatty acid levels, a common finding in heart failure and chronic ischemia are associated with decreased conversion of T_4 to T_3. However, this is a common finding in many noxious states and the basis of the euthyroid low T_3 syndrome. Cardiac surgery is another acute low output state in which the administration of thyroid hormones or analogues may prove protective.[43] The findings of Spinale who found that acute T_3 administration improves myocyte contractile function after cardioplegic arrest are in accordance.[44] Very recently Mackie et al[45] showed a better clinical outcome scores in neonatal heart surgery in a double-blind placebo-controlled trial of tri-iodothyronine. They suggest that these findings should be tested in larger studies. However, these agents have not really found consistent clinical application in cardiac surgery.

Thyroid hormones and analogues may also find a role in reversing the unfavorable effects of ageing, Kimura et al[46] have actually shown that in elderly patient with congestive heart failure TSH was positively correlated with the fT3/fT4 ratio. They may offset the absence of some protective substances such as desmin by providing cytoskeletal protective proteins, such as Hsp27, which has been found to increase the stability of the cytoskeleton and protect against ischemia[47]. Desmin absence is specifically associated with loss of cytoskeleton stability.[48] .

2.1.4. Hypothyroidism

Induction of hypothyroidism was a last-ditch approach to the management of intractable angina many decades ago.[49, 50] That it did not stand the test of time strongly suggests that it was not effective. Hypothyroidism causes an elevation in plasma lipids,[51] an increased arterial resistance[52] and attenuates flow mediated dilatation.[53] We have found that thyroid hormone plays a significant role in vascular physiology.[54] However, we have been strongly impressed by the profound protection against global ischemia that hypothyroidism confers to the myocardium. Recovery values up to 80% against 45-55% seen in the control after 20 minutes of global ischemia are common in the hypothyroid rat.[55] However, nobody would accept a hypothyroid state in current practice. A new concept which may emerge is cardio-selective hypothyroidism. This is effected by drugs which selectively inhibit the TRα1 receptor. Such a new substance is dronedarone which has both antiarrhythmic and cardioprotective effects.[56] Amiodarone was many years ago actually introduced as a cardioprotective drug although its potential for causing clinical hypo – or hyperthyroidism has hampered its use as an anti-ischemic medication, which actually was its initial indication. An interesting finding with the use of this drug is that it creates cardiac transcript changes very similar to those of hypothyroidism, i.e. SERCA2 reduction and phospholamban increase, while those of dronedarone were much milder,[57] as we also showed[56] (see also chapter 2).

2.2. Myocardial status

It should be concretely appreciated that the findings emerging from laboratory animals, within their overwhelming majority – normal hearts, cannot be reasonably extrapolated to the human with coronary or myocardial disease. The various plights afflicting the myocardium in these conditions should be addressed.

2.2.1. Myocardial hypertrophy

A large percentage of patients show this abnormality. Data concerning its influence on myocardial protection are scant. Basically, myocardial hypertrophy renders the myocardium more vulnerable to ischemia. This has been abundantly shown many years and studies since. Apstein et al have given a very detailed account 15 years ago.[58] Both in the global and regional rat model of ischemia,[59, 60] and after cardiac surgery in the human, many workers have shown that the hypertrophied hearts are more sensitive to ischemic injury. The "stone heart" after aortic valve replacement is well known.[61] Schaper et al[62] have actually shown a significant correlation between the degree of hypertrophy and the magnitude of intraoperative ischemic injury in man. However, most authors agree that very careful attention to the avoidance of low perfusion pressure should be drawn, a difficult state to avoid in the hypertrophied heart.[63]

However, an interesting and somewhat unexpected finding is that preconditioning is not affected by myocardial hypertrophy. This was initially proven by Speechly – Dick in Yellon´s group in DOCA – salt induced hypertrophy[64] and subsequently by our group in the abdominal aortic banding rat model.[65] However, Moolman et al[66] in the genetically hypertensive New Zealand Wistar rat model showed that preconditioning does not protect the hypertrophied myocardium against ischemia. An aspect which has not been further examined is the modality of producing hypertrophy. Is banding the same as salt-induced hypertension? Does preconditioning weaken when hypertrophy evolves into heart failure as in the ascending – aorta banded rat? However, in the hyperthyroid rat we have shown that both propranolol and irbesartan inhibit the emergence of hypertrophy but not the cardioprotection produced by this intervention.[67] The findings of Chang et al[68] are interesting in the aspect; they found that in hypertrophied rat hearts Ca^{2+} turnover is impaired. This untoward effect is restored after thyroxine administration.

2.2.2. Myocardial dysfunction

It is surprising that the influence of the main element complicating coronary artery disease, myocardial decompensation, has not been adequately studied as regards its influence on cardioprotection. Findings are scarce and sometimes contradictory. Miki et al found that rat hearts[69] after a large myocardial infarct followed by remodeling manifest a loss of preconditioning which is re-instated with the use of angiotensin converting enzyme inhibition. Ghosh et al[70] also found that the pathological human myocardium cannot be adequately preconditioned. Dekker et al[71] found that in rabbit papillary muscles ischemic preconditioning is actually harmful and not protective; probably even the mild ischemic burden necessary for protection may be too heavy for the diseased heart. However, no serious work can be found as to how different stages of cardiac decompensation affect not only tolerance to ischemia but also protective mechanisms such as preconditioning. Here it should be mentioned that on the whole the failing heart is more vulnerable to ischemia and reperfusion.[72] Furthermore, another aspect is more favorable. This concerns the myocardium remote from a previous myocardial infarction. Here a caveat should be mentioned: The findings to be described concern otherwise normal laboratory animals in whom an area of myocardial necrosis has been produced through ligation of a coronary artery but whose unaffected myocardium is otherwise completely healthy. In this myocardium, favorable processes take place: The Na^+/H^+ exchanger is inhibited, thus rendering the heart more resistant to ischemia.[73] We have also found that these hearts manifest better recovery of function against global ischemia. Again, in this setting a huge amount of information is missing. We do not know the stage of remodeling or decompensation of these hearts. If this information is difficult to attain in the laboratory setting, it is vastly more impractical to judge in the clinical set up. One might postulate, that as in diabetes mellitus, the decompensating and remodeling heart slowly begins to lose its varying and diverse cardioprotective mechanisms. Efstathiou et al[72] showed differential effects of preconditioning depending on the presence or absence of extensively infarcted myocardial mass. Furthermore, as has been discussed in the case of left ventricular hypertrophy, the process which creates this decompensation may differ as regards its influences. Is the post-infarcted heart different from the ascending aorta-banded heart or from the Dahl salt-sensitive rat or the spontaneously hypertensive rat which at some stage deteriorates into decompensation? These questions have been largely unanswered.

3. THE STAGE OF THE ISCHEMIA-REPERFUSION INJURY CASCADE

It has long been appreciated that the main event of an acute myocardial infarction is the occlusion of a coronary artery. A vast number of efforts have been addressed to the attainment of the goal of the fastest possible reperfusion either through thrombolysis or through the "mechanical" effects of interventional techniques. However, most of the protective mechanisms currently studied and employed concern the pre-reperfusion phase. Only very recently has the search for agents protecting the myocardium at or after reperfusion, reached respectable proportions. An intriguing concept has recently emerged – that of post-conditioning.

According to this phenomenon, brief flow interruptions (10 seconds each) very early after the onset of reperfusion produce an improvement in myocardial recovery.[74, 75] This improvement is less robust than that of pre-conditioning but still can be considered of clinical significance. Diaz and Wilson[74] postulate that the brief periods of reperfusion prevent the endogenous mechanisms scavenging the reactive oxygen species (ROS) from being overwhelmed. Kin et al[75] state that they were able to produce less myocardial salvage in the rat than in the dog. Rats have greater xanthine oxidase activity than the dog, rabbit and man. The effect of post-conditioning in the rabbit[75] is also stronger than that of the rat, which gives hopes that this technique may be successful in the human. Technically it should be easy to apply during primary angioplasty. Analogs to this phenomenon have been reported. Thus, in the cerebral experimental ischemic model, if reperfusion is carried out with lower oxygen concentrations recovery is better.[76] However, its evident counterpart, employment of free oxygen radical scavengers although promising in the experimental setting, has not given significant practical solutions in the clinical setting, as will be further described.

Piper et al[77] in a recent review try to identify the mechanisms of reperfusion-induced cell death. They stress the importance of reoxygenation-induced contractile dysfunction which has two main causes: Ca^{2+} overload, and a rigor type mechanism. To counteract the first mechanism, they postulate that simultaneous inhibition of both the Na^+/H^+ exchanger (NHE) and the Na^+/HCO_3 symporter (NBS) is needed, to preserve ischemic intracellular acidosis since isolated NHE inhibition has not proven effective, either experimentally[78, 79] or clinically.[80] (See also Table) For the rigor contracture to occur, low ATP concentrations are required, while Ca^{2+} overload is not a consideration. Mitochondrial energy substrates may prove effective such as succinate, and ways to protect mitochondria from compulsory Ca^{2+} uptake, such as cyclosporine A.[81] The same authors postulate that activation of PKG dependent and PI3 Kinase signaling can be effective, the former by NO donors, members of the natriuretic peptide family, such as ANP[82] and urodilatin[83] and the latter by insulin, which has been widely used by Yellon´s group[84] and Fischer-Rasokat.[85] The latter authors showed that insulin can improve recovery of function even after ischemia. Yellon´s group has also shown that statins are very effective in preventing reperfusion injury.[86] Both these agents will be described later. A very detailed and lucid description of reperfusion injury and the ways to prevent it is given by Verma et al.[87]

The discussion of drugs has up to now been conscientiously avoided, reserved for the latter part of this essay. However, it is interesting to note that different teams have advised parallel solutions. Thus, the group of Sutherland[88] working with the experimental infarct setting in the dog have concluded that the most significant myocardial salvage can be achieved if the first technique to be applied is thrombolysis followed within days by interventional artery opening. If these results are further verified, one can postulate that the initial, although incomplete opening of the artery allows the area of the myocardium subtended by it to avoid extensive necrosis but also to be spared of the gush of free radicals which would follow the abrupt mechanical opening. This latter technique applied at a later stage would further relieve any ongoing hibernation due to low flow. This theory has not been proven but its attractiveness cannot be denied.

One cannot however resist the temptation at this point of becoming philosophical and succumbing to the lure of the obscure philosophical concepts of eastern philosophy. Taoism has expanded on the "yin and yang" theory, that of the co-existence and complementation of opposites. Even the most concretely and practically experimental scientific executive cannot but ponder however that a small amount of ischemia preconditions-protects but a larger kills the cell. The same can be said of the free radicals which when "employed in moderation", like alcohol, protect[89-91] but, when overwhelmingly inundating the tissues, cause destruction. The ROS are also considered as an essential step of the preconditioning process.[89,92] Actually H_2O_2 activates p38 MAPK and Hsp27 phosphorylation; they also activate the mitochondrial K_{ATP} channels.[90] A similar interesting interaction has been noted with the use of antioxidant interventions. Thus, not only do the ROS induce cardioprotection, but some of the best players in this field the K_{ATP} openers induce ROS protection.[93] Accordingly, N-acetylcysteine has been found to abolish the ischemic preconditioning protection, as well as that induced by diazoxide.[94] Roth and Jaberansari[95] gave an elegant review a few years ago on this subject. They advance the proposal that when low quantities of ROS are produced, the administration of antioxidants is unfavorable, because they inhibit preconditioning. However, when very high ROS production is the main characteristic, antioxidants prevent the ensuing necrosis.

Another paradox must be mentioned here: In some instances a "protected" heart will not allow the beneficial effects of preconditioning to be fully appreciated.[96, 97] Immature hearts are such an example; as already stated, they are better intrinsically protected, but they manifest the benefits of preconditioning to a lesser degree.[18, 19] Khatkevich et al[98] showed that if shorter (in their experimental setup 20 minutes) periods of ischemia are used the protection of preconditioning is less evident than with longer periods-up to 35 minutes. But if preconditioning is such potent stuff how can it be harnessed[99] to protect the myocardium into a wider adapted way and to achieve greater applicability than that afforded by chance occurrence of prodromal pre-infarction myocardial ischemia? Here the additional clinical situations where preconditioning or other means of myocardial protection can be meaningfully employed will be enumerated.

The occurrence of "walkthrough" or "warm-up" angina has been noted since many years ago,[100] and has been during the last decade[101] ascribed to the "early" or "classic" preconditioning. According to this concept if an individual undergoes two consecutive exercise tests within approximately one hour, the second test will show fewer and less severe ischemic manifestations.[102] However, the practical advantages afforded by this process cannot be significant. On the contrary, exercise – induced ischemia can be appreciable as a protective measure through the mechanism of delayed preconditioning which can extent for up to 24-72 hours, in the animal[103] and the human.[104] Further clinical proof by Holter monitoring may broaden our understanding of this phenomenon. However, it can be envisaged as one of the salutary mechanisms of regular exercise training programs.[105]

Of course, late preconditioning was very early manifested by both ischemia and heat shock in the rat.[106] It would be very difficult to exert this mechanism in the human outside a Nazi concentration camp, although drugs producing fever, notably amphetamines,[107] have been tried in the animal. However, a large variety of drugs can cause or "mimick" late preconditioning as will be discussed later.

The phenomenon of preconditioning was noted very early during the implementation of angioplasty. It is manifested deviation during the second or third balloon inflation as compared to the first.[108, 109] However, it is hard to envisage how this phenomenon can be of appreciable clinical importance, apart from the recording of CK-MB and/or troponin elevation which can more reliably by ascribed to debris "showers" emanating from interventions on a frequently unstable plaque.[110] Some authors have described[111] preconditioning at a distance.[112] This could have an application nowadays when patients with compromised ventricular function are undergoing multivessel interventions: First opening an artery subtending a normal area of myocardium could protect the more dysfunctional region when opening of the stenotic vessel subtending it is attempted.[113] Stunning during PCI has been described,[114] but its clinical significance remains to be elucidated. Few instances of acute cardiac decompensation during PCI have been described and the actual reasons are difficult to determine. Still, pharmaceutical cardioprotection could be considered as an adjunct in the patient with significant myocardial compromise undergoing coronary interventions in the chronic setting. The considerations concerning reperfusion in acute myocardial infarction have already been discussed.

Ischemic preconditioning by intermittent cessation of flow was demonstrated in bypass surgery by Yellon in 1993.[115, 116] However, since then very few efforts with significant clinical implications have been made.[117] Here it should be mentioned that stunning has also been seen after bypass surgery.[118-121] It may prove critical in the patient with compromised cardiac function and preoperatively could be prevented by preconditioning. Probably surgeons regard the procedure as too tedious and time consuming. However, although somewhat anecdotally, preconditioning is being applied in the off-pump surgery where, in the absence of cardioplegia, preservation of the myocardium during the LAD occlusion period is of paramount importance. Still in most of the large reported series this approach is not mentioned.[122] Thus, one can see that the most valuable technique of myocardial protection that has been discovered in the current era, is not practically being applied in everyday practice. The prevailing effort is to confirm myocardial protection by drugs, either mimicking or replacing/duplicating ischemic preconditioning. As could be expected these agents are legion, constantly augmenting in numbers. The more important ones which have had at least some clinical applications will be mentioned here, with a concomitant discussion of drugs with an opposite action, i.e. abrogation of preconditioning effects, either in the experimental or in the clinical setting.

4. CARDIOPROTECTIVE AGENTS

I will not follow the very elegant protection "step" classification with mainly research implications followed by Baines,[123] but will approach their classification in a clinical sequence.

Adenosine is one of the basic components of myocardial preconditioning. Some questions exist as to whether all animal species are subject to adenosine-induced protection. Most studies have been carried out in rabbit. In this animal, Liu et al[124] first described the early protective effects of 5 min infusion of this agent. However, A_1 adenosine receptors can also cause delayed preconditioning both in rabbits[125] and in mice.[126]

The drug itself has been clinically tested during PTCA,[127] in a dose of 20 mg by the intracoronary route, with prevention of the deterioration of left ventricular function (LVEF). The same dose was employed by Leesar et al.[128] The action of adenosine was indirectly confirmed by Claeys et al[129] who showed that aminophylline an inhibitor of the action of adenosine inhibits the adaptation to ischemia during angioplasty. Adenosine has also been shown to diminish the no-reflow phenomenon in the setting of acute myocardial infarction.[130] (See also Table). However, the clinical application of adenosine in the thousands of percutaneous coronary interventions performed daily is negligible. I cannot but wonder that if indeed the use of adenosine had given outstanding results its use would have become universal. Similarly, although adenosine antagonists were shown to abolish the effect of adenosine during PCI,[129] very few clinicians actually ask their patients if they are indeed using such agents.

Adenosine has also been given during aortocoronary bypass surgery. Indeed, it has been shown to diminish enzyme production after surgery. However, its routine use during cardiac surgery has not become established, although the results in the animal model have been encouraging.[131]

Adenosine is probably not operative in the rat heart. The exact mechanism for this finding has not been adequately elucidated. A_1 receptors are postulated by Yao and Gross[132] to act through K_{ATP} channels.

Opening of the K_{ATP} controlled channel of – predominantly – the mitochondria has been associated with significant cardioprotection in the experimental animal. Many of the drugs employed for this purpose have also been used in the clinical setting. Diazoxide is such an agent, as well as cromakalim. Grover and Garlid, the main researchers of this family of drugs[133-137] and Liu[138] gave elegant reviews a few years ago.

Tamargo et al gave a very recent review.[139] They point out that K_{ATP} channels are inhibited by ATP and activated by Mg ADP, so that the channel activity is influenced by the ATP/ADP ratio. They also draw attention to the fact that mitochondrial K_{ATP} channel is responsible for ischemic preconditioning. They suggest that these channels are not blocked only by sulfonylureas, but also by many antiarrhythmic drugs, such as bretylium, disopyramide, flecainide and propafenone, and also by diltiazem and verapamil, but not by amiodarone or dronedarone, which will be addressed later.

Cleveland et al[140] have shown that isolated human atria from patients treated long-term with oral hypoglycemic agents were resistant to ischemic preconditioning. They postulated that this finding may explain the excess cardiovascular mortality noted by some authors in these patients. However, while an increase of mortality by the use of these drugs have been postulated, Brady and Terzie[141] point out that the mortality effect of oral hypoglycemic therapy in diabetic patients is still uncertain. However, the main drawback of these drugs is that they are effective only when given at the onset of ischemia and not at reperfusion. This obviously limits their applicability. Indeed, they are very sparingly used in the clinical setting for this purpose.[142] Thus Auchampach et al[143] showed that bimakalim, a typical representative, does not result in protection when it was administered during the reperfusion period only. However, they are effective in producing late preconditioning also,[142] which may advocate their chronic use. Another problem already stated, is that many drugs, with the sulfonylureas as a prime example, inhibit their action.[144] Notably, less selective inhibitors such as glimepiride[145, 146] do not appreciably express this action. However, in the clinical setting neither are K_{ATP} channel openers used before the interventions, nor is glibenclamide expressly avoided or glimepiride advised to be selectively employed instead.

Nicorandil is hybrid nitrate with K_{ATP} channel opening properties.[147] It has been shown to mimic preconditioning in the angioplasty setting.[148] Very recently, it has been shown that this drug can re-instate the preconditioning effect after the time interval for its occurrence has elapsed,[149] and in elderly patients.[150] It must be admitted however, that despite these very favorable qualities nicorandil is used very sparingly in chronic angina where it can be expected that given on a regular basis it may protect the myocardium against extensive necrosis when the onset of acute myocardial infarction occurs. In this context the results of the IONA randomized trial[151] which showed a reduction of major coronary events by therapy with nicorandil in patients with stable angina may be particularly relevant. (See also Table).

These drugs have also been found to be very effective in preventing myocardial injury when given before the onset of ischemia. They have not been used in the clinical setting before percutaneous coronary interventions.[78, 79] However, these drugs have been given in the setting of acute myocardial infarction. In the ESCAMI trial cariporide[80] was given at the time of hospital admission of patients with acute myocardial infarction. The results of this well planned and conducted study were disappointing. It is indeed doubtful if this class of drugs will be used again in myocardial infarction. However, Buerke et al[152] in a small pilot trial in 100 patients undergoing angioplasty in acute myocardial infarction showed a modest improvement in LV function and regional wall motion. (See also Table).

Hill et al in the experimental setting in the rabbit[153] and Leesar et al in coronary angioplasty[154] in the human elegantly showed that nitrates cause late preconditioning. Heusch stresses that these drugs typically cause delayed preconditioning.[155] These results complement the findings of Bolli et al[155] that late preconditioning is triggered by the generation of nitric oxide. Of course, they are drugs very widely used: In the ESC Survey of acute coronary syndromes, they were used in 44.5%, 48.9% and 64.8% at discharge for surviving patients after Q and non Q wave myocardial infarction and unstable angina respectively.[156] However, the chronic use of nitrates has not been associated with a decrease in mortality or the emergence of acute episodes or the need for revascularization. Thus, these drugs continue to be used as antianginal agents and obviously not with the indication of decreasing morbidity and mortality.

In many studies the administration of estrogens has been shown to diminish infarct size in the rabbit model in which the LAD was ligated.[157,158] This result has been ascribed to a Ca^{2+}-activated potassium channel opening effect of these agents. These data may explain the relative immunity from the complications of CAD in women at the menstruating age. More recently, the "synthetic" estrogen-action product raloxifene has also shown favorable effects in the canine heart,[159] despite its lack of effect in the rabbit.[158]

A completely divergent finding comes as a surprise. Complementing clinical studies in which administration of testosterone can cause coronary artery vasodilatation[160] this hormone improved recovery of myocardial function after ischemia/reperfusion injury in the orchectomized rats.[161] Furthermore, in a cellular model of ischemia, the hormone decreased the rate of ischemia-induced death of cardiomyocytes. This effect was attributed to a mitochondrial K_{ATP} channel opening effect.[162] However, androgens may stimulate oxidative stress[162] and promote the development of hypertension,[163] and hypertrophy.[164] Pham et al[165] also found that testosterone protects against proarrhythmia produced by dofetilide in normal female rabbits.

It is difficult to envisage, however, that hormone replacement therapy, after having given very conflicting results in the female sex[163] will find a strong following in the male population.

ACE inhibitors are by now very widely used in hypertension, heart failure and coronary artery disease. As already mentioned earlier in this review in rabbits whose heart is undergoing remodeling after an acute myocardial infarction, ischemic preconditioning is weakened or abolished. Thus, Ghosh et al[70] showed that hearts in failure could not be preconditioned. The administration of valsartan was found to re-instate preconditioning by preventing remodeling at two weeks.[69] In this model the hearts had not failed yet. Similarly, the acute administration of quinaprilat protects the post-infarction failing rat heart, at 10 weeks after ischemia.[166] Since these drugs are used very widely, almost universally in heart failure, after an acute myocardial infarction and after aortocoronary bypass surgery, their beneficial cardioprotective action may be more widespread than assessed by our clinical methods.

Sato et al[167] in the isolated rat heart in the working mode showed that losartan reduced myocardial ischemia/reperfusion injury by blocking AT_1 receptors. These beneficial effects were inhibited by a bradykinin B_2 receptor blocker. They postulate that ACE inhibition potentiate preconditioning through bradykinin B_2-receptor activation. Accordingly, Leesar et al[168] showed that in human intracoronary infusion of bradykinin reproduces the cardioprotective effects of ischemic preconditioning. It is interesting that Valen et al[169] also found that bradykinin plasma levels increased at cardiopulmonary bypass during open heart syrgery. Schwarz et al[170] in the open-chest pig undergoing left anterior descending coronary artery occlusion an angiotensin II receptor antagonist infusion not only reduced infarct size but also augmented the infarct size-limiting effects of preconditioning by ischemia. Nozawa et al[171] and Jaberansari et al[172] showed another very interesting effect of ACE inhibition, a lowering of the threshold preconditioning stimulus. The former authors studied rabbits who received an ACE inhibitor for 14 days and underwent a 2 min only period of preconditioning. The latter group from Yellon´s laboratory studied the effects of perindopril in a late preconditioning protocol in the pig. Bartling et al[173] showed that ACE inhibitors improved recovery after preconditioning in patients with severe angina, while nitrates and β-blockers did not have a significant effect.

β-blockers are also used very widely. They have not been found to mimic preconditioning. However, there is no doubt that they are protective against ischemia. These drugs are strong anti-apoptotic agents and thus modifiers of the ischemia-reperfusion injury,[174] In ischemia-reperfusion, after 30 minutes of global isolated heart ischemia and 2 hours reperfusion 24% of the cells are found to have undergone apoptosis versus 35% which have suffered necrosis.[175] Veronese et al[176] studying anesthetized dogs under total ischemia found that propranolol delayed the onset of ischemic contracture, but also decreased the rate of anaerobic glycolysis during ischemia, suggesting that with β-blockade the myocardium is allowed to survive with lower levels of ATP.

Probably not all β-blockers are created equal. Thus, Cargnoni et al[177] showed that carvedilol protects against ischemia/reperfusion to a greater degree than propranolol. They ascribe this differential action to the anti-oxidant effects of the former drug. Yue et al[178] also showed that carvedilol reduces reperfusion injury in the rabbit heart, while inhibiting the activation of JNK at reperfusion.

The possible cardiac functions of amiodarone are attributed to tissue hypothyroidism.[55] Ide et al[177] showed that this drug protect cardiac myocytes from the canine left ventricular free wall against oxidative stress-mediated injury by H_2O_2, while disopyramide and atenolol had no such effects.

Calcium blockers have mostly been studied in the clinical context. They protect the myocardium from deleterious ischemia-induced Ca^{2+} intake.[180] They have been used experimentally in ischemia with success. All drugs have been found to be successful, but verapamil[181] and diltiazem[182] analogues are used more often in research. They have been found more effective than nifedipine in inhibiting ischemic contracture, improving postischemic left ventricular function, and preserve high energy phosphates.[181, 183] Many authors stress that these drugs have a very significant effect against post-ischemic stunning, both in the clinical[184] and experimental setting.[185-190] Garrett et al[191] mentioned another very interesting effect of verapamil, that it prevents the development of alcoholic dysfunction in harmster myocardium. This finding is analogous to the effects of this drug in preventing the development of heart failure in the inherited cardiomyopathy of the Syrian hamster.[192] (See also Table).

Free fatty acid (FFA) are the main substances used as fuel by the myocardium, normally preferentially over glucose. However, they need more oxygen than glucose to produce equal amounts of ATP. Moreover, their increased oxidation concomitantly results into a diminution of the oxidation of glucose with an increase of lactic acid production and protons, which in their turn need greater ATP consumption. Thus, cardiac efficiency is diminished, while FFA toxicity is also postulated. A way to interrupt this vicious cycle is to employ substances that selectively "switch" the cell metabolism to glucose, by stimulating the enzymic complex of pyruvate dehydrogenase. The following agents have been used to this purpose:

Dichloroacetate, which however is clinically not practical, since it has a short half-life and needs to be administered in large doses.[193]

Ranolazine is a drug which has been already used clinically. This drug increases glucose oxidation both under normoxic and hypoxic conditions or low flow ischemia.[193, 194]

Etomoxir[195] diminishes the uptake of fatty acids by the mitochondria and thus stimulates glucose oxidation. It has been successfully used in idiopathic cardiomyopathy.

Trimetazidine has been widely used as an antianginal drug.[196] It has also been found to be protective during coronary artery graft surgery[197] and angioplasty.[198] Mody et al[199] using positron emission tomography showed that it enhances myocardial glucose utilization in normal and ischemic myocardial tissue. We have shown that in the isolated rat heart, when the drug is given before ischemia it significantly protects against necrosis,[200] while when given at reperfusion it ameliorates stunning.

L-carnitine and its derivative, propionyl L-carnitine, have both anti-ischemic and cardioprotective functions. Broderick et al[201] perfused isolated rat hearts with glucose, palmitate and insulin, and randomized them to a control group or to those receiving 10mM L-carnitine before ischemia. Glucose oxidation rates were significantly elevated during reperfusion, together with an improvement in mechanical recovery. The authors point out that not only do FFA decrease glucose oxidation but have also been shown to potentiate ischemic injury in the experimental animal and increase infarct size in the human. The same drug is widely used clinically in heart failure[202] and in pediatric cardiomyopathy.[203, 204] Iliceto et al[205] reported another very interesting finding. They randomized 472 patients within 24 hours after a first acute myocardial infarction to placebo or L-carnitine 9g/day IV for 5 days and 6g/day orally thereafter for 12 months. They found a significant attenuation of left ventricular dilation but no significant change in LVEF; a small but nonsignificant decrease in mortality was seen with carnitine. (See also Table). However, the authors point out that the study was not designed to show differences in clinical end-points. In an editorial,[206] I referred to two clinical studies showing an improvement in prognosis with the use of trimetazidine in ischemic cardiomyopathy, and to the potential of these drugs to re-instate viability in this entity.

Of course when metabolic interventions affecting glucose metabolism are considered, insulin comes under discussion. This drug, together with glucose and potassium was used many years ago by the group of Sodi-Pallares. It has gained clinical rebirth[207, 208] and has also been employed in recent years by important teams. (See also Table). In the open-chest rat, Jonassen et al[209] showed that the glucose-insulin-potassium solution (GIK) administered only during the reperfusion phase was equally effective as when given during the entire ischemia/reperfusion period in reducing infarct size, and improving left ventricular function. GIK infusion also resulted in reduced plasma concentrations of FFA. These authors recapitulate the possible FFA toxicity on the myocardium through proton accumulation and possibly calcium overload.[210] Chaudhuri et al[211] offer another explanation for the favorable effects of insulin in acute ST-segment-elevation myocardial infarction. They showed that insulin diminishes the absolute increase of CRP and serum amyloid A(SAA) and an increase of PAI-1; the monocyte p47 phox subunit of NADPH oxidase, which mediates oxidative stress was also suppressed. However, the main characteristic of insulin administration seems to be its capacity to protect the myocardium even when given at reperfusion.

Another family of metabolically active drugs are statins. As already mentioned, Bell and Yellon[86] have shown that it is very effective in reducing reperfusion injury. Di Napoli et al[212] also showed that simvastatin reduces reperfusion injury in the isolated working rat heart. These authors showed that the drug significantly increased eNOS mRNA and protein, while it decreased iNOS mRNA and protein, as well as nitrite production after ischemia-reperfusion. The authors stress that this NO-dependent mechanism is cholesterol independent. Actually, Feng et al[213] have shown that increased iNOS expression in mice results in myocardial dysfunction and higher mortality after experimental infarction. These authors point out that although increased NO production from iNOS may decrease vascular resistance, excessively high NO levels may decrease myocardial contractility and even cause myocardial damage through peroxynitrite formation.[214] However, Arnaud et al[215] showed that iNOS is a mediator of the heat stress-induced preconditioning. The statins may also be beneficial in reversing the lipid hydroperoxide modification of proteins (generation of LOOH-proteins) a characteristic of ischemia-reperfusion.[216]

Calcium channel blockers have been already mentioned as exerting their beneficial effect through preventing Ca^{2+} overload. It is interesting that diltiazem has been found to reduce lipid peroxidation in the reperfused isolated rabbit heart.[217] In this context it should be noted that according to Eaton et al[216] lipid peroxidation products are formed when omega-6 polyunsaturated fatty acids react with free radical species. Thus, it comes as no surprise that omega-3 fatty acids protect against ischemia[218] and reperfusion. Eicosipentanoic acid was additionally found to attenuate p38 MAPK phosphorylation, augmentation of lipid peroxidation and importantly upregulation of MMP-1 produced by hypoxia-reoxygenation in adult rat myocytes. Ander et al[219] found that flaxseed, a rich plant source of alpha-linolenic acid protects against ventricular fibrillation induced by ischemia-reperfusion in rabbits.

The quest for naturally occurring antioxidants continues. Resveratrol,[220] a natural antioxidant present in red wine has been found to protect against ischemia-reperfusion arrhythmias and mortality in rats. Thus, the French paradox may have another counterpart besides favorable lipid modification. The emergence of cross-tolerance has already been described. Consequently, it comes as no surprise that regular exercise, apart from protecting against ischemia-reperfusion has been found to protect against the direct oxidative injury produced by H_2O_2, as already mentioned.[1]

The effects of oxidant stress in ischemia reperfusion thus come again into prominence. ROS and peroxynitrite produce cellular injury through diverse mechanisms. As already mentioned many antioxidants have been tried but none has come into clinical prominence. In addition to previously employed antioxidants, newer proposed substances are N-acetylcysteine[221] which has also been found beneficial in protecting against renal damage during coronary angiography/angioplasty,[222, 223] through inactivation of oxygen-free radicals. In this context our group has shown that vitamin C is renoprotective.[224] It might be advisable to re-study if this substance is cardioprotective in the clinical context. Nespereira et al[225] showed that it can prevent lipid peroxidation, which as will be further described is a main product of ischemia-reperfusion. However, it is not clear whether antioxidants can protect when given after occlusion. Thus Bolli et al[226] showed that N-(2-mercaptopropionyl)- glycine given 1 minute before reperfusion enhanced myocardial recovery, but was ineffective when given 1 minute after reperfusion. As Werns et al[227] and Kloner et al[228] point out the main free radical scavengers are superoxide dismutase, catalase and their combination, allopurinol and desferrioxamine.

Many of these agents have found clinical application, especially desferrioxamine perioperatively.[229] It is very interesting that allopurinol, while found to decrease experimental infarct size,[230, 231] also increases survival in murine postischemic cardiomyopathy, most probably by diminishing oxidative cardiac load.[232]

The number of protective influences reported is constantly increasing. Both endogenous and exogenous opioids, acting through opioid receptors δ and ϰ have been found to be cardioprotective.[233] Peart and Gross[234] recently reported that morphine-tolerant mice exhibit a profound and persistant cardioprotective phenotype. The authors point out that chronic opioid treatment produces an increase in the release of endogenous substance P, calcitonin gene-related peptide and adenosine. δ_1-opioid receptor stimulation induces delayed cardioprotection possibly through mitochondrial K_{ATP} stimulation. While not advocating morphine addiction as a means to cardioprotect, this finding should prompt for the quest of ways to enhance endogenous opioid receptors such as exercise – or develop new drugs with similar actions.

Since a narcotic drug such as morphine is mentioned, an anesthetic drug, i.e. propofol should be considered. This widely used substance has been found to be cardioprotective against oxidative stress and reperfusion injury.[235, 236] Javadov et al[237] showed that this drug confers a significant protection against both normothermic global ischemia and during cold cardioplegic arrest. The authors ascribe this beneficial effect to a decrease of the mitochondrial permeability transition pores.[238] Moreover, the authors point out that the appropriate dosage is very important: Higher doses may impair oxidative phosphorylation of isolated mitochondria.

The prototype of mitochondrial pore opening inhibitor is cyclosporine. Weinbrenner et al already in 1998 stressed that this drug can limit myocardial infarct size even when administered after onset of ischemia.[81] This finding is very important because, as already described, most drugs are effective only when given before the onset of ischemia. Borutaite et al[239] reported similar results, also stressing that this drug prevents ischemia-induced apoptosis. Niemann et al[240] gave further detailed data on this subject: They showed a dose-response effect of cyclosporine on the reduction in myocardial energy metabolism, by reducing oxidative phosphorylation. The capacity of cyclosporine to reduce myocardial injury even when given after ischemia is evidently very important. A search is on-going for other agents sharing this quality. Thus, cardiotrophin-1, a cytokine family member can protect myocytes when added both prior to ischemia and at re-oxygenation.[241]

Suzuki et al[242] from Yacoub´s group reported that rat hearts overexpressing an interleukin-1 receptor antagonist demonstrate cardioprotection. These superficially conflicting results help to bring into focus the widely divergent effects of the various cytokines, which may exhibit both beneficial and noxious effects.

Levosimendan is widely used in recent years as an inotrope with very favorable properties. It has actually been shown to be beneficial in ischemia-reperfusion in the isolated heart,[243] in distinct contrast to dobutamine which by itself has an unfavorable effect.[244]

Erythropoietin is a drug beginning to be widely used in cardiac failure, both for combatting the anemia associated with this syndrome and for its beneficial myocardial action. It was initially to prevent neurological damage.[245] Bogoyevitch gave a very recent review on this subject.[246] She points out that the drug is anti-apoptotic and protects against infarct expansion. Shi et al[247] point out that this drug mimicks preconditioning by activating protein kinases and potassium channels. Cai et al[248] showed that it protects against ischemia-reperfusion injury. Rui et al[249] also showed that it prevents the acute myocardial inflammatory response produced by ischemia-reperfusion via induction of AP-1.The ease of administration of this drug and its lack of side effects makes its use a very attractive proposition.

Another drug which has attracted great attention is melatonin. It is used for many disorders, from the jet lag to the fatigue syndrome. Dobsak et al[250] reported that melatonin protects both against ischemia-reperfusion injury and apoptosis, presumably via its antioxidant properties. Sahna et al[251] also attribute these beneficial effects to attenuation of lipid peroxidation by this drug. Reiter and Tan[252] in a very detailed review also point out that melatonin has a major role against oxidative injury. Again, the ease of administration and low toxicity of this drug make it a very attractive agent. The authors point out that the drug has antiarrhythmic effects. Moreover, exogenously given melatonin does not inhibit its endogenous production.

A caveat should also be noted. Shinmura et al[253] from Bolli's group found that high doses of aspirin (25mg/kg) abrogate late preconditioning in conscious rabbits. As Heusch[254] in an accompanying editorial points out further research is needed on this point. However, such doses are irrelevant in man.

After having enumerated all the interventions producing cardioprotection it should be pointed out that frequently it is difficult to differentiate between myocardium and endothelium. Ischemic injury affects the endothelium as well.[255] Microvascular dysfunction, expressed as slow flow, is of great prognostic value after a myocardial infarction and can be attributed to endothelial dysfunction.[256] Moreover, the endothelium produces Hsp70 by itself[257] which decreases i.e IL-6 and i-NOS but upgrades e-NOS;[258] endothelium itself is a main source of NO.[259] It is of interest however that myocardium and endothelium share the same friends and foes.[260]

5. SYNTHESIS

Finally, in view of all the aforementioned protective mechanisms many of which still belong to the "concept" what can be the practical considerations of a clinician in advancing myocardial protection? Of course it must be realized that a single patient cannot be expected to consume an unlimited number of medications.

In the patient with chronic angina, the drugs commonly used seem to offer important myocardial protection: Thus, β-blockers, ACE inhibitors and most probably angiotensin receptor blockers, statins, Ca^{2+} channel blockers, all are in their way cardioprotective. Nitrates and more importantly nicorandil are worthwhile options. Trimetazidine and drugs producing a shift towards preferential glucose oxidation would also be a consideration. A number of studies stress that they may produce an improvement in ischemic cardiomyopathy, probably through an anti-inflammatory action.[261]

If the patient with angina is diabetic, certain considerations apply. Insulin is eminently cardioprotective, as already described, while the sulfonylureas have an unfavorable profile. Probably less selective blockers as glimepiride should be preferred to glibenclamide.[146] PPARγ agonists such as rosiglitazone have been found to be cardioprotective[262, 263] and to have an antiapoptotic effect in hypercholesterolemic rabbits subjected to myocardial ischemia/reperfusion.[264]

The value of statins has already been described. Recent work shows that they may reduce infarct size through an anti-inflammatory effect.[265] Their action in heart failure is

Table 1. Clinical studies conducted with cardioprotective agents.

Reference	Characteristics	Size (n)	Primary end-points	Results
Van Horst et al.[208]	GIK infusion, 15-20 min after hospital admission, in patients with AMI subjected to PTCA	940	Mortality	Significant reduction after 30 days in patients without signs of heart failure
Malmberg et al.[207] "DIGAMI"	GIK infusion in diabetic patients with AMI	306	Mortality	Significant reduction after 1 year (18.6% vs 26.1%) and after a mean of 3.4 years (33% vs 44%)
Mehta et al.[266] "CREATE-ECLA"	GIK infusion for 24 h in AMI patients with ST-segment elevation	20201	Mortality, cardiac arrest, cardiogenic shock, and reinfarction	No difference in any end-point at 30 days
Theroux et al.[267] "GUARDIAN"	Cariporide administration at different doses in patients with unstable angina or non-ST-AMI or subjected to PTCA, CABG	11590	Mortality, AMI	A significant reduction was observed after 36 days and 6 months only in patients subjected to CABG
Zeymer et al.[80] "ESCAMI"	Enaporide administration as early reperfusion therapy in patients with AMI	1411	Infarct size, mortality	Reduction in infarct size after 72 h in patients with AMI<30 min. Trend towards excess death due to stroke in enaporide group
Mentzer[268] "EXPEDITION"	Cariporide administration in patients before and after CABG	5761	Perioperative AMI, mortality	Significant reduction in perioperative AMI but increase in mortality, stroke and renal failure in cariporide group
Sochman et al.[269] "ISLAND"	N-acetyl-cysteine administration in patients with AMI subjected to thrombolysis	30	Infarct size, LV function	Reduction in infarct size and improved LV function after 2-weeks

GIK, glucose-insulin-potassium solution; AMI, acute myocardial infarction; PTCA, percutaneous transluminal coronary angioplasty; CABG, coronary artery bypass graft; cariporide and enaporide are sodium/proton exchanger inhibitors; N-acetyl-cysteine is an anti-oxidant agent.

Reference	Characteristics	Size (n)	Primary end-points	Results
"IONA"[151]	Nicorandil administration in patients with stable angina	5126	Mortality, coronary events	Significant reduction in mortality and frequency of coronary events after a mean of 1.6 years.
Marangelli et al.[270] "VAMI"	Verapamil infusion in patients with 1st anterior AMI before thrombolysis	88	Left ventricular remodeling, NYHA class	A trend towards smaller left ventricular volunes and significant reduction in heart failure symptoms after 3 months
Theroux et al.[271] "DATA"	Diltiazem infusion in patients with AMI before thrombolysis	59	Cardiac events (death, AMI or recurrent ischemia)	Significant reduction in cardiac events
Kopecky et al.[272] "ADMIRE"	AMP579 infusion in patients with AMI subjected to PTCA	311	Infarct size	No difference
Ross et al.[273] "AMISTAD II"	Adenosine infusion for 3 h in AMI patients subjected to PTCA or thrombolysis	2084	Infarct size, HF, mortality	Significant reduction in infarct size, trend towards a decrease in mortality
Quintana et al.[274] "ATTACC"	Adenosine infusion for 6 h in AMI patients subjected to thrombolysis	608	LV systolic and diastolic function	No difference in LV function, trend towards reduced mortality
Iliceto et al.[205] "CEDIM"	L-carnitine administration within 24 h and for 12 months in AMI patients	472	LV remodeling, LV ejection fraction	Significant reduction in LV dilation, no difference in LV ejection fraction

AMI, acute myocardial infarction; PTCA, percutaneous transluminal coronary angioplasty; CABG, coronary artery bypass graft; HF, heart failure; LV, left ventricular; Niconradil is a K_{ATP} channel opener;

being increasingly discussed.[275] It is very difficult to determine if the above mentioned agents have additive effects, however in most cases they are used in combination.

If the patient with coronary artery disease also develops cardiac dysfunction, the same medications would be expected to apply, but for additional reasons. The re-instation of preconditioning mechanisms by ACEI administration has already been described. β-blockers have additional mechanisms, such as an antiapoptotic and antioxidant action.[276] In this situation oxidative stress is also predominant and may further exacerbate apoptotic mechanisms.[277] The only drugs predictably diminishing oxidative stress in clinical usage are carvedilol and statins. The latter drug family is also used in heart failure. Exercise is also a standard preventive and therapeutic intervention in both the above categories.

After the value of drugs has been praised, a very simple remedy should not be forgotten: Exercise rehabilitation. This modality has been found to reduce mortality after a myocardial infarction[278] and in heart failure.[279] A host of beneficial effects has been cited of which preconditioning may not be the least. Very recently, prior training has been shown to improve outcome of myocardial infarction in the rat, probably through improvement in remodeling.[280]

Three main potential applications of cardioprotection currently apply in the interventional treatment of the coronary patient:

Protection of the patient undergoing high risk angioplasty/stent placement. In this context, the site of the stenosis is not the sole consideration. Patients with compromised left ventricular function are especially vulnerable. Apart from the aforementioned medications which are by now a staple management, the following medications should be considered: Nitrates or alternatively nitrodil given before the procedure.

In the setting of cardial surgery, levosimendan given preoperatively would also be a consideration. Of the various antoxidants, desferrioxamine could be a candidate. Erythropoietin would be another strong candidate; it is already widely used in heart failure.

The most dramatic moment in cardiology is the performance of primary angioplasty in the setting of acute myocardial infarction. In this situation the main effort up to now is to achieve rapid opening of the occluded coronary artery. However, up to now efforts at preventing or reversing the ischemia/reperfusion injury have been meager. Of course, one must remain on the practical side. Luckily, statins which have been advocated to be very efficacious are given to almost all patients anyway.

What drugs could be given before angioplasty? Cyclosporine or analogues could be a consideration. Antioxidants might be expected to be effective, but the right agent is difficult to define. Desferrioxamine has not been used. Erythropoietin may be another consideration, with its antioxidative action. β-blockers, acting as antiapoptotic agents may be expected to subacutely salvage myocardium. Graded arterial opening could be considered, but it would be difficult to convince an invasive interventionist to defer complete opening of the artery and defer stent placement. In a very thoughtful recent state-of-the-art paper, Kloner and Rezkalla[281] believe that adenosine, K_{ATP} channel openers, Na^+/H^+ exchanger inhibitors and hypothermia, tried in small trials, deserve larger future studies.

Thus, the effort of protecting the myocardium should continue with the aim of diminishing cardiac attrition and presenting myocardial integrity. The search for new agents should further evolve with the pragmatic approach always remaining a prime consideration.

REFERENCES

1. R. P. Taylor, J. T. Ciccolo, J. W. Starnes, Effect of exercise training on the ability of the rat heart to tolerate hydrogen peroxide, *Cardiovasc Res* **58**, 575–581 (2003).
2. J. L. Martin, R. Mestril, R. Hilal-Dandan, L. L. Brunton, W. H. Dillmann, Small heat shock proteins and protection against ischemic injury in cardiac myocytes, *Circulation* **96**, 4343–4348 (1997).
3. C. E. Murry, RB. Jennings, K. A. Reimer, Preconditioning with ischemia: a delay of lethal cell injury in ischemic myocardium, *Circulation* **75**, 1124–1136 (1986).
4. F. Ottani, M. Galvani, D. Ferrini, F. Sorbello, P. Limonetti, D. Pantoli, F. Rusticali, Prodromal angina limits infarct size. A role for ischemic preconditioning, *Circulation* **91**, 291–297 (1995).
5. Y. Nakagawa, H. Ito, M. Kitakaze, H. Kusuoka, M. Hori, T. Kuzuya, Y. Higashino, K. Fujii, T. Minamino, Effect of angina pectoris on myocardial protection in patients with reperfused anterior wall myocardial infarction : retrospective clinical evidence of «preconditioning», *J Am Coll Cardiol* **25**, 1076–1083 (1995).
6. N. A. Ruocco, B. A. Bergelson, A. K. Jacobs, M. M. Frederick, D. P. Faxon, T. J. Ryan, Invasive versus conservative strategy after thrombolytic therapy for acute myocardial infarction in patients with antecedent angina. A report from Thrombolysis in Myocardial Infarction phase II study (TIMI II), *J Am Coll Cardiol* **20**,1445–1551 (1992).
7. D. W. M. Muller, E. J. Topol, R. M. Califf, K. N. Sigmon, L. Gorman, B. S. George, D. L. Kereiakis, K. L. Lee, S. G. Ellis, TAMI study Group. Relationship between antecedent angina pectoris and short term prognosis after thrombolytic therapy for acute myocardial infarction, *Am Heart J* **119**. 224–31 (1990).
8. R. A. Kloner, T. Shook, K. Przyklenk, V. G. Davis, L. Junio, R. V. Matthews, S. Burstein, C. M. Gibson, W. K. Poole, C. P. Cannon, C. H. McCabe, E. Brawnwald, for the TIMI 4 investigators, Previous angina alters in-hospital outcome in TIMI 4. A clinical correlate to preconditioning? *Circulation* **91**, 37–45 (1995).
9. M. Ishihara, H. Sato, H. Tateishi, T. Kawagoe, Y. Shimatani, S. Kurisu, K. Sakai, K. Ueda, Implications of prodromal angina pectoris in anterior wall acute myocardial infarction: acute angiographic findings and long-term prognosis, *J Am Coll Cardiol* **31**, 1701 (1998).
10. P. Taggart, D. M. Yellon, Preconditioning and arrhythmias, *Circulation* **106**, 2999–3001 (2002).
11. G. I. Barbash, H. D. White, M. Modan, F. Van de Werf, Antecedent angina pectoris predicts worse outcome after myocardial infarction in patients receiving thrombolytic therapy: experience gleaned from the International Tissue Plasminogen Activator/Streptokinase Mortality Trial, *J Am Coll Cardiol* **20**, 6–41 (1992).
12. F. Ottani, M. Galvani, D. Ferrini, Angina and Cardiac adaptation. In: Delayed preconditioning and adaptive cardioprotection. G. F. Baxter, D. M. Yellon, eds Kluwer Academic Publishers, *Dordrecht*, pp. 209–224 (1998).
13. A. D. Cokkinos, S. Tzeis, P. Moraitis, C. Pantos, H. Carageorgiou, D. Panousopoulos, D. D. Varonos, D. V. Cokkinos, Loss of cardioprotection induced by ischemic preconditioning after an initial ischemic period in isolated rat hearts, *Exp Clin Cardiol* **8**, 5–9 (2003).
14. P. Abete, N. Ferrara, A. Cioppa, P. Ferrara, S. Bianco, C. Calabrese, F. Cacciatore, G. Longobardi, F. Rengo, Preconditioning does not prevent postischemic dysfunction in ageing heart, *J Am Coll Cardiol* **27**, 1777–86 (1996).
15. M. Tani, Y. Honma, H. Hasegawa, K. Tamaki, Direct activation of mitochondrial K_{ATP} channels mimics preconditioning but protein kinase C activation is less effective in middle-aged rat hearts, *Cardiovascular Research* **49**, 56–68 (2001).
16. P. Abete, C. Calabrese, N. Ferrara, A. Cioppa, P. Pisanelli, F. Cacciatore, G. Longobardi, C. Napoli, F. Rengo, Exercise training restores ischemic preconditioning in the ageing heart, *J Am Coll Cardiol* **36**, 643–50 (2000).
17. E. J. Baker, LE. Boerboom, G. N. Olinger, J. E. Baker, Tolerance of the developing heart to ischemia: impact of hypoxemia from birth, *Am J Physiol* **268**, H1165–73 (1995).
18. K. Iwaki, S. Chi, W. H. Dillmann, R. Mestril, Induction of Hsp70 in cultured rat neonatal cardiomyocytes by hypoxia and metabolic stress, *Circulation* **87**, 2023–2032 (1993).
19. J. E. Baker, P. Holman, G. J. Gross, Preconditioning in immature rabbit hearts: Role of K_{ATP} channels, *Circulation* **99**,1249–1254 (1999).
20. W. I. Awad, M. J. Shattock, D. J. Chambers, Ischemic preconditioning in immature myocardium, *Circulation* **98**, II-206–II-213 (1998).

21. G. Hadour, R. Ferrera, L. Sebbag, R. Forrat, J. Delaye, M. de Lorgeril, Improved myocardial tolerance to ischemia in the diabetic rabbit, *J Mol Cell Cardiol* **30**, 1869–75 (1998).
22. A. Tosaki, D. T. Engelman, R. M. Engelman, D. K. Das, The evolution of diabetic response to ischemia/reperfusion and preconditioning in isolated working rat hearts, *Cardiovasc Res* **31(4)**, 526–36 (1996).
23. T. Ravingerova, J. Neckar, F. Kolar, R. Stetka, K. Volkovova, A. Ziegelhoffer, J. Styk, Ventricular arrhythmias following coronary artery occlusion in rats: is the diabetic heart less or more sensitive to ischemia? *Basic Res Cardiol* **96**, 160–168 (2001).
24. P. Ferdinandy, Z. Szilvassy, G. F. Baxter, Adaptation to myocardial stress in disease states: is preconditioning a healthy heart phenomenon? *Trends Pharmacol Sci* **19**, 223–9 (1998).
25. L. Szekeres, Z. Szilvassy, P. Ferdinandy, I. Nagy, S. Karscu, S. Csati, Delayed cardiac protection against harmful consequences of stress can be induced in experimental atherosclerosis in rabbits, *J Mol Cell Cardiol* **129**, 1977–83 (1997).
26. D. Kremastinos, E. Bofilis, G. Karavolias, A. Papalois, L. Kaklamanis, E. Iliodromitis, Preconditioning limits myocardial infarct size in hypercholesterolemic rabbits, *Atherosclerosis* **150**, 81–85 (2000).
27. C. Pantos, V. Malliopoulou, D. Varonos, D. V. Cokkinos, Thyroid hormone and phenotypes of cardioprotection, *Basic Res Cardiol* **99**, 101–120 (2004).
28. C. Pantos, V. Malliopoulou, I. Mourouzis, E. Karamanoli, S. M. Tzeis, H.C. Carageorgiou, D.D. Varonos, D.V. Cokkinos, Long-term thyroxine administration increases Hsp70 mRNA expression and attenuates p38MAP kinase activity in response to ischemia, *J Endocrinol* **170**, 207–215 (2001).
29. C. Pantos, V. Malliopoulou, I. Mourouzis, E. Karamanoli, I. Paizis, N. Steinberg, D.D. Varonos, D.V. Cokkinos, Long-term thyroxine administration protects the heart in a similar pattern as ischemic preconditioning, *Thyroid* **12**, 325–329 (2002).
30. C. Pantos, V. Malliopoulou, I. Paizis, P. Moraitis, I. Mourouzis, S. Tzeis, E. Karamanoli, D. D. Cokkinos, H.C. Carageorgiou, D.D. Varonos, D.V. Cokkinos, Thyroid hormone and cardioprotection; study of p38 MAPK and JNKs during ischemia and at reperfusion in isolated rat heart, *Mol Cell Biochem* **242**, 173–180 (2003).
31. J. Zhao, O. Renner, L. Wightman, P. H. Sugden, L. Stewart, A. D. Miller, D S. Latchman, M. S. Marber, The expression of constitutively active isotypes of protein kinase C to investigate preconditioning, *J Biol Chem* **273** 23072–79 (1998).
32. D. Salter, C. Dyke, A. Wechsler, Triodothyronine (T3) and cardiovascular therapeutics: a review, *J Card Surg* **4**, 363–374 (1992).
33. P. Moruzzi, E. Doria, P. G. Agostoni, V. Capacchione, P. Saganzerla. Usefulness of L-thyroxine to improve cardiac, and exercise performance in idiopathic dilated cardiomyopathy. *Am J Cardiol* **73**, 374–378 (1994).
34. P. Moruzzi, E. Doria, P. G. Agostoni, Medium term effectiveness of l-thyroxine treatment in idiopathic dilated carrdiomyopathy, *Am J Med* **101**, 461–467 (1996).
35. M. A. Hamilton, L. W. Stevenson, G. C. Fonarow, Safery and hemodynamic effect of intravenous triiodothyronine in advanced congestive heart failure, *Am J Cardiol* **81**, 443–447 (1998).
36. K. W. Mahaffay, T. Raya, G. Pennock, E. Morkin, S. Goldman, Left ventricular performance and remodelling in rabbits after myocardial infarction : effects of a thyroid hormone analogue, *Circulation* **91**, 794–801 (1995).
37. K. Ojamaa, A. Kenessey, R. Shenoy, I. Klein, Thyroid hormone metabolism and cardiac gene expression after acute myocardial infarction in the rat, *Am J Physiol Endocrinol Metab* **279**, E1319–1324 (2000).
38. L. Friberg, V. Drvota, A. H. Bjelak, Association between increased levels of reverse triiodothyronine and mortality after acute myocardial infarction, *Arch Intern Med* **162** 1388–94 (2002).
39. G. Iervasi, A. Pinagitore, P. Landi, M. Raciti, A. Ripoli, M. Scarlattini, A. L´Abbate, L. Donato, Low T3 syndrome, *Circulation* **107**, 708–713 (2003).
40. M. A. Hamilton, L. W. Stevenson, M. Luu, J. A. Walden, Altered thyroid hormone metabolism in advanced heart failure, *J Am Coll Cardiol* **16**, 91–95 (1990).
41. D. Psirropoulos, N. Lefkos, F. Boudonas, A. Efthimiadis, V. Vogas, C. Keskilidis, G. Tsapas, Heart failure accompanied by sick euthyroid syndrome and exercise training, *Curr Opinion Cardiol* **17**, 266–70 (2002).
42. Y. Suzuki, M. Nanno, R. Gemma, T. Yoshimi, Plasma free fatty acids, inhibitor of extrathyroidal conversion of T4 to T3 and thyroid hormone binding inhibitor in patients with various nonthyroidal illness,*Endocrinol Jpn* **39**, 445–53 (1992).
43. D. Novitzky, P. A. Human, D. K. Cooper, Inotropic effect of triiodothyronine following myocardial ischemia and cardiopulmonary bypass: an experimental study in pigs, *Ann Thorac Surg* **45**, 50–55 (1988).

44. F. G. Spinale, Cellular and molecular therapeutic targets for treatment of contractile dysfunction after cardioplegic arrest, *Ann Thorac Surg* **68**, 1934–41 (1999).
45. A. Mackie, K. Booth, J. Newburger, et al, A randomized, double-blinded, placebo-controlled trial of triiodothyronine in neonatal heart surgery (Abstr.), *J Am Coll Cardiol* **45**, 321A (2005).
46. T. Kimura, T. Kanda, A. Kuwabara, H. Shinohara, I. Kobayashi, Participation of the pituitary-thyroid axis in the cardiovascular systemic elderly patients with congestive heart failure, *J Med* **28**, 75–80 (1997).
47. C. Pantos, V. Malliopoulou, I. Mourouzis, E. Karamanoli, P. Moraitis, S. Tzeis, I. Paizis, H. Carageorgiou, D. Varonos, D. V. Cokkinos, Thyroxine pre-treatment increases basal myocardial Hsp27 expression and accelerates translocation and phosphorylation of this protein upon ischemia, *Eur J Pharmacol* **478**, 53–60 (2003).
48. F. Chen, R. Chang, M. Trivedi, Y. Capetanaki, V. L. Cryns, Caspase proteolysis of desmin produces a dominant-negative inhibitor of intermediate filaments and promotes apoptosis, *J Biol Chem* **278**, 6848–53 (2003).
49. H. L. Blumgart, A. S. Freedberg, G. S. Kurland, Radioactive iodine treatment of angina pectoris and congestive heart failure, *Circulation* **16**, 110–18 (1957).
50. J. P. Stroraasli, E. L. Schoeniger, H. K. Hellerstein, H. L. Friedell, Thyroid ablation with I^{131} in euthyroid cardiac patients with special reference to preparation with antithyroid drugs, *Radiology* **4**, E10–21 (1960).
51. M. Gomberg-Maitland, W. H. Frishman, Thyroid hormone and cardiovascular disease, *Am Heart J* **135**, 187–196 (1998).
52. I. Klein, K. Ojamaa, Thyroid hormone and the cardiovascular system, *N Engl J Med* **344**, 501–509 (2001).
53. J. Lekakis, C. Papamichael, M. Alevizaki, G. Piperingos, P. Marafelia, J. Mantzos, S. Stamatelopoulos, D. A. Koutras, Flow-mediated, endothelium-dependent vasodilation is impaired in subjects with hypothyroidism, borderline hypothyroidism, and high-normal serum thyrotropin (TSH) values, *Thyroid* **7**, 411–4 (1997).
54. C. I. Pantos, V. Tzilalis, S. Giannakakis, D. D. Cokkinos, S. M. Tzeis,V. Malliopoulou, I. Mourouzis, P. Asimakopoulos, H.C. Carageorgiou, D.D. Varonos, D.V. Cokkinos, Phenylephrine induced aortic vasoconstriction is attenuated in hyperthyroid rats, *Int Angiol* **20**, 181–186 (2001).
55. C. Pantos. V. Malliopoulou, I. Mourouzis, K. Sfakianoudis, S. Tzeis, P. Doumba, C. Xinaris, A.D. Cokkinos, H.C. Carageorgiou, D.D. Varonos, D.V. Cokkinos, Propylthiouracil induced hypothyroidism is associated with increased tolerance of the isolated rat heart to ischemia-reperfusion, *J Endocrinol 178*, 427–735 (2003).
56. C. Pantos, I. Mourouzis, V. Malliopoulou, I. Paizis, S. Tzeis, P. Moraitis, K. Sfakianoudis, D.D. Varonos, D.V. Cokkinos, Dronedarone administration prevents body weight gain and increases tolerance of the heart to ischemic stress: A Possible involvement of thyroid hormone receptor α1. *Thyroid* **15**, 16–23 (2005).
57. R.-G. Shi, J.-K. Lee, Y. Takeuchi, M. Horiba, F. Kambe, H. Sea, I Murata, I Kodama, Remodeling of T_3-responsive gene transcription in rat hearts by chronic amiodarone (Abstr), *Circulation* **10**, III–99 (2004).
58. C. S. Apstein, P. Menasche, B. H. Lorell, Hypoxia, ischemia, and the hypertrophied myocardium: basic medical and surgical considerations. In: *Cardiac hypertrophy and failure. Swynghedauw B, ed. Editions INSERM*, Paris pp 65–87 (1990).
59. L. F. Wexler, B. H. Lorell, S. Momomura, E. O. Weinberg, J. S. Ingwall, C. S. Apstein, Enhanced sensitivity to hypoxia-induced diastolic dysfunction in pressure-overload left ventricular hypertrophy in the rat: role of high-energy phosphate depletion, *Circ Res* **62**, 766–75 (1988).
60 S. Koyanagi, C. L. Eastham, D. G. Harrison, M. L. Marcus, Increased size of myocardial infarction in dogs with chronic hypertension and left ventricular hypertrophy, *Circ Res* **50**, 55–62 (1982).
61. D. A. Cooley, G. J. Reul, D. C. Wukash, Ischemic contracture of the heart "stone heart", *Am J Cardiol* **29**, 575–77 (1972).
62. J. Schaper, F. Schwarz, W. Flameng, F. Hehrlein, Tolerance to ischemia of hypertrophied human hearts during valve replacement, *Basic Res Cardiol* **73**, 171–87 (1978).
63. M. L. Marcus, S. Koyanagi, D. G. Harrison, D. B. Doty, L. F. Hiratzka, C. L. Eastham, Abnormalities in the coronary circulation that occur as a consequence of cardiac hypertrophy, Am J Med 1983;75:62–66.
64. M. E. Speechly-Dick, G. F. Baxter, D. M. Yellon, Ischemic preconditioning protects hypertrophied myocardium, *Cardiovasc Res* **8**, 1025–1029 (1994).

65. C. I. Pantos, C. H. Davos, H. C. Carageorgiou, D. V. Varonos, D. V. Cokkinos, Ischemic preconditioning protects against myocardial dysfunction caused by ishaemia in isolated hypertrophied rat hearts, *Basic Res Cardiol* **91**, 444–449 (1996).
66. J. A. Moolman, S. Genade, E. Tromp, L. H. Opie, A. Lochner, Ischemic preconditioning does not protect hypertrophied myocardium against ischemia, *S Afr Med J* **87**, C151–6 (1997).
67. C. Pantos, I. Mourouzis, S. Tzeis, V. Malliopoulou, D. D. Cokkinos, Asimakopoulos, H.C. Carageorgiou, D.D. Varonos, D.V. Cokkinos, Propranolol diminishes cardiac hypertrophy but does not abolish acceleration of the ischemic contracture in hyperthyroid hearts, *J Cardiovasc Pharmacol* **36**, 384–389 (2000).
68. K. C. Chang, V. M. Figueredo, J. H. M. Schreur, K. Kariya, M. W. Weiner, P. C. Simpson, S. A. Camacho, Thyroid hormone improves function and Ca^{2+} handling in pressure overload hypertrophy. Association with increased sarcoplasmic reticulum Ca^{2+}-ATPase and alpha-myosin heavy chain in rat hearts, *J Clin Invest* **100**, 1742–1749 (1997).
69. T. Miki, T. Miura, A. Tsuchiada, A. Nakano, T. Hasegawa, T. Fukuma, K. Shimamoto, Cardioprotective mechanism of ischemic preconditioning is impaired by postinfarct ventricular remodeling through angiotensin II type receptor activation, *Circulation* **102**, 458–63 (2001).
70. S. Ghosh, N. B. Standen, M. Galinanes, Failure to precondition pathological human myocardium, *J Am Coll Cardiol* **37**, 711–8 (2001).
71. L. R. Dekker, H. Rademaker, J. T. Vermeulen, T. Opthof, R. Coronel, J. A. Spaan, M. J. Janse,. Cellular uncoupling during ischemia in hypertrophied and failing rabbit ventricular myocardium: effects of preconditioning, *Circulation* **97**, 1724–30 (1998).
72. A. Efstathiou, S. Seraskeris, C. Papakonstantinou, A. Aidonopoulos, A. Lazou, Differential effect of preconditioning on post-ischemic myocardial performance in the absence of substantial infarction and in extensively infarced rat hearts, *Eur J Cardiothorac Surg* **19**, 493–499 (2001).
73. T. Shimohama, Y. Suzuki, C. Noda, H. Niwano, K. Sato, T. Masuda, K. Kawahara , T. Izumi, Decreased expression of Na^+/H^+ exchanger isoform 1 (NHE1) in non-infarced myocardium after acute myocardial infarction, *Jpn Heart J* **3**, 273–82 (2002).
74. R. J. Diaz, G. J. Wilson, Modifying the first minute of reperfusion: potential for myocardial salvage. Editorial, *Cardiovasc Res* **62**, 4–6 (2004).
75. H. Kin, Z.-Q. Zhao, H.-Y. Sun, N.-P. Wang, J. S. Corvera, M. E. Halkos, F. Kerandi, R. A. Guyton, J. Vinten-Johansen, Postconditioning attenuates myocardial ischemia-reperfusion injury by inhibiting events in the early minutes of reperfusion, *Cardiovasc Res* **62**, 9–85 (2004).
76. H. S. Mickel, Y. K. Vaishnav, O. Kempski, D. von Lubitz, J. F. Weiss, G. Feuerstein, Breathing 100% oxygen after global brain ischemia in Mongolian gerbils redults in increased lipid peroxidation and increased mortality, *Stroke* **18**, 426–30 (1987).
77. H. M. Piper, Y. Abdallah, C. Schofer, The first minutes of reperfusion: a window of opportunity for cardioprotection, *Cardiovasc Res* **61**, 365–71 (2004).
78. J. Inerte, D. Garcia-Dorado, M. Ruiz-Meana, F. Padilla, JA. Barrabes, P. Pina. L. Agullo, H. M. Piper, J. Soler-Soler, Effect of inhibition of Na^+/Ca^{2+} exchanger at the time of myocardial reperfusion on hypercontracture and cell death, *Cardiovasc Res* **55**, 739–48 (2002).
79. H. H. Klein, S. Pich, R. M. Bohle, J. Wollenweber, K. Nebendahl, Na^+/H^+ exchange inhibitor caripovide attenuates cell injury precominantly during ischemic and not on onset of reperfusion in porcine hearts with low residual blood flow, *Circulation* **92**, 912–7 (1995).
80. U. Zeymer, H. Suryapranata, J. P. Monassier, G. Opolski, J. Davies, G. Rasmanis, G. Linssen, U. Tebbe, R. Schroder, R. Tiemann, T. Machnig, K.L. Neuhaus; ESCAMI Investigators, The Na^+/H^+ exchange inhibitor eniporide as an adjunct to early reperfusion therapy for acute myocardial infarction. Results of the evaluation of the safery and cardioprotective effects of eniporide in acute myocardial infarction (ESCAMI trial), *J Am Coll Cardiol* **38**, 645–50 (2001).
81. C. Weinbrenner, G. S. Liu, J. M. Downey, M. V. Cohen, Cyclosporine A limits infarct size even when administered after onset of ischemia, *Cardiovasc Res* **38**, 678–84 (1998).
82. A. Hempel, M. Friedrich, K. D. Schlóter, W. G. Forssmann, M. Kuhn, H. M. Piper, ANP protects against reoxygenation-induced hypercontracture in adult cardiomyocytes, *Am J Physiol* **273**, H244–9 (1997).
83. F. Padilla, D. Garcia-Doprado, L. Agullo, J. A. Barrabes, J. Inserte, N. Escalona, M. Meyer, M. Mirabet, P. Pina, J. Soler-Soler, Intravenous administration of the natriuretic pepride urodilatin at low doses during coronary reperfusion limits infarct size in anesthetized pigs, *Cardiovasc Res* **51**. 592–600 (2001).

84. M. N. Sack, D. M. Yellon, Insulin therapy as an adjunct to reperfusion after acute coronary ischemia proposed direct myocardial cell survival effect independent of metabolic modulation, *J Am Coll Cardiol* **41**, 1404–7 (2003).
85. U. Fischer-Rasokat, F. Beyersdorf, T. Doenst, Insulin addition after ischemia improves recovery of function equal to ischemic preconditioning in rar heart, *Basic Res Cardiol* **8**, 329–36 (2003).
86. R. M. Bell, D. M. Yellon, Atorvastatin administered at the onset of reperfusion, and independently of lipid lowering, protects the myocardium by up-regulating a pro-survival pathway, *J Am Coll Cardiol* **41**, 508–15 (2003).
87. S. Verma, P. Fedak, R. D. Weisel, J. Butany, V. Rao, A. Maitland, R.-K. Li, B. Dhillon, and T. M. You, Fundamentals of reperfusion injury for the clinical cardiologist, *Criculation* **105**, 2332–36 (2002).
88. O. Turschner, J. D'hooge, C. Dommke, P. Claus, E. Verbeken, I. De Scheerder, B. Bijnens, and G. R. Sutherland, The sequential changes in myocardial thickness and thickening which occur during acute transmural infarction, infarct reperfusion and the resultant expression of reperfusion injury, *Eur Heart J* **25**, 794–803 (2004).
89. I. Tritto, D. D'Andrea, N. Eramo, A. Scognamiglio, C. De Simone, A. Violante, A. Esposito, M. Chiariello, G Ambrosio, Oxygen radicals can induce preconditioning in rabbit hearts, *Circ Res* **80**, 743–748 (1997).
90. D. X.Zhang, Y.-F. Chen, W. B. Campbell, A.-P. Zou, G. J. Gross, P.-L. Li, Characteristics and superoxide-induced activation of reconstituted myocardial mitochondrial ATP-sensitive potassium channels, *Circ Res* **89**, 177–83 (2001).
91. J. Huot, F. Houle, F. Marceau, J. Landry, Oxidative stress-induced actin reorganization mediated by the p38 mitogen-activated protein kinase/heat shock protein 27 pathway in vascular endothelial cells, *Circ Res* **80**, 383–392 (1997).
92. X. L. Tang, H. Takano, A. Rizvi, J. F. Turrens, Y. Qiu, W. J. Wu, Q. Zhang, R. Bolli, Oxidant species trigger late preconditioning against myocardial stunning in conscious rabbits, *Am J Physiol Heart Circ Physiol* **282**, H281–91 (2002).
93. K. D. Garlid, Opening mitochondrial K_{ATP} in the heart-what happens, and what does not happen, *Basic Res Cardiol* **95**, 275–279 (2000).
94. R. A. Forbes, C. Steenbergen, E. Murphy, Diazoxide-induced cardioprotection requires signaling through a redox-sensitive mechanism, *Circ Res* **88**, 802–09 (2001).
95. E. Roth, M. T. Jaberansari, Reactive oxygen species in early and delayed cardiac adaptation, *Exp Clin Cardiol* **6**, 81–86 (2001).
96. C. S. Carr, D. Yellon, Ischemic preconditioning may abolish the protection afforded by ATP-sensitive potassium channel openers in isolated human atrial muscle, *Basic Res Cardiol* **92**, 252–60 (1997).
97. J. Minners, E. J. van den Bos, D. M. Yellon, H. Schwalb, L. H. Opie, M. N. Sack, Dinitrophenol, cyclosporin A, and trimetazidine modulate preconditioning in the isolated rat heart: support for a mitochondrial role in cardioprotection, *Cardiovasc Res* **47**, 68–73 (2000).
98. A. N. Khatkevich, S. N. Dvoryantsev, V. Kapelko, E. K. Ruuge, The protective effect of ischemic preconditioning depends on the duration of prolonged ischemia, *Exp Clin Cardiol* **4**, 186–190 (1999).
99. M. V. Cohen, J. M. Downey. Ischemic preconditioning: can the protection be bottled? *Lancet* **342**, 8862–66 (1998).
100. R. N. MacAlpin, A. A. Kattus, Adaptation to exercise in angina pectoris, *Circulation* **33**, 183–201 (1966).
101. F. Tomai, Warm up phenomenon and preconditioning in clinical practice, *Heart* **87**, 91–100 (2002).
102. Y. Okazaki, K. Kodama, H. Sato, M. Kitakaze, A. Hirayama, M. Mishima, M. Hori, M. Inoue, Attenuation of increased regional myocardial consumption during exercise as a major cause of warm-up phenomenon, *J Am Coll Cardiol* **21**, 1597–604 (1993).
103. N. Yamashita, S. Hoshida, K. Otsu, M. Asahi, T. Kuzuya, M. Hori, Exercise provides direct biphasic cardioprotection via manganese superoxide dismutase activation, *J Exp Med* **189**, 699–1706 (1999).
104. P. D. Lambiase, R. J. Edwards, M. R. Cusack, C. A. Bucknall, S. R. Redwood, M. S. Marber, Exercise – induced ischemia initates the second window of protection in humans independent of collateral recruitment, *J Am Coll Cardiol* **41**, 1174–82 (2003).
105. A. D. Kelion, T. P. Webb, M. A. Gardner, The warm-up effect protects against ishcemic left ventricular dysfunction in patients with angina, *J Am Coll Cardiol* **37**, 705–10 (2001).
106. M. S. Marber, D. S. Latchman, J. M. Walker, D. M. Yellon, Cardiac stress protein elevation 24 hours after brief ischemia or heat stress is associated with assistance to myocardial infarction, *Circulation* **88**, 1264–72 (1993).

107. N. Maulik, R. M. Engelman, Z. Wei, X. Liu, J. A. Rousou, J. E. Flack, D. Deaton, D. K. Das, Ischemic preconditioning reduces apoptosis by upregulating anti-death gene Bcl-2, *Circulation* **100**, II-369–75 (1999).
108. E. Deutsch, M. Berger, W. G. Kussmaul, J. W. Hirshfeld, H. C. Herrmann, W. L. Laskey, Adaptation to ischemia during percutaneous transluminal coronary angioplasty. Clinical hemodynamic and metabolic features, *Circulation* **82**, 044–51 (1990).
109. A. Cribier, L. Korsatz, R. Koning, P. Path, H. Gamra, G. Stix, S. Merchant, C. Chan, B. Letac, Improved myocardial ischemic response and enhanced collateral circulation with long repetitive coronary occlusion during angioplasty, J *Am Coll Cardiol* **20**, 578–586 (1992).
110. L. W. Klein, M. J. Kern, P. Berger, T. Sanborn, P. Block, J Babb, C. Tommaso, J. M. Hodgson, T. Feldman, Society of cardiac angiography and interventions; suggested management of the no-reflow phenomenon in the cardiac catheterization laboratory, *Catheter Cardiovasc Interv* **60**, 194–201 (2003).
111. K. Przyklenk, B. Bauer, M. Ovize, R. A. Kloner, P. Whittaker, Regional ischemic preconditioning protects remote virgin myocardium from subsequent sustained coronary occlusion, *Circulation* **87**, 893–899 (1993).
112. Y. Birnbaum, S. L. Hale, R. A. Kloner, Ischemic preconditioning at a distance: reduction of myocardial infarct size by partial reduction of blood supply combined with rapid stimulation of the gastrocnemius muscle in the rabbit, *Circulation* **96**, 641–6 (1997).
113. K. Przyklenk, C. E. Darling, E. W. Dickson, P. Whittaker, Cardioprotection «outside the box», *Basic Res Cardiol* **98**, 149–57 (2003).
114. I. Sheiban, S. Tonni, P. Benussi, A. Marini, G.P. Trevi, Left ventricular dysfunction following transient ischemia induced by transluminal coronary angioplasty, *Eur Heart J* **4**, (Suppl A):14–21 (1993).
115. D. M. Yellon, A. M. Alkulaifi, W. B. Pugsley, Preconditioning the human myocardium, *Lancet* **42**, 276–277 (1993).
116. D. P. Jenkins, W. B. Pugsley, M. Kemp, J. Hooper, D. M. Yellon, Ischemic preconditioning reduces troponin-T release in patients undergoing cardiac surgery, *Heart* **77**, 14–318 (1997).
117. P. Szmagala, K. T. Gbure, N. Morawski, et al, A clinical assessment of ischemic preconditioning for aorto-coronary bypass surgery, *Cor Europaeum* **7**, 107–111 (1999).
118. R. Gray, J. Maddhai, D. Berman, M. Raymond, A. Waxman, W. Ganz, J. Matloff, H. J. C. Swan, Scintigraphic and hemodynamic demonstration of transient left ventricular dysfunction immediately after uncomplicated coronary artery bypass grafting, *J Thorac Cardiovasc Surg.* **77**, 504–10 (1979).
119. D. T. Mangano, Biventricular function after myocardial revascularization in humans. Deterioration and recovery patterns during the first 24 hours, *Anesthesiology* **62**, 571–577 (1985).
120. C. M. Ballantyne, M. S. Verani, H. D. Short, C. Hyatt, G. P. Noon, Delayed recovery of severely "stunned" myocardium with the support of a left ventricular assist device after coronary artery bypass graft surgery, *J Am Coll Cardiol* **10**, 710–712 (1987).
121. L. Czer, A. Hamer, F. Murphy, J. Bussell, A. Chaux, T. Bateman, J. Matloff, R. J. Gray, Transient hemodynamic dysfunction after myocardial revascularization, *J Thorac Cardiovasc Surg* **86**, 226–234 (1983).
122. S. Verma, P. W. Fedak, R. D. Weisel, P. E. Szmitko, M. V. Badiwala, D. Bonneau, D. Latter, L. Errett, Y. LeClerc, Off-pump coronary artery bypass surgery: fundamentals for the clinical cardiologist, *Circulation* **109**, 1206–11 (2004).
123. C. P. Baines, J. M. Pass, P. Ping, Protein kinases and kinase-modulated effectors in the late phase of ischemic preconditioning, *Basic Res Cardiol* **96**, 207–218 (2001).
124. G. S. Liu, J. Thornton, D. M. van Winkle, A. W. H. Stanely, R. A. Olsson, J. M. Downey, Protection against infarction afforded by preconditioning is mediated by A1 adenosine receptors in rabbit heart, *Circulation* **84**, 350–6 (1991).
125. A. Dana, M. Skarli, J. Papakrivopoulou, D. M. Yellon, Adenosine A(1) receptor induced delayed preconditioning in rabbits: induction of p38 mitogen-actibated protein kinase activation and Hsp27 phosphorylation via a tyrosine kinase and protein kinase C-dependent mechanism, *Circ Res* **86**, 921–2 (2000).
126. T. C. Zhao, D. S. Hines, R. C. Kukreja, Adenosine-induced late preconditioning in mouse hearts: role of p38 MAP kinase and mitochondrial K_{ATP} channels, *Am J Physiol Heart Circ Physiol* **280**, H1278–85 (2001).
127. U. E. Heidland, M. P. Heintzen, B. Schwartzkopff, B. E. Strauer, Preconditioning during percutaneous transluminal coronary angioplasty by endogenous and exogenous adenosine, *Am Heart J* **140**, 813–20 (2000).

128. M. A. Leesar, M. Stoddard, M. Ahmed, J. Broadbent, R. Bolli, Preconditioning of human myocardium with adenosine during coronary angioplasty, *Circulation* **95**, 2500–7 (1997).
129. M. J. Claeys, C. J. Vrints, J. M. Bosmans, V. M. Conraads, J. P. Snoeck, Aminophylline inhibits adaptation to ischemia during angioplasty, *Eur Heart J* **17**, 539–44 (1996).
130. M. Quintana, T. Kahan, P. Hjemdahl, Pharmacological prevention of reperfusion injury in acute myocardial infarction, A potential role for adenosine as a therapeutic agent. *Am J Cardiovasc Drugs* **4**, 159–67 (2004).
131. V. H. Thourani, R. S. Ronson, D. G. L van Wylen, S. T. Shearer, S. L. Katzmark, Z.-Q. Zhao, D. C. Han, RA Guyton, J. Vinten-Johansen, Adenosine-supplemented blood cardioplegia attenuates postischemic dysfunction after severe regional ischemia, *Circulation* **100**, II 376–83 (1999).
132. Z. Yao, G. J. Gross, Glibenclamide antagonizes adenosine A_1 receptor-mediated cardioprotection in stunned canine myocardium, *Circulation* **88**, 235–44 (1993).
133. G. J. Grover, A. J. D'Alonzo, S. Dzwonczyk, C. S. Parham, R. B. Darbenzio, Preconditioning is not abolished by the delayed rectifier K^+ blocker dofetilide, *Am J Physiol* **271**, H1207–H1214 (1996).
134. K. D. Garlid, P. Paucek, V. Yarov-Yarovoy, H. N. Murray, R. B. Darbenzio, A. J. D'Alonzo, N. J. Lodge, M. A. Smith, G. J. Grover, Cardioprotective effect of diazoxide and its interaction with mitochondrial ATP-sensitive K^+ channels, Possible mechanism of cardioprotection, *Circ Res* **81**, 1072–1082 (1997).
135. K. D. Garlid, P. Paucek, B. Yarov-Yarovoy, H. N. M. Murray, R. B. Darbenzio, A. J. D'Alonzo, N..J. Lodge, M. A. Smith, G. J. Grover, Cardioprotective effect of diazoxide and its interaction with mitochondrial ATP-sensitive potassium channels: possible mechanism of cardioprotection, *Circ Res* **1**, 1072–1082 (1997).
136. G. Grover, J. Newburger, P. Sleph, S. Dzwonczyk, S. Taylor, S. Ahmed, K. Atwal, Cardioprotective effects of the potassium channel opener cromakalim: stereoselectivity and effects on myocardial adenine nucleotides, *J Pharmacol Exp Ther* **257**, 156–162 (1991).
137. G. J. Grover, K. D. Garlid. ATP-sensitive potassium channels: a review of their cardioprotective pharmacology. *J Mol Cell Cardiol* **32**, 677–695 (2000).
138. Y. Liu, T. Sato, B. O'Rourke, E. Marban, Mitochondrial K_{ATP}-dependent potassium channels: novel effectors of cardioprotection? *Circulation* **97**, 2463–2469 (1998).
139. J. Tamargo, R. Caballero, R. Gomez, C. Valenzuela, E. Delpon, Pharmacology of cardiac potassium channels, *Cardiovasc Res* **62**, 9–33 (2004).
140. J. C. Cleveland, D. R. Meldrum, V. S. Cain, A. Banerjee, A. Harken, Oral sulfonylurea hypoglycemic agents prevent ischemic preconditioning in human myocardium. Two paradoxes revisited, *Circulation* **96**, 29–32 (1997).
141. P. Brady, A. Terzie, The sulfonylurea controversy: more questions from the heart, *J Am Coll Cardiol* **131**, 950–6 (1998).
142. B. O'Rourke, Mitochondrial K_{ATP} channels in preconditioning, *Circ Res* **87**, 845–855 (2000).
143. J. A. Auchampach, M. Maruyama, G. J. Gross, Cardioprotective actions of potassium channel openers, *Eur Heart J* **15**, 81–84 (1994).
144. F. Tomai, F. Crea, A. Gaspardone, F. Versaci, R. De Paulis, A. Penta de Peppo, L. Chiariello, P.A. Gioffre, Ischemic preconditioning during coronary angioplasty is prevented by glibenclamide, a selective ATP-sensitive K^+ channel blocker, *Circulation* **90**, 700–5 (1994).
145. M. M. Mocanu, H. L. Maddock, G. F. Baxter, C. L. Lawrence, N. B. Standen, D. M. Yellon, Glimepiride, a Novel Sulfonylurea, does not abolish myocardial protection afforded by either ischemic preconditioning of diazoxide, *Circulation* **103**, 111–3116 (2001).
146. H. Klepzig, G. Kober. C. Matter, H. Luus, H. Scheneider, K. H. Boedeker, W. Kiowski, Amman, F. W. D. Gruber, S. Harris, W. Burger, Sulfonylureas and ischemic preconditioning, *Eur Heart J* **20**, 439–46 (1999).
147. T. Matsubara, S. Minatoguchi, H. Matsuo, K. Hayakawa, T. Segawa, Y. Matsuno, S. Watenabe, M. Arai, Y. Uno, M. Kawasaki, T. Noda, G. Takemura, K. Nishigaki, H. Fujiwara, Three minutes, but not one minute, ischemia and nicorandil have a preconditioning effect in patients with coronary artery disease, *J Am Coll Cardiol* **35**, 345–51 (2000).
148. N. Taira, Nicorandil as a hybrid between nitrates and potassium channel activators, *Am J Cardiol* **3**, 18J–24J (1989).
149. E. K. Iliodromitis, P. Cokkinos, A. Zoga, I. Steliou, A. R. Vrettou, D. T. Kremastinos, Nicorandil recaptures the waned protection from preconditioning in vivo, *Br J Pharmacol* **138**, 1101–06 (2003).
150. T.-M. Lee, S.-F. Su, T.-F. Chou, Y. T. Lee, C.-H. Tsai, Loss of preconditioning by attenuated activation of myocardial ATP-sensitive potassium channels in elderly patients undergoing coronary angioplasty, *Circulation* **105**, 334–40 (2002).

151. The IONA study group. Effect of nicorandil on coronary events in patients with stable angina: The impact of Nicorandil in Angina (IONA) randomized trial, *Lancet* **359**, 1269–7 (2002).
152. M. Buerke, H.-J. Rupprecht, J. vom Dahl, W. Terres, M. Seyfurth, H.-P. Schultheiss, G. Richardt, F. H. Sheehan, H. Dexlet, Sodium-hydrogen exchange inhibition: Novel strategy to prevent myocardial injury following ischemia and reperfusion, *Am J Cardiol* **83**, 19G–22G (1999).
153. M. Hill, H. Takano, X.-L. Tang, E. Kodani, G. Shirk, R. Bolli, Nitroglycerin induces late preconditioning against myocardial infarction in conscious rabbits despite development of nitrate tolerance, *Circulation* **104**, 694–699 (2001).
154. M. A. Leesar, M. F. Stoddard, B. Dawn,V. G. Jasti, R. Masden, R Bolli, Delayed preconditioning-mimetic action of nitroglycerin in patients undergoing coronary angioplasty, *Circulation* **103**, 2935–2941 (2001).
155. G. Heusch, Nitroglycerin and delayed preconditioning in humans, *Circulation* **103**, 2876–2878 (2001).
156. D. Hasdai, S. Behar, L. Wallentin. N. Danchin, A. K. Gitt, E. Boersma, P. M. Fioretti, M. L. Simoons, A. Battler, A prospective survey of the characteristics, treatments and outcomes of patients with acute coronary syndromes in Europe and the Mediterranean basin, *Eur Heart J* **23**, 1190–1201 (2002).
157. E. Sbarouni, E. K. Iliodromitis, E. Bofilis, Z. S. Kyriakides, D. T. Kremastinos, Short-term estrogen reduces myocardial infarct size in oophororectomized female rabbits in a dose-dependent manner, *Cardiovasc Drugs Ther* **12**, 457–62 (1998).
158. E. Sbarouni, E. K. Iliodromitis, E. Bofilis, ZS. Kyriakides, D. T. Kremastinos, Estrogen alone or combined with medroxyprogesterone but not raloxifene reduce myocardial infarct size, *Eur J Pharmaco*l **467**, 163–8 (2003).
159. H. Ogita, K. Node, H. Asanuma, S. Sanada, Y. Liao, S. Takashima, M. Asakura, H. Mori, Y. Shizonaki, M. Hori, M. Kitakazo, Amelioration of ischemia and reperfusion-induced myocardial injury by the selective estrogen receptor modulator, raloxifene, in the canine heart, *J Am Coll Cardol* **40**, 998–1005 (2002).
160. K. M. English, R. D. Jones, T. H. Jones, A. H. Morice, K. S. Channer, Testosterone acts as a coronary vasodilator by a calcium antagonistic action, *J Endocrinol Invest* **25**, 455–8 (2002).
161. F. Callils, H. Stromer, R. H. Schwinger, B. Bolck, K. Hu, S. Frantz, A. Leupold, S. Beet, B. Allolio, A. M. Bonz, Administration of testosterone is associated with a reduced susceptibility to myocardial ischemia, *Endocrinology* **144**, 4478–83 (2003).
162. F. Er, G. Michels, N. Gassanov, F. Rivero, U. C. Hope, Testosterone induces cytoprotection by activating K^+ channels in the cardiac mitochondrial inner membrane, *Circulation* **110**, 3100–07 (2004).
163. JF. Reckelhoff, Sex steroids, cardiovascular disease, and hypertension, *Hypertension* **45**, 170–4 (2005).
164. R. B. Melchert, A. A. Weider. Cardiovascular effects of androgenic anabolic steroids. *Med Sci Sports Exerc* 7, 1252–62 (1995).
165. T. V. Pham, E. A. Sosunov, E. P. Anyukhorsky, P Jr Danilo, M. R. Rosen, Testosterone diminishes the proarrhythmic effects of dofetilide in normal female rabbits, *Circulation* **06**, 2132–6 (2002).
166. B. K. Podesser, J. Schirnhofer, O. Y. Bernecker, A. Kroner, M. Franz, S. Semsroth, B. Fellner, J. Neumóller, S. Hallstrom, and E. Wolner, Optimizing ischemia/reperfusion in the failing rat heart-improved myocardial protection with acute ACE inhibition, *Circulation* **106**, Suppl I:277–283 (2002).
167. M. Sato, R. M. Engelman, H. Otani, N. Maulik, J. Rousou, J. Flack, D. W. Deaton, D. K. Das, Myocardial protection by preconditioning of heart with losartan, an angiotensin II type 1-receptor blocker. Implication of bradykinin-dependent and bradykinin-independent mechanisma, *Circulation* **120**, suplIII: III–346–III–351 (2000).
168. M. Leesar, M. F. Stoddard, S. Manchikalapudi, R. Bolli, Bradykinin-induced preconditioning in patients undergoing coronary angioplasty, *J Am Coll Cardiol* **34**, 639–50 (1999).
169. G. Valen, S. Takeshima, M. Ahmad, J. Zeitlin, J. Parratt, J. Baage, Bradykinin in open heart surgery: Metabolism of bradykinin in the coronary circulation during reperfusion, *Exp Clin Cardiol* **2**, 223–227 (1997).
170. E. R. Schwarz, H. Montino, J. Fleischhauer, H. G. Klues, J. vom Dahl, P. Hanrath, Angiotensin II receptor antagonist EXP 3174 reduces infarct size comparable with enalaprilat and augments preconditionng in the pig heart, *Cardiovasc Drugs Ther* **11**, 687–9 (1997)5.
171. Y. Nozawa, T. Miura, A. Tsuchida, H. Kita, T. Fukuma, K. Shimamoto, Chronic treatment with an ACE inhibitor, temocapril, lowers the threshold for the infarct size-limiting effect of ischemic preconditioning, *Cardiovasc Drugs Ther* **13**, 151–7 (1999).
172. M. T. Jaberansari, G. F. Baxter, C. A. Muller, S. E. Latouf, E. Roth, L. H. Opie, D. M. Yellon, Angiotensin-converting enzyme inhibition enhances a subthreshold stimulus to elicit delayed preconditioning in pig myocardium, *J Am Coll Cardiol* **37**, 1996–2001 (2001).

173. B. Bartling, I. Friedrich, R. E. Silber, A. Simm, Ischemic preconditioning is not cardioprotective in senescent human myocardium, *Ann Thorac Surg* **76**, 105–11 (2003).
174. K. Hayakawa, G. Takemura, M. Kanoh, Y. Li, M. Koda, Y. Kawase, R. Marwyama, H. Okada, S. Minatoguchi, T. Fujiwara, H. Fujiwara, Inhibition of granulation tissue cell apoptosis during the subacute stage of myocardial infarction improves cardiac remodeling and dysfunctio nat the chronic stage, *Circulation* **108**, 104–09 (2003).
175. N. Maulik, R. M. Engelman, J. A. Rousou, J.E. Flack 3rd, D. Deaton, D.K. Das, Ischemic preconditioning reduces apoptosis by upregulating anti-death gene bcl-2, *Circulation* **100**, Suppl II-369–375 (1999).
176. C. D. Veronsee, W. R. Lewis, M. W. Takla, E. A. Hull-Ryde, J. E. Lowe, Protective metabolic effects of propranolol during total myocardial ischemia, *J Thorac Cardiovasc Surg* **92**, 425–33 (1986).
177. A. Cargnoni, C. Ceconi, P. Bernocchi, A. Boraso, G. Parrinello, S. Curello, R. Ferrari, Reduction of oxidative stress by carvedilol: role in maintenance of ischemic myocardium viability, *Cardiovasc Res* **47**, 556–566 (2000).
178. T. L. Yue, X. L. Ma, R. Gu, R. R. Jr Ruffolo, G. Z. Feuerstein, Carvedilol inhibits activation of stress-activated protein kinase JNK and reduces reperfusion injury in perfused rabbit heart, *Eur J Pharmacol* **345**, 61–5 (1998).
179. T. Ide, H. Tsutsui, S. Kinugawa, H. Utsumi, A. Takeshita, Amiodarone protects cardiac myocytes against oxidative injury by its free radical scavenging action, *Circulation* **100**, 690–692 (1999).
180. R. Gasser, G. Frey, G. Fleckenstein-Grón, Y. K. Byon, A. Fleckenstein, Some observations on Ca-overload in rat ventricular tissue, *J Clin Basic Cardiol* **2**, 255–8 (1999).
181. M. J. Daly, J. S. Elz, W. G. Nayler, The effect of verapamil on ischemia-induced changes to the sarcolemma, *J Mol Cell Cardiol* **7**, 667–74 (1985).
182. K. Inagaki, Y. Kihara, T. Izumi, S. Sasayama, The cardioprotective effects of a new 1,4-benzothiazepine derivative, JTV519, on ischemia/reperfusion-induced Ca^{2+} overload is isolated rat hearts, *Cardiovasc Drug Ther* **14**, 489–95 (2000).
183. R. Sato, J. Yamazaki, T. Nagao, Temporal differences in actions of calcium channel blockers on K^+ accumulation, cardiac function, and high-energy phosphate levels in ischemic guinea pig hearts, *J Pharmacol Exp Ther* **89**, 831–9 (1999).
184. D. V. Fitzpatrick, M. Karmazyn, Comparative effects of calcium channel blocking agents and varying extracellular calcium concentration on hypoxia/reoxygenation and ischemia/reperfusion-induced cardiac injury, *J Pharmacol Exp Ther* **28**, 761–768 (1984).
185. K. Herbaczynska-Cedro, W. Gordon-Makszak, Nisoldipine inhibits lipid peroxidation induced by coronary occlusion in pig myocardium, *Caridiovasc Res* **24**, 683–687 (1990).
186. A. J. Higgins, K. J. Blackburn, Prevention of reperfusion damage in working rat hearts by calcium antagonists and calmodulin antagonists, *J Mol Cell Cardiol* **16**, 127–138 (1984).
187. W. W. Holt, M. F. Wendland, N. Derugin, C. Wolfe, M. Saeed, C. B. Higgins, Effects of nicardipine, a calcium antagonist, on myocardial salvage and high energy phosphate stores in reperfused myocardial injury, *J Am Coll Cardiol* **16**, 1736–1744 (1990).
188. K. Przylenk, R. A. Kloner, Effect of verapamil on postischemic "stunned" myocardium. Importance of the timing of treatment, *J Am Coll Cardiol* **11**, 614–623 (1988).
189. L. H. Opie, Reperfusion injury and its pharmacological modification. *Circulation* **80**, 1049–1062 (1989).
190. L. H. Opie, Reperfusion injury and calcium antagonists, *Cardiologia* **35(Suppl 1)**, 213–221 (1990).
191. J. S. Garrett, J. Wikman-Coffelt, R. Sievers, W. E. Finkbeiner, W. W. Parmley, Verapamil prevents the development of alcoholic dysfunction in hamster myocardium, *J Am Coll Cardiol* **9**, 1326–31 (1987).
192. R. Sievers, W. W. Parmley, T. James, J. Wikman-Coffelt, Energy levels at systole vs diastole in normal hamster hearts vs myopathic hamster hearts, *Circ Res* **53**, 759–66 (1983).
193. J. J. McVeigh, G. D. Lopaschuk, Dichloroacetate stimulation of glucose oxidation improves recovery of ischemic rat hearts, *Am J Physiol* **259**, H1079–H1085 (1990).
194. M. R. Graslinski, S. C. Black, K. S. Kilgore, A. Y. Chou, J. G. McCormack, B. R. Lucchesi, Cardioprotective effects of ranolazine (RS-43285) in the isolated perfused rabbit heart, *Cardiovasc Res* **28**, 1231–1237 (1994).
195. S. Schmidt-Schweda, C. Holubarsch, First clinical trial with etomoxir in patients with chronic congestive heart failure, *Clin Sci* **99**, 7–35 (1999).
196. J. M. Detry, P. Sellier, S. Pennaforte, D. Cokkinos, H. Dargie, P Mathes, Trimetazidine: a new concept in the treatment of angina. Comparison with propranolo in patients with stable angina, *Br J Clin Pharmacol* **37**, 279–88 (1994).

197. J. N. Fabiani, O. Ponzio, I. Emerit, S. Massonet-Castel, M. Paris, P. Chevalier, V. Jebara, A. Carpentier, Cardioprotective effect of trimetazidine during coronary artery graft surgery, *J Cardiovasc Surg* **3**, 486–491 (1992).
198. S. Schmidt-Schweda, C. Holubarsch, First clinical trial with etomoxir in patients with chronic congestive heart failure, *Clin Sci* **99**, 27–35 (1999).
199. F. V. Mody, B. N. Singh, I. H. Mohiuddin, K. B. Coyle, D. B. Buxton, H. W. Hansen, R. Sumida, H. R. Schekber, Trimetazidine-induced enhancement of myocardial glucose utilization in normal and ischemic myocardial tissue: An evaluation by positron emission tomography, *Am J Cardiol* **82**, 42K–49K (1998).
200. C. Pantos, A. Bescond-Jacket, S. Tzeis, I. Paizis, I. Mourouzis, P. Moraitis, V. Malliopoulou, E.D. Politi, H. Karageorgiou, D. Varonos, D.V. Cokkinos, Trimetazidine protects isolated rat hearts against ischemia-reperfusion injury in an experimental timing-dependent manner, *Basic Res Cardiol* **100(2)**, 154–160 (2005).
201. T. L. Broderick, A. Quinney, C. Barker, G. Lopaschuk, Beneficial effect of carnitine on mechanical recovery of rat hearts reperfused after a transient period of global ischemia is accompanied by a stimulation of glucose oxidation, *Circulation* **87**, 972–981 (1993).
202 . I. Rizos, Three-year survival of patients with heart failure caused by dilated cardiomyopathy and L-carnitine administration, *Am Heart J* **139**, S120–3 (2000).
203. S. Winter, K. Jue, J. Prochazka, P. Francis, W. Hamilton, L. Linn, E. Helton, The role of L-carnitine in pediatric cardiomyopathy, *J Child Neurol* **10**, 2S45–2S51 (1995).
204. E. Helton, R. Darragh, P. Francis, J. Fricker, K. Jue, G. Koch, D. Mair, M. E. Pierpont, J. V. Prochazka, S. C. Winter, Metabolic aspects of myocardial disease and a role for L-carnitine in the treatment of childhood cardiomyopathy, *Pediatrics* **105**, 1260–1270 (2000).
205. S. Iliceto, D. Scrutinio, P. Bruzzi, G. D'Ambrosio, L. Boni, M. Di Biase, G. Biasco, P. Hugenholtz, P. Rizzon, on behalf of the CEDIM Investigators. Effects of L-carnitine administration on left ventricular remodeling after acute anterior myocardial infarction: The L-carnitine ecocardiografia digitalizzata infarto miocardico (CEDIM) trial, *J Am Coll Cardiol* **26**, 380–7 (1995).
206. D. V. Cokkinos, Can metabolic manipulation reverse myocardial dysfunction? *Editorial Eur Heart J* **22**, 2138–2139 (2001).
207. K. Malmberg, L. Ryden, S. Efendic, J. Herlitz, P. Nicol, A. Waldenstrom, H. Wedel. Randomized trial of insulin-glucose infusion followed by subcutaneous insulin treatment in diabetic patients with acute myocardial infarction (DIGAMI study): effects on mortality at 1 year. *J Am Coll Cardol* **26**, 57–65 (1995).
208. I. C. Van der Horst, F. Zijlstra, A. W. van't Hof, C. J. Doggen, M. J. de Boer, H. Suryapranata, J. C. Hoorntje, J. H. Dambrink, R. O. Gans, H. J. Bilo; Swolle Infarct Study Group, Glucose-insulin potassium infusion in patients treated with primary angioplasty for acute myocardial infarction: the glucose-insulin-potassium study: a randomised trial, *J Am Coll Cardiol 42*, 784–91 (2003).
209. A. K. Jonassen, E. Aasum, R. A. Riemersma, O. D. Mjos, T. S. Larsen, Glucose-insulin-potassium reduces infarct size when administered during reperfusion, *Cardiovasc Drugs Ther* **14**, 615–23 (2001).
210. M. Tani, J. R. Neely, Role of intracellular Na^+ in Ca^{2+} overload and depressed recovery of ventricular function of reperfused ischemic rat hearts, *Circ Res* **65**, 1045–56 (1989).
211. A. Chaudhuri, D. Janicke, M. F. Wilson, D. Tripaty, R. Garg, A. Bandypadhyay, J. Calieri, D. Hoffmeyer, T. Syed, H. Ghanim, A. Aljada, P. Dandona, Anti-inflammatory and profibrinolytic effect of insulin in acute ST-segment-elevation myocardial infarction, *Circulation* **109**, 849–54 (2004).
212. P. Di Napoli, A. A. Taccardi, A. Grilli, R. Spina, M. Felaco, A. Barsotti, R. De Caterina, Simvastatin reduces reperfusion injury by modulating nitric oxide synthase expression : an ex-vivo study in isolated working rat hearts, *Cardiovasc Res* **1**, 283–93 (2001).
213. Q. Feng, X. Lu, D. L. Jones, J. Shen, J. M. O. Arnold, Increased inducible nitric oxide synthase expression contributes to myocardial dysfunction and higher mortality after myocardial infarction in mice, *Circulation* **104**, 700–04 (2001).
214. P. Ferdinandy, H. Danial, I. Ambrus, R. A. Rothery, R. Schulz, Peroxynitrite is a major contributor to cytokine-induced myocardial contractile failure, *Circ Res* **87**, 170–2 (2000).
215. C. Arnaud, D. Godin-Ribuot, S. Bottari, A. Reinnequin, M. Joyeux, P. Demenge, C. Ribuot, iNOS is a mediator of the heat stress-induced preconditioning against myocardial infarction in vivo in the rat, *Cardiovasc Res* **58**, 118–25 (2003).
216. P, Eaton, D. J. Hearse, M. J. Shattock, Lipid hydroperoxide modification of proteins during myocardial ischemia, *Cardiovasc Res* **51**, 294–303 (2001).

217. P. T. Koller, SR. Bergmann, Reduction of lipid peroxidation in reperfused isolated rabbit hearts by diltiazem, *Circ Res* **65**, 838–45 (1989).
218. H. Chen, D. Li, G. J. Roberts, T. Saldeen, JL. Mehta, Eicosipentanoic acid inhibits hypoxia-reoxygenation-induced injury by attenuating upregulation of MMP-1 in adult rat muyocytes, *Cardiovasc Res* **59**, 7–13 (2003).
219. B. P. Ander, A. R. Weber, P. P. Rampersad, J. S. Gilchrist, G. N. Pierce, A. Lukas, Dietary flaxseed protects against ventricular fibrillation induced by ischemia-reperfusion in normal and hypercholesterolemic rabbits, *JU Nutr* **134**, 3250–6 (2004).
220. L.-M. Hung, J.-K. Chen, S.-S. Huang, R.-S. Lee, M.-J. Su, Cardioprotective effect of resveratrol a natural antioxidant derived from grapes, *Cardiovasc Res* **47**, 549–55 (2000).
221. S. Cuzzocrea, E. Mazzon, G. Constantino, I. Serraino, A. De Sarro, A. Caputi, Effects of n-acetylcysteine in rat model of ischemia and reperfusion injury, *Cardiovasc Res* **47**, 537–48 (2000).
222. M. Tepel, M. van der Giet, C. Schwarzfeld, U. Laufer, D. Liermann, W. Zidek, Prevention of radiographic-contrast-agent-induced reductions in renal function by acetylcysteine, *N Engl J Med* **343**, 180–4 (2000).
223. J. Kay, W. H. Chow, T. M. Chan, S.K. Lo, O.H. Kwok, A. Yip, K. Fan, C.H. Lee, W.F. Lam, Acetylcysteine for prevention of acute deterioration of renal function following elective coronary angiography and intervention: a randomised controlled trial, *JAMA* **289**, 553–8 (2003).
224. K. Spargias, E. Alexopoulos, S. Kyrzopoulos, P. Iakovis, D. C. Greenwood, A. Manginas, V. Voudris, G. Pavlides, C. E. Buller, D. Kremastinos, D. V. Cokkinos, Ascorbic acid prevents contrast-mediated nephropathy in patiens with renal dysfunction undergoing coronary angiography or intervention, *Circulation* **110**, 2837–2842 (2004).
225. B. Nespereira, M. Perez-Ilzarbe, P. Fernandez, A. M. Fuentes, J. A. Paramo, J. A. Rodriguez, Vitamins C and E downregulate vascular VEGF and VEGFR-2 expression in apolipoprotein-E-deficient mice, *Atherosclerosis* **171**, 67–73 (2003).
226. R. Bolli, M. O. Jeroudi, B. S. Patel, O. I. Aruoma, B. Halliwell, E. K. Lai, P. B. McCay, Marked reduction of free radical generation and contractile dysfunction by antioxidant therapy begun at the time of reperfusion. Evidence that myocardial "stunning" is a manifestation of reperfusion injury, *Circ Res* **65**, 607–22 (1989).
227. S. W. Werns, M. J. Shea, B. R. Lucchesi, Free radicals and myocardial injury: pharmacologic implications, *Circulation* **74**, 1–5 (1986).
228. R. A. Kloner, K. Przyklenk, S. H. Rahimtoola, E Braunwald, Myocardial stunning and hibernation: mechanisms and clinical implication. In: Stunning, hibernation and calcium in myocardial ischemia and reperfusion, Opie LH, ed. Kluwer Academic Publishers, *Boston pp* 251–280 (1992).
229. I. A. Paraskevaidis, E. K. Iliodromitis, D. Vlahakos, D. P. Tsiapras, A. Nikolaids, A. Marathias, A. Michalis, D. T. Kremastinos, Deferoxamine infusion during coronary artery bypass grafting ameliorates lipid peroxidation and protects the myocardium against reperfusion injury: immediate and long-term significance, *Eur Heart J* **26**, 263–270 (2005).
230. D. E. Chambers, D. A. Parks, G. Patterson, R. Roy, J. M. McCord, S. Yoshida, L. F. Parmley, J. M. Downey. Xanthine oxidase as a source of free radical damage in myocardial ischemia. *J Mol Cell Cardiol* **17**, 145–52 (1985).
231. S. W. Werns, M. J. Shea, S. E. Mitsos, R. C. Dysko, J. C. Fantone, A. Schork, G. D. Abrams, H. B. Pi, B. R. Lucchesi, Reduction of the size of infarction by allopurinol in the ischemic-reperfused canine heart, *Circulation* **73**, 518–524 (1986).
232. L. B. Stull, M. K. Leppo, L. Szweda, D. Gao, E. Marban, Chronic treatment with allopurinol boosts survival and cardiac contractility in murine postischemic cardiomyopathy, *Circ Res* **95**, 1005–11 (2001).
233. R. M. Fryer, A. K. Hsu, J. T. Eells, H. Nagase, G. J. Gross, Opioid-induced second window of cardioprotection: potential role of mitochondrial K_{ATP} channels., *Circ Res* **84**, 846–51 (1999).
234. J. N. Peart, G. J. Gross, Morphine-tolerant mice exhibit a profound and persistant cardioprotective phenotype, *Circulation* **109**, 1219–22 (2004).
235. N. Kokita, A. Hara, Propofol attenuates hydrogen-peroxide induced mechanical and metabolic derangements in the isolated rat heart, *Anesthesiology* **84**, 117–27 (1996).
236. S. H. Ko, C. W. Yu, S. K. Lee, H. Choe, M. J. Chung, Y. G. Kwak, S. W. Chae, H. S. Song, Propofol attenuates ischemic-reperfusion injury in the isolated rat heart, *Anesth Analg* **85**, 719–24 (1997).
237. S. A. Javadov, K. H. H. Lim, P. M. Kerr, S. Suleiman, G. D. Angelini, A. P. Halestrap, Protection of hearts from reperfusion injury by propofol is associated with inhibition of the mitochondrial permeability transition, *Cardiovasc Res* **45**, 360–69 (2000).

238. D. Branca, E. Vincenti, G. Scutari, Influence of the anesthetic 2,6 – diisopropylphenol (propofol) on isolated rat heart mitochondria, *Comp Biochem Physiol C: Pharmacol Toxicol Endocrinol* **110**, 41–45 (1995).
239. V. Borutaite, A. Jekabsone, R. Morkuniene, G. C. Brown, Inhibition of mitochondrial permeability transition prevents mitochondrial dysfunction, cytochrome C release and apoptosis induced by heart ischemia, *J Moll Cell Cardiol* **35**, 357–366 (2003).
240. C. U. Niemann, M. Saeed, H. Akbari, W. Jacobsen, L. Z. Benet, U. Christinas, N. Serkova, Close association between the reduction in myocardial energy metabolism and infarct size: dose – response assessment of cyclosporine, *Pharmacol Exp Ther* **302**, 1123–8 (2002).
241. B. K. Brar, A. Stephanou, Z. Liao, R. M. O'Leary, D. Rennica, D. M. Yellon, D. S. Latchman, Cardiotrophin-1 can protect cardiac myocytes from injury when added both prior to simulated ischemia and at reoxygenation, *Cardiovasc Res* **51**, 265–74 (2001).
242. K. Suzuki, B. Murtuza, R. T. Smolenski, I. A. Sammut, N. Suzuki, Y. Kaneda, M. H. Yacoub, Overexpression of interleukin-1 receptor antagonist provides cardioprotection against ischemia-reperfusion injury associated with reduction in apoptosis, *Circulation* **104**, I308–13 (2001).
243. E. F. Du Toit, C. A. Muller, J. McCarthy, L. H. Opie, Levosimendan: effects of a calcium sensitizer on function and arrhythmias and cyclic nucleotide levels during ischemia/reperfusion in the Langendorff-perfused guinea pig heart, *J Pharmacol Exp Ther* **290**, 505–14 (1999).
244. C. Pantos, I. Mourouzis, S. Tzeis, P. Moraitis, V. Malliopoulou, D.D. Cokkinos, H. Karageorgiou, D. Varonos, D.V. Cokkinos, Dobutamine administration exacerbates postischemic myocardial dysfunction in isolated rat hearts; an effect reversed by thyroxine pre-treatment, *Eur J Pharmacol* **460**, 155–61 (2003).
245. G. Calapai, M. C. Marciano, F. Corica, A. Allegra, A. Parisi, N. Frisina, A. P. Caputi, M. Buemi, Erythropoietin protects against brain ischemic injury by inhibition of nitric oxide formation, *Eur J Pharmacol* **401**, 349–56(2000).
246. M. A. Bogoyevitch, Review: An update on the cardiac effects of erythropoietin cardioprotection by erythropoietin and the lessons learnt from studies in neuroprotection, *Cardiovasc Res* **63**, 208–16 (2004).
247. Y. Shi, P. Rafiee, J. Su, K. A. Jr Pritchard, J. S. Tweddell, J. E. Baker, Acute cardioprotective effects of erythropoietin in infant rabbits are mediated by activation of protein kinases and potassium channels, *Basic Res Cardiol* **99**, 173–82 (2004).
248. Z. Cai, D. Manalo, G. Wei, E. R. Rodriguez, K. Fox-Talbot, H. Lu, JL. Zweier, G. L. Semenza, Hearts from rodents exposed to intermittent hypoxia or erythropoietin are protected against ischemia-reperfusion injury, *Circulation* **108**, 79–85 (2003).
249. T. Rui, Q. Fenf, M. Lei, T. Peng, J. Zhang, M. Xu, E. Dale Abel, A. Xenocostas, P. R. Kvietys, Erythropoietin prevents the acute myocardial inflammatory response induced by ischemia/reperfusion via induction of AP-1, *Cardiovasc Res* **65**, 19–27 (2005).
250. P. Dobsak, J. Siegelova, J. C. Eicher, K. Jancik, H. Svacinova, J. Vascu, S. Kuchtickova, M. Horky, J. E. Wolf. Melatonin protect against ischemia-reperfusion injury and inhibits apoptosis in isolated working rat heart. *Physiology* **9**, 179–87 (2003).
251. E. Sahna, H. Parlakpinar, Y. Turkoz, A. Acet, Protective effects of melatonin on myocardial ischemia reperfusion induced infarct size and oxidative changes, *Physiol Res* (Epub ahead of print) (2005).
252. R. J. Reiter, D.-X. Tan, Melatonin: a novel protective agent against oxidative injury of the ischemia reperfused heart, *Cardiovasc Res* **58**, 10–19 (2003).
253. K. Shinmura, E. Kodani, Y.-T. Xuan, B. Dawn, X.-T. Tang, R. Bolli, Effect of aspirin on late preconditioning against myocardial stunning in conscious rabbits, *J Am Coll Cardiol* **41**, 1183–94 (2003).
254. K. Przyklenk, G. Heusch, Late preconditioning against myocardial stunning. Does aspirin close the "second window" of endogenous cardioprotection? *J Am Coll Cardiol* **41**, 1195–7 (2003).
255. J. F. Bouchard, D. Lamontagne, Protection afforded by preconditioning to the diabetic heart against ischemic injury, *Cardiovasc Res* **37**, 82–90 (1998).
256. Z. Yang, S. S. Berr, W. D. Gilson, M.-C. Toufektsian, B. A. French, Simultanous evaluation of infarct size and cardiac function in intact mice by contrast-enhanced cardiac magnetic resonance imaging reveals contractile dysfunction in noninfarcted regions early after myocardial infarction, *Circulation* **09**, 1161–67 (2004).
257. M. Amrani, N. Latif, K. Morrison, C. C. Gray, J. Jayakumar, J. Corbett, A. T. Goodwin, M. J. Dunn, M. H. Yacoub, Relative induction of heat shock protein in coronary endothelial cells and cardiomyocytes : implications for myocardial protection, *J Thorac Cardiovasc Sirg* **115**, 200–9 (1998).

258. Y. Hayashi, Y. Sawa, N. Fukuyama, H. Nakazawa, H. Matsuda, Preoperative glutamine administration induces heat-shock protein 70 expression and attenuates cardiopulmonary bypass-induced inflammatory response by regulating nitric oxide synthase activity, *Circulation* **106**, 2601–07 (2002).
259. H. Duplain, R. Burcelin, C. Sartori, S. Cook, M. Egli, M. Lepori, P. Vollenweider, T. Pedrazzini, P. Nicod, B. Thorens, U. Scherrer, Insulin resistance, hyperlipidemia, and hypertension in mice lacking endothelial nitric oxide synthase. *Circulation* **104**, 342–5 (2001).
260. M. E. Widlansky, N. Gokce, J. F. Keaney, J. A. Vita, The clinical implications of endothelial dysfunction, *J Am Coll Cardiol* **42**, 1149–60 (2003).
261. P. Di Napoli, A. A. Taccardi, A. Barsotti, Long term cardioprotective action of trimetazidine and potential effect on the inflammatory process in patients with ischemic dilated cardiomyopathy, *Heart* **91**, 161–65 (2005).
262. T. M. Lee, T. F. Chou, Troglitazone administration limits infarct size by reduced phosphorylation of canine myocardial connexin 43 proteins, *Am J Physiol. Heart Circ Physiol* **85**, H1650–59 (2003).
263. T. L. Yue, J. Chen, W. Bao, P. K. Narayanan, A. Bril, W. Jiang, P. G. Lysko, J. L. Gu, R. Boyce, D. M. Zimmerman, T. K. Hart, R. E. Buckingham, E. H. Ohlstein, In vivo myocardial protection from ischemia/reperfusion injury by the peroxisome proliferator-activated receptor -gamma agonist rosiglitazone, *Circulation* **104**, 2588–94 (2001).
264. H.-R. Liu, L. Tao, E. Gao, B. L. Lopez, T. A. Christopher, R. N. Willette, E. H. Ohlstein, T. L. Yue, X. L. Ma, Anti-apoptotic effects of rosiglitazone in hypercholesterolemic rabbits subjected to myocardial ischemia and reperfusion, *Cardiovasc Res* **62**, 135–44 (2004).
265. E. O.Weinberg, M. Scherrer-Crosbie, M. H. Picard, B. A. Nasseri, MacGillivray, J. Cannon, Q. Lian, K. D. Bloch, R. T. Lee, Rosuvastatin reduces experimental left ventricular infarct size after ischemia-reperfusion injury but not total coronary occlusion, *Am J Physiol-Heart and Circulatory Physiology* **288**, H1802–H1809 (2005).
266. S.R. Mehta, S. Yusuf, R. Diaz, J. Zhu, P. Pais, D. Xavier, E. Paolasso, R. Ahmed, C. Xie, K. Kazmi, J. Tai, A. Orlandini, J. Pogue, L. Liu; CREATE-ECLA Trial Group Investigators, Effect of glucose-insulin-potassium infusion on mortality in patients with acute ST-segment elevation myocardial infarction: the CREATE-ECLA randomized controlled trial, *JAMA*. **293(4)**, 437–446 (2005).
267. P. Theroux, B.R. Chaitman, L. Erhardt, A. Jessel, T. Meinertz, W.U. Nickel, J.S. Schroeder, G. Tognoni, H. White and J.T. Willerson, Design of a trial evaluating myocardial cell protection with cariporide, an inhibitor of the transmembrane sodium-hydrogen exchanger: the Guard During Ischemia Against Necrosis (GUARDIAN) trial, *Curr Control Trials Cardiovasc Med.* **1(1)**, 59–67 (2000).
268. R.M. Mentzer Jr, Sodium-proton exchange inhibition to prevent coronary events in acute cardiac conditions trial, *Paper presented at the American Heart Association Scientific Sessions*. November **12**, (2003).
269. J. Sochman, J. Vrbska, B. Musilova and M. Rocek, Infarct Size Limitation: acute N-acetylcysteine defense (ISLAND trial): preliminary analysis and report after the first 30 patients, *Clin Cardiol.* **19(2)**, 94–100 (1996).
270. V. Marangelli, C. Memmola, M.S. Brigiani, L. Boni, M.G. Biasco, D. Scrutinio, S. Iliceto and P. Rizzon, Early administration of verapamil after thrombolysis in acute anterior myocardial infarction. Effect on left ventricular remodeling and clinical outcome. VAMI Study Group. Verapamil Acute Myocardial Infarction, *Ital Heart J.* **1(5)**, 336–343 (2000).
271. P. Theroux, J. Gregoire, C. Chin, G. Pelletier, P. de Guise and M. Juneau, Intravenous diltiazem in acute myocardial infarction. Diltiazem as adjunctive therapy to activase (DATA) trial, *J Am Coll Cardiol.* **32(3)**, 620–628 (1998).
272. S.L. Kopecky, R.J. Aviles, M.R. Bell, J.K. Lobl, D. Tipping, G. Frommell, K. Ramsey, A.E. Holland, M. Midei, A. Jain, M. Kellett and R.J. Gibbons, A randomized, double-blinded, placebo-controlled, dose-ranging study measuring the effect of an adenosine agonist on infarct size reduction in patients undergoing primary percutaneous transluminal coronary angioplasty: the ADMIRE (AmP579 Delivery for Myocardial Infarction REduction) study, *Am. Heart J.* **146(1)**, 146–152 (2003).
273. S.L. Kopecky, R.J. Aviles, M.R. Bell, J.K. Lobl, D. Tipping, G. Frommell, K. Ramsey, A.E. Holland, M. Midei, A. Jain, M. Kellett and R.J. Gibbons, A randomized, double-blinded, placebo-controlled, dose-ranging study measuring the effect of an adenosine agonist on infarct size reduction in patients undergoing primary percutaneous transluminal coronary angioplasty: the ADMIRE (AmP579 Delivery for Myocardial Infarction REduction) study, *Am. Heart J.* **146(1)**, 146–152 (2003).

274. M. Quintana, P. Hjemdahl, A. Sollevi, T. Kahan, M. Edner, N. Rehnqvist, E. Swahn, A.C. Kjerr, P. Nasman; ATTACC investigators, Left ventricular function and cardiovascular events following adjuvant therapy with adenosine in acute myocardial infarction treated with thrombolysis, results of the ATTenuation by Adenosine of Cardiac Complications (ATTACC) study, *Eur J Clin Pharmacol.* **59(1)**, 1–9 (2003).
275. S. Von Haehling, S. D. Anker, Statins for heart failure: at the crossroads between cholesterol reduction and pleiotropism? *Heart* **91**, 1–2 (2005).
276. C. Communal, W. S. Colucci, The control of cardiomyocyte apoptosis via the β-adrenergic signaling pathways, *Arch Mol Coeur* **98**, 236–41 (2005).
277. D. V. Sawyer, D. A. Siwik, L. Xiao, D. R. Pimentel, K. Singh, W. S. Colucci, Role of oxidative stress in myocardial hypertrophy and failure, *J Mol Cell Cardiol* **34**, 379–88 (2002).
278. G. T. O'Connor, J. E. Buring, S. Yusuf, S. Z. Goldhaber, E. M. Olmstead, R. S. Jr Paffenbarger, C. H. Hennekens, An overview of randomized trials of rehabilitation with exercise after myocardial infarction, *Circulation* **80**, 234–45 (1989).
279. R. Bellardinelli, D. Georgiou, G. Cianci, A. Purcaro, Randomized, controlled trial of long-term moderate exercise training in chronic heart failure: effect on functional capacity, quality of life, and clinical outcome, *Circulation* **99**, 1173–82 (1999).
280. S. Freimann, Scheinowitz, D. Yekutieli, M. S. Feinberg, M. Eldar, G. Kessler-Icekson, Prior exercise training improves the outcome of acute myocardial infarction in the rat: Heart structure, funation, and gene expression, *J Am Coll Cardiol* **45**, 931–8 (2005).
281. R. A. Kloner, S. H. Rezkalla, Cardiac protection during acute myocardial infarction: Where do we stand in 2004? *J Am Coll Cardiol* **44**, 276–86 (2004).

CHAPTER 8
A SYNOPSIS

Dennis V. Cokkinos

Over the past years, research in the cardiovascular field has been fruitful and experimental work has contributed to better understanding of the pathophysiology of myocardial ischemia, enabling new therapeutic treatments to emerge. In this book some important conceptual advances are highlighted in self- contained mini- reviews.

An extended role of metabolism, beyond of being a process of energy transfer is described in an elegant way in the Introduction. Metabolism has pleiotropic actions providing signals for function, growth, gene expression and viability. Healthy hearts are functionally and structurally adapted to environmental changes thanks to metabolic flexibility. This advantage though is lost in diseased hearts. In addition, an important role for metabolism is suggested in stressed myocardium; metabolic remodeling precedes, triggers and sustains functional and structural remodeling of the heart.

Various aspects of myocardial ischemia are highlighted in Chapter 1. Reperfusion, generally a pre-requisite for tissue survival may increase injury over and above that sustained during ischemia. In this context, the role of apoptosis is appreciated. Mitochondrion seems to be the site of 'life' or 'death'. This organelle that provides ATP to sustain cell life is converted to an instrument of programmed cell death or necrosis upon stress depending on the severity of the insult.

An extensive role for oxygen beyond that in energy metabolism is now recognized. Oxygen appears to be a major determinant of myocardial gene expression, and as myocardial oxygen levels decrease, either in isolated hypoxia or ischemia associated hypoxia, gene expression patterns are altered. In addition, oxygen is a critical participant in the formation of reactive oxygen species which can trigger detrimental or survival signaling depending on the amount produced. Reactive oxygen species production in moderation switches death signaling to cell survival signaling. Ischemic preconditioning or sublethal heat stress appear to adapt the heart to ischemia by modulating reactive oxygen species production. Thus, agents with a modulatory effect on reactive oxygen species production may prove effective treatments for ischemic heart disease.

Complex intracellular signaling has been identified to be in operation in the setting of ischemia and reperfusion. A delicate balance between pro-death and survival pathways exists and determines the fate of the stressed cell. This signaling can be pharma-

Professor of Cardiology, Medical School, University of Athens, Greece
Address for correspondence: Chairman, department of Cardiology, Onassis Cardiac Surgery Center, 356 Sygrou Ave. 176 74 Kallithea, Athens, Greece. E-mail: cokkino1@otenet.gr

cologically manipulated either at pre-ischemia or at reperfusion phase with important therapeutic implications.

The pathophysiology of contractile dysfunction observed in stunning and hibernation has been better characterized. Stunning may explain much delayed contractile recovery after thrombolytic therapy. Hibernation is searched for in efforts to improve left contractile function by revascularization.

Lastly, it is now recognized that the diseased myocardium can adapt to ischemic stress and is not always a vulnerable substrate to ischemia.

The role of hormone signaling in the context of ischemia and reperfusion is emphasized in Chapter 2. Hormones have pleiotropic actions in cell metabolism, growth and survival through their genomic or non genomic actions. Hormones can target cardioprotective signaling protecting the heart against ischemia. Hormones signaling can be selectively manipulated and hormone analogs have been synthesized making their use in clinical practice feasible. Hormones may prove to be the 'poor man's' gene therapy.

The complex mechanisms of ischemic preconditioning are unraveled in Chapter 3. Ischemic preconditioning is one of the most striking discoveries over the past years.'Ischemia' can adapt the heart to 'ischemia'. Unstable angina is an example of a clinical counterpart of this phenomenon.

Further insight into mechanisms of preconditioning is given in Chapter 4. Connexin (Cx43), which has a regulatory effect on the cell to cell communication, appears to play a critical role for the preconditioning response. Loss of Cx43 occurs in certain diseased states and that may, in part, offer an explanation why preconditioning may not operate in some pathological conditions.

The pharmacological implications of the ischemic preconditioning are described in Chapters 3 and 7. A pharmacologically induced permanent preconditioned state may be feasible and justified in high risk patients. However, there are some limitations; the mechanisms of preconditioning are not operable under certain pathological conditions and concurrent medications may prevent the action of preconditioning mimetic agents. Aspirin or beta-blockers are some examples. Furthermore, in the setting of acute ischemic events, pre-ischemic strategies mimicking preconditioning effect may be difficult to institute.

A clinically relevant phenomenon is described in Chapter 5. Coronary microembolization which is a frequent event in ischemic heart disease due to plaque ruptures may compromise the microcirculation with subsequent events such as arrhythmias, cardiac dysfunction, infarcts and reduced coronary reserve. Furthermore, microembolization of coronary vasa vasorum may contribute to plaque instability and propagation of atherosclerosis into the more distal coronary vascular tree. Microembolization may offer an interpretation for some unexplained manifestations of ischemic heart disease in clinical practice.

An approach to tissue regeneration is attempted in Chapter 6. Accumulating evidence shows that the adult heart contains small populations of myocytes, derived from a local renewal pool, or homing in from the bone marrow that are capable of proliferating and replacing lost tissue. This process may be accelerated by growth factors. FGF-2 seems to be an example. Its safety and efficacy is being under investigation in clinical studies.

All this new advances find now their way to clinical practice. Promising data from early clinical studies are presented in Chapter 7. The list of therapeutic options is growing rapidly and their efficacy is awaited to be tested by conducting large clinical trials.

INDEX

MIX
Papier aus verantwortungsvollen Quellen
Paper from responsible sources
FSC® C105338

If you have any concerns about our products,
you can contact us on
ProductSafety@springernature.com

In case Publisher is established outside the EU,
the EU authorized representative is:
Springer Nature Customer Service Center GmbH
Europaplatz 3, 69115 Heidelberg, Germany

Printed by Libri Plureos GmbH
in Hamburg, Germany